The German Spa in the
Long Eighteenth Century

Shifting the focus from the medical use of spas to their cultural and social functions, this study shows that eighteenth- and early nineteenth-century German spas served a vital role as spaces where new ways of perceiving the natural environment and conceptualizing society were disseminated. Although spas continued to be places of health and healing, their function and perception in central Europe changed fundamentally around the middle of the eighteenth century. This transformation of the role of the spa occurred in two ways. First, the spa popularized a new perception of the landscape with a preference for mountains and the seacoast, forming the basis for the cultural assumptions underlying modern tourism. Second, contemporaries perceived spas as meeting places comparable to institutions of Enlightenment sociability like coffeehouses, salons, and Masonic lodges. Spas were conceived as spaces where the nobility and the bourgeoisie could interact on an equal footing, thereby overcoming the constraints of early modern social boundaries. These changes were negotiated through both personal interactions at spas and an increasingly sophisticated published spa discourse. The late eighteenth- and early nineteenth-century German spa thus helped to bring about social and cultural modernity.

Ute Lotz-Heumann is Heiko A. Oberman Professor in the Division for Late Medieval and Reformation Studies (DLMRS) and the Department of History and Director of DLMRS at the University of Arizona.

Routledge Studies in Cultural History

101 British Concepts of Heroic "Gallantry" and the Sixties Transition
The Politics of Medals
Matthew J. Lord

102 Cultural Histories of Ageing
Myths, Plots and Metaphors of the Senescent Self
Edited by Margery Vibe Skagen

103 Coding and Representation from the Nineteenth Century to the Present
Edited by Anne Chapman and Natalie Hume

104 Disability and Tourism in Nineteenth- and Twentieth-Century Italy
Luciano Maffi and Martino Lorenzo Fagnani

105 De-Illustrating the History of the British Empire
Preliminary Perspectives
Edited by Annamaria Motrescu-Mayes

106 Contact, Conquest and Colonization
How Practices of Comparing Shaped Empires and Colonialism Around the World
Edited by Eleonora Rohland, Angelika Epple, Antje Flüchter and Kirsten Kramer

107 The German Spa in the Long Eighteenth Century
A Cultural History
Ute Lotz-Heumann

108 The Formal Call in the Making of the Baltic Bourgeoisie
Kekke Stadin

For more information about this series, please visit: www.routledge.com/Routledge-Studies-in-Cultural-History/book-series/SE0367

The German Spa in the Long Eighteenth Century
A Cultural History

Ute Lotz-Heumann

Routledge
Taylor & Francis Group

NEW YORK AND LONDON

First published 2022
by Routledge
605 Third Avenue, New York, NY 10158

and by Routledge
2 Park Square, Milton Park, Abingdon, Oxon, OX14 4RN

Routledge is an imprint of the Taylor & Francis Group, an informa business

© 2022 Taylor & Francis

Library of Congress Cataloging-in-Publication Data
A catalog record for this title has been requested

ISBN: 978-0-367-44095-4 (hbk)
ISBN: 978-1-032-04571-9 (pbk)
ISBN: 978-1-003-00752-4 (ebk)

Typeset in Sabon
by Apex CoVantage, LLC

Contents

List of Figures		vii
Preface		ix
Acknowledgments		xi
A Note on Translations		xii

Introduction   1

PART I
Foundations   23

1   Spas from the Late Middle Ages to the Eighteenth Century   25

2   Spas as Centers of Communication: Face-to-Face Interactions and Print Culture   58

PART II
Space and Time   97

Introduction to Part II   99

3   Reinventing the Eighteenth-Century Spa as a Leisure Space   104

4   Spas and Seaside Resorts on the Cusp of Modern Tourism: New Perceptions of Nature and a Daily Routine   142

PART III
Meeting Place   189

Introduction to Part III   191

5   The Spa in the Eighteenth Century: From Social
    Hierarchy to New Demands for Equality   199

6   Nobility and Bourgeoisie at the Spa: Creating Unity
    and Maintaining Differences   227

Conclusion   283

  *Map: Teutsche Spas in the Published
  Spa Discourse, c. 1700–c. 1820*   294
  Bibliography   296
  Index   341

Figures

1.1   Plombières or Plummers in Lorraine, engraving, 1553   26

1.2   Aachen, therapeutic showers, engraving, 1688   27

1.3   Aachen, drinking wells, engraving, 1688   28

2.1   Pyrmont, main avenue, engraving by C.G. Geyser after a drawing by J.F. Weitsch, 1784   62

2.2   Pyrmont, communal breakfast, colored drawing by a French spa guest, 1795   83

2.3   Liebenstein, cave, engraving by F. Rosmäsler junior, 1819   83

3.1   Pfäfers in Switzerland, engraving by Matthäus Merian the Elder, 1654   105

3.2   Fold-out map of Aachen, engraving, 1688   106

3.3   Wiesbaden, engraving by Matthäus Merian the Elder, 1655   108

3.4   Schwalbach, engraving by Matthäus Merian the Elder, 1655   109

3.5   Ems, engraving by Matthäus Merian the Elder, 1655   110

3.6   Ems, colored lithography, mid-nineteenth century   110

3.7   Fold-out map of Karlsbad (today Karlovy Vary), engraving, 1754   112

3.8   Aachen, tree-lined walks, engraving, 1737   113

3.9   Pyrmont, engraving, 1698   113

3.10   Boll, engraving, 1602   114

3.11   Adelholzen, engraving by Matthäus Merian the Elder, 1644   115

3.12   Map of Pyrmont, colored copperplate engraving by J.C. Dammert and F. Cöntgen, 1790   118

3.13   Lauchstädt, pond and avenue, colored etching by Friedrich August Scheureck, c. 1790   120

3.14   Lauchstädt, assembly hall (ballroom) and healing well, colored etching by Friedrich August Scheureck, c. 1790   121

3.15   Lauchstädt, pavilion, colored etching by Friedrich August Scheureck, c. 1790   122

3.16 Lauchstädt, avenue with pond on left and sales boutiques on right, colored etching by Friedrich August Scheureck, c. 1790   122

3.17 Wilhelmsbad, colored engraving, 1780   123

3.18 Wilhelmsbad, avenue, painting by Anton Wilhelm Tischbein, c. 1783   124

3.19 Wilhelmsbad, equipment for landscape garden including games and exercise, drawing, c. 1777   125

3.20 Wilhelmsbad, pond and island with pyramid, painting by Anton Wilhelm Tischbein, c. 1783   125

3.21 Bertrich, leisure facilities along the Üßbach, colored drawing by H. Kirn, 1778   127

3.22 Map of Bocklet, engraving, 1793   128

3.23 Teplitz (today Teplice), princely palace   131

3.24 Brückenau, princely palace   131

4.1 Monastery Hagenrode near Alexisbad, engraving by Johann Friedrich Klusemann, 1812   152

4.2 Griesbach, engraving by F. Rosmäsler junior, 1819   153

4.3 Castle Daubersberg (today Doubravská hora) near Teplitz (today Teplice), engraving by F. Rosmäsler junior, 1819   154

4.4 Castle Rosenburg (today Hrad Krupka) in Graupen (today Krupka) near Teplitz (today Teplice), engraving by F. Rosmäsler junior, 1819   154

4.5 Map of the surroundings of Baden-Baden and the Murg river valley, engraving by Carl Ausfeld (one half of a two-part map), 1810   156

4.6 Heiligendamm, painting, first quarter of nineteenth century   161

4.7 Doberan, engraving by F. Rosmäsler junior, 1819   163

6.1 General spa uniform for ladies, colored engraving, 1792   236

Preface

This book has been in the making for a long time. I first conceived of it in 1997, when I was still working on finishing my Ph.D. in early modern Irish history. My father celebrated his seventieth birthday at a spa – Wilhelmsbad – and I made a little speech in his honor. Ever the historian, I included historical information about the venue – and the topic of my next book project emerged.

Habent sua fata libelli. This book has had a varied fate, even before its publication. I started to work on it in earnest in 2000, and its first iteration was a *Habilitation* in German, submitted at Humboldt University of Berlin in 2009. Since then, many things have happened in my life, and revising and publishing the manuscript as a book was on the backburner for a long time. I eventually decided to publish it in English, the language I work and write in most of the time now.

It has been a long road since that first beginning. When I became Heiko A. Oberman Professor at the University of Arizona in Tucson in 2008, my husband Dirk and I discovered that an international move is not for the faint-hearted. After long illnesses, my father passed away in 2015, and my mother in 2019, but I'm glad that they both read the original German version. They were the most supportive parents any child could ever hope for, and I will be eternally grateful for everything they did for me. My husband Dirk has been equally supportive over many years and has helped me enormously to get this book over the finish line during a pandemic. He is the best life and pandemic partner anyone could ever imagine.

Over the years, friends and colleagues have given me a lot of encouragement, advice, and support. I would like to express my special thanks to Heinz Schilling, my doctoral advisor and *Habilitation* mentor in Berlin; Stefan Ehrenpreis and Matthias Pohlig, my former colleagues in Berlin; Susan Karant-Nunn, Director Emerita of the Division for Late Medieval and Reformation Studies and a friend and mentor for many years; Beth Plummer, my colleague in the Division; Susan Crane, Linda Darling, Laura Tabili, and Doug Weiner, my colleagues in the Department of History; and Karl and Sue Bottigheimer, friends and mentors since my days as a Ph.D. student. I am also grateful to Mary Lindemann for providing important advice on how to proceed with my book at a crucial moment in time.

In 2005/2006 and 2008, I was awarded fellowships by the Leibniz-Institut für Geschichte und Kultur des östlichen Europa (GWZO) in Leipzig, the Leibniz Institute of European History (IEG) in Mainz, and the Kommission für Frauenförderung in Berlin to work on my *Habilitation*. I am grateful to these institutions for their support.

Isabel Atzl and Jacob Schilling in Berlin and Dean Messinger in Tucson helped with collecting sources, asking for copyright permissions, and other practical matters. Nick O'Gara produced the map at the end of this volume. Sabine Schmidt and Hannah McClain helped with polishing the manuscript and eliminating as many Germanisms as possible. Many thanks to all of them.

Ute Lotz-Heumann
Tucson, October 2020

Acknowledgments

Some material in the Introduction and in Chapters 1, 2, and 4 was originally published in German in the following articles and chapters:

Ute Lotz-Heumann. "Kurorte im Reich des 18. Jahrhunderts – ein Typus urbanen Lebens und Laboratorium der bürgerlichen Gesellschaft: Eine Problemskizze." In *Bäder und Kuren in der Aufklärung: Medizinaldiskurs und Freizeitvergnügen*, edited by Raingard Eßer and Thomas Fuchs, 15–35. Berlin: Berliner Wissenschafts-Verlag, 2003. By permission of Berliner Wissenschafts-Verlag.

Ute Lotz-Heumann. "Unterirdische Gänge, oberirdische Gänge, Spaziergänge: Freimaurerei und deutsche Kurorte im 18. Jahrhundert." *Aufklärung* 15 (2003): 159–186. By permission of Felix Meiner Verlag.

Ute Lotz-Heumann. "Daheim und auf Reisen: Fürst Franz im Bade – Heterotopie und fürstliche Repräsentation an der Wende vom 18. zum 19. Jahrhundert." In *Das Leben des Fürsten: Studien zur Biografie von Leopold III. Friedrich Franz von Anhalt-Dessau (1740–1817)*, edited by Holger Zaunstöck, 109–120. Halle: Mitteldeutscher Verlag, 2008. By permission of Mitteldeutscher Verlag.

Ute Lotz-Heumann. "Wie kommt der Wandel in den Diskurs? Die Heterotopie Kurort in der Sattelzeit." In *Diskursiver Wandel*, edited by Achim Landwehr, 281–308. Wiesbaden: VS Verlag, 2010. By permission of VS Verlag für Sozialwissenschaften.

A Note on Translations

All translations from primary and secondary sources are my own unless otherwise indicated. The punctuation in translated primary source quotations has been changed to modern English-language conventions. Quotations in the original language are provided in the notes, with the spelling and punctuation preserved. I have included original German terms (in brackets and italics) in translated quotations if these terms are important for my argument.

Introduction

In his 1815 book *Practical Overview of the Most Prominent Healing Springs in Germany* (*Praktische Uebersicht der vorzüglichsten Heilquellen Teutschlands*), the physician Christoph Wilhelm Hufeland remarked about the spa of Pyrmont:

> Since it is one of the most popular spas, and the upper and richest classes visit it regularly, the way of life is naturally boisterous, luxurious, expensive, and grand, and therefore often constraining and oppressive for the lesser estates. One may hope, however, that this will fade out and people will finally realize that one main appeal of these institutions is and should be to step out of the ordinary conditions and rigid restrictions of civil life, so that for once one may enjoy in the open air the freedom of life and find delight in pure nature and its gifts in a natural way.[1]

Why did a physician writing a book about healing waters feel compelled to comment on the social atmosphere and the natural surroundings of a spa?

Shifting the focus from the medical use of the spa to its cultural and social functions, this study shows that the eighteenth- and early nineteenth-century German spa served a vital role as a space where new ways of perceiving the natural environment and conceptualizing society were disseminated. Although spas continued to be places of health and healing, their function and perception in central Europe changed fundamentally around the middle of the eighteenth century. Reports from spa-goers, spa guides, and other published materials about spas, including images, increasingly emphasized spa amenities, cultural consumption, enjoyment of the landscape, and especially the spa's role as a meeting place. As physicians complained, laypeople decided to go to a spa not because of their physician's recommendation but rather because of the spa's reputation, or because their friends and colleagues frequented the same spa. Eighteenth-century spas, therefore, can be characterized as spaces that existed as concepts in people's minds well before guests set foot in them.

These concepts were based on both personal correspondence and published reading material.

During the second half of the eighteenth century, central European spas thus took on a new quality. While they continued to serve as places where guests sought to maintain and restore their health, spas also became multipliers of Enlightenment ideas. As such, the late eighteenth- and early nineteenth-century German spa helped to bring about social and cultural modernity. This fundamental transformation of the role of the spa occurred in two ways. First, the spa popularized a new perception of the landscape with a preference for mountains and the seacoast, forming the basis for the cultural perceptions underlying modern tourism. Second, contemporaries perceived spas as meeting places comparable to salons and Masonic lodges, where the nobility and the bourgeoisie (*Bürgertum*) were supposed to interact on an equal footing, thereby overcoming the constraints of early modern social boundaries. These changes were negotiated through both personal interactions at the spa and an increasingly sophisticated published spa discourse.

Central European spas occasionally receive attention in works about health, diseases, and medicine,[2] about cities and towns,[3] and about leisure and consumption,[4] but only a limited number of research monographs and essay collections have been devoted to individual spas or to the phenomenon as a whole in early modern and eighteenth-century Germany.[5] Much more research has been done on the nineteenth and early twentieth centuries, when German spas like Baden-Baden, Ems, and Wiesbaden grew exponentially and gained international fame.[6] However, research on nineteenth-century spas often does not explore the important transformations spas underwent during the long eighteenth century. This study focuses on the cultural history of the German spa in order to describe how spas gradually transformed from places with an emphasis on healing to places with an emphasis on sociability, leisure, and early tourist experiences.

In recent decades, the concept of cultural history has gained widespread acceptance in historiography. Cultural history is no longer understood to cover a specific aspect of history, as is the case with urban history or the history of medicine. Rather, cultural history refers to a comprehensive historiographical interest in the history of perception and "the collective production of meaning."[7] This development in historiography toward cultural history has made a significant impact on all the areas of research touched upon in this study. Traditional fields of research in social history, such as research on the bourgeoisie, the nobility, and Enlightenment societies, have been redefined by cultural historical approaches.[8] At the same time, topics that used to be part of the older cultural history, such as research on the perception of the landscape and the study of leisure, have received more attention in historiography as a result of the broader range of questions and approaches introduced by the new cultural history.[9] In fact, this study fuses two thematic aspects of the spa, namely landscape perception and social interaction, previously regarded as separate historiographical fields. From a cultural historical perspective, however, both are vital aspects of the construction of the eighteenth-century spa in the eyes of contemporaries.

One might be inclined to think that the geographical location of successful spas in the eighteenth century was determined by geological conditions and the resulting existence of scientifically proven healing waters. This is only partially the case, however. While it cannot be denied that the age of the so-called scientific revolution led to a surge in scientific and medical knowledge and resulted in considerable advances in the chemical analysis of healing waters,[10] the healing power of spa waters was still primarily a matter of successful attribution and social consensus, even at the beginning of the nineteenth century.[11] Spa physicians continued to claim as many therapeutic benefits as possible in their spa guides, with the cure of childlessness and hypochondria included at the top of every list. In addition, spa physicians went so far as to deny the curative qualities of other spa waters or at least to claim a better quality for their own water through comparative advertising.[12]

Spa guides and other works commissioned by German princes to advertise the spas in their territories attributed a wide variety of curative powers to these healing waters. In the most extreme cases, healing powers were ascribed to spa waters later shown to be ineffective or even harmful. Advertising campaigns praised the quality of the waters of spas such as Lauchstädt near Halle and Wilhelmsbad near Hanau, although contemporaries already questioned their efficacy.[13] These spas were sufficiently successful in the late eighteenth and early nineteenth centuries, however, that they continued to be included in spa guides and travelogues published in the early nineteenth century.[14] The architectural ensembles of these spas are preserved today because they stopped attracting visitors later in the nineteenth century.

Moreover, to the chagrin of contemporary physicians, eighteenth-century spa visitors did not necessarily heed the advice of medical experts for their choice of one spa over another. Thus, Friedrich Christian Gottlieb Scheidemantel complained in 1792, "So the reason why they select a certain water over others is none other than that they have promised friends to take the waters together at a certain spa."[15] And Rasmus Frankenau sarcastically admonished his readers in 1799, "Those who feel the urge to visit a spa, especially ladies, should not invite gossiping friends to a tea party in order to use this opportunity – with much Oh! and Ah! – to collectively vote on which spa the lady may honor with her presence."[16]

While individuals based their decisions on which spa to visit on different types of input, such as consulting with family and friends, reading spa guides, seeking medical advice, or a combination thereof, the creation and promotion of spas in the eighteenth century were not determined

by geological conditions or curative powers in a modern sense. Therefore, many therapeutic water springs never became spas, and not all spas
had curative springs. The established definition of a spa required a water
spring that was marketed as healing water, but the success of a spa was
determined by its reputation, itself the result of a complex combination
of assumed health benefits, advertising and presence in the print media,
a resort-like space offering various leisure activities, and, as a result, an
increasing number of spa visitors from the nobility and the bourgeoisie.

The long-standing tradition of spa-going in Europe began in Roman
times and was revived in the late Middle Ages. By the end of the sixteenth
century, spa visits had become an established practice in central Europe.
The famous essayist Michel de Montaigne and the Nuremberg merchant
Balthasar Paumgartner frequented spas in the sixteenth century. By the
second half of the seventeenth century, Hans Jacob Christoph von Grimmelshausen in his novel *Simplicius Simplicissimus (Der Abentheuerliche
Simplicissimus)* could make extensive references to spas and the practice
of spa-going in the firm knowledge that his readers knew how to contex-
tualize these references. His hero, Simplicissimus, even imagines himself
in the role of a successful spa-founder.

By the second half of the eighteenth century, regular spa visits lasting
several weeks during the summer became an integral part of the nobility's
and the bourgeoisie's lifestyle. A combination of amusements, health care,
and sometimes work was characteristic of these visits. The names of well-
known and lesser-known spa visitors of the eighteenth century are legion:
Johann Wolfgang von Goethe, his partner and later wife Christiane Vulpius, the law professor Johann Stephan Pütter, the Baltic German writer
Elisa von der Recke, Prince Franz of Anhalt-Dessau, King Frederick II of
Prussia, Queen Louise of Prussia, the law student and later Hanoverian
archivist and privy councillor Johann Christian Kestner, the bailiff and
town councillor Ludwig Friedrich Christoph Schmid from Uffenheim, not
to mention fictional characters such as "Dr. Katzenberger"[17] and "the
judge from Lüda."[18] Accordingly, Friedrich Christian Gottlieb Scheidemantel stated in 1792 that spas were "used by a great many people, especially those of the higher and middle classes, every summer."[19]

Bathing cures in thermal waters prevailed in the late Middle Ages and
at the beginning of the sixteenth century. In the late sixteenth century, the
advent of cold mineral waters and drinking cures led to an expansion of
the number of spas. The Thirty Years' War disrupted the development of
spas in central Europe, but by the end of the seventeenth century spas saw
a steady increase in visitors. Despite further disruptions during the Seven
Years' War and the Napoleonic Wars, the number of spas proliferated in
the second half of the eighteenth century and again at the beginning of
the nineteenth century.

In her memoirs written in the 1830s, Johanna Schopenhauer described
the development of spas since the second half of the eighteenth century:

"In general, the number of spas in Germany was very small at that time because they were very poorly equipped. Now it would be difficult to travel more than ten miles without encountering a larger or smaller spa created by human ingenuity or nature. Fifty or sixty years ago, many of the now very popular spas were yet unknown, some of them were poorly equipped and only frequented by people living nearby, and nobody even considered the establishment of seaside resorts."[20] Schopenhauer highlights the considerable increase in the number of spas from the 1770s onward and the fundamental change of the map of summer resorts in Germany brought about by the creation of seaside resorts at the end of the eighteenth and the beginning of the nineteenth centuries. Starting in the 1810s, a further major expansion occurred. On the one hand, spas like Baden-Baden, Ems, and Wiesbaden, which were middling spas in the eighteenth century, became world-famous and attracted unprecedented numbers of visitors. On the other hand, the number of spas rose sharply because many of the salt-producing towns were now converted into spas. From the middle of the nineteenth century onward, mass transportation facilitated by railroads once again transformed the spas.[21]

The majority of German spas were founded by princes who ruled over small and medium-sized territories. Nevertheless, the eighteenth-century spas came in many shapes and sizes, from a royal town such as Karlsbad in Bohemia[22] (today Karlovy Vary in the Czech Republic) and a spa district in the imperial city of Aachen on one end of the spectrum to small towns, villages, and even facilities in the open countryside on the other. The latter, however, were generally located in the immediate vicinity of towns and were often associated with a princely summer residence. Examples of small spa towns include Lauchstädt, Wiesbaden, and Baden in Swabia (today Baden-Baden); Schlangenbad and Godesberg were villages; Wilhelmsbad near Hanau, the "health spring" (*Gesundbrunnen*) near Hofgeismar, Driburg, and the "healing spring" (*Kurbrunnen*) near Brückenau are typical examples of spas close to small and medium-sized towns.

Most spas remained places where everyone, from prince to beggar, could seek a cure, because healing waters were supposed to be available to all social classes.[23] Accordingly, spas, albeit often reluctantly, provided spaces for the lower middle class, the peasantry, and the poor for the use of the healing waters. However, a spa visit lasting several weeks and dedicated not only to maintaining or regaining one's health but also – or even exclusively – to pleasure required financial resources. During the second half of the eighteenth century, the German middle classes (*Bürgertum*)[24] increasingly had these necessary financial means at their disposal. Furthered by other developments in the Holy Roman Empire, such as improved roads and stagecoaches,[25] this led to an increased presence of the bourgeoisie at the spas. The so-called "Spa Chronicle" ("Badechronik") in the *Journal of Luxury and Fashions* (*Journal des Luxus und der Moden*) stated in

1805, "In this regard, as everywhere in the field of luxury and fashion, the example of the great and the rich influences those on a lower [social] level. Hence the mania of the middle classes [*mittleren Stände*] to visit spas, even without being sick, simply because it is fashionable."[26]

Spas fulfilled multiple functions in the late eighteenth and early nineteenth centuries. This is reflected in the way spas were represented in the print media. A typical spa guide deals with all or most of the following aspects of a summer visit to a spa: travel routes to the spa; the topography of its architecture and gardens; the surrounding landscape; services and cultural consumption such as theater performances and balls; the spa's health function, including facilities like baths and drinking fountains; and social interactions at the spa. In sum, spas aspired to be all things to all people – "every need is met, both of the sick and of the healthy, both for necessity and for pleasure," as the "Spa Chronicle" put it in 1800[27] – with the important caveat that, in reality, access to the leisure spaces of the spas was restricted to the upper middle class and the nobility.

In the 1780 travelogue *News from a Spa Visit to Karlsbad* (*Nachrichten von einer Carlsbader Brunnenreise*) by Johann Peter Willebrand, the narrator comments in a fictitious letter to a friend:

> But do not think, my dearest friend, that all the people who come here are really sick and that they are spa guests in the true sense of the word. No – heaven forbid! Many people travel here to escape boredom, to spend several weeks without work *cum privilegio* [with permission from their employers] and rid themselves of worries about the duties of their offices, to seek domestic peace and quiet, to rinse their livers in order to indulge in more feasts. Many of them here seek admiration for their horses, their grooms in modern liveries, also their lackeys etc., and they want to show off their new medals of knighthood, they want to be envied and called a baron.[28]

In short, the spa provided a striking combination of an allegedly worry-free space and a place where the motto was "see and be seen" – not unlike modern luxury resorts.

Letters, diaries, and autobiographies confirm this picture. Activities to preserve or regain one's health were combined with a variety of other activities – communal meals, walks, attending balls, concerts, and the theater, shopping, meetings in small circles of friends, and more. Leisure activities and medical treatments, pleasure and work, noble privilege and the bourgeois demand for equality combined at the spa in various ways. People made professional contacts, met friends, and made new acquaintances. The spa also functioned as a marriage market and provided an opportunity to consume art, fashion, and other luxury goods.[29] In 1789, the *Journal of Luxury and Fashions* (*Journal des Luxus und der Moden*) thus remarked critically, "In our time they [the spas] are considered and visited by most people as places of pleasure, so for them balneotherapy is a mere luxury. Most of the guests at the spas do not drink water or bathe. Their intention is merely to go on a pleasure trip, to meet friends, to dance, to play, to amuse themselves, etc."[30] Spa guests, however, did not perceive this as a reason for reproach but rather as an important consideration in favor of a spa visit. Justus Möser enthusiastically wrote to Friedrich Nicolai in 1789, "On the evening of 4 July, at 9 o'clock, God willing, I will be in Pyrmont, and the pleasure of seeing you there will have a better effect on my health than the bath and the spring, neither of which I [will] use."[31]

The original *raison d'être* of the spa was the healing of illnesses, but subsequently its *raison d'être* in the public sphere of the late eighteenth and early nineteenth centuries changed so dramatically that actual, visible illness became a problem. The spa effectively had to be a meeting place for healthy people in order to fulfill its manifold functions. Strikingly, it became commonplace, especially in spa guides that served as advertisements for specific spas, to claim that the number of sick people was low or nonexistent.[32] Accordingly, Deneken stated in his 1796 description of Rehburg, "Everyone wants to forget his business here and lift his spirits. All spa guests, who otherwise live in very different circumstances, share the common goal of promoting each other's pleasure. Corpse-like sick people staggering toward the grave are rarely to be found at Rehburg. Many come here simply to enjoy themselves."[33] And Hoser warned in his spa guide of Franzensbad, "A spa that lacks amusements will scare away every healthy person, who is only looking for diversion for his money and who . . . is really the soul of entertainment and of the free, cheerful social atmosphere in such places."[34] This was not wishful thinking by authors trying to promote a spa but reflected the reality at many spas, as is confirmed by Friedrich Wilhelm von Ketelhodt, who kept a travel diary for the princes of Schwarzburg-Rudolstadt in 1789–1790. He remarked about Lauchstädt, "This spa is lively and fun because very few people come here to restore their health, but most come for pleasure."[35]

Contemporary observers recognized the fundamental discrepancy between the original definition and the actual functioning of spas. For example, Justus Möser in his 1746 *Letter by the Author to His Sister* (*Schreiben des Verfassers an seine Schwester*) commented with a dash of irony about Pyrmont, "Whoever is ill here is lost in paradise."[36] The 1805 "Spa Chronicle" ("Badechronik") in the *Journal of Luxury and Fashions* (*Journal des Luxus und der Moden*) did not mince words: "We live in an age of contradictions. Even where the sufferer seeks relief and healing for the ailments of his body, the sybarite builds temples of joy and well-being for himself, and the healing springs that nature has allowed to flow in order to help the sick are transformed by the pleasure-seeking and never-satisfied man of the world into sources of the finest, but not always innocent pleasures."[37]

As the number of visitors to the spas increased after 1750, so did the discussion of the spa as a topic in contemporary print media. This played out against the backdrop of the "rise of the public sphere."[38] During the eighteenth century – and especially its second half – the spread of Enlightenment ideas, the expansion of readership, and the long-term rise of the bourgeoisie were reflected in the expansion of the print media.[39] We will probably never know the exact number of readers in Germany in the eighteenth century or the size of the audience reached by the increasing number of publications, but researchers give an estimate of about 300,000 readers by the end of the eighteenth century. A large proportion of this readership were educated members of the bourgeoisie and the nobility, many of whom were writers themselves.[40]

In the "bourgeois media society"[41] of the eighteenth century, the older market with its books, pamphlets, and broadsheets diversified fundamentally. In consequence, newspapers, intelligencers (*Intelligenzblätter*), and almanacs gained in importance. The moral weeklies gave rise to a journal market covering a broad range of topics, from political-economic journals and literary reviews to educational and fashion journals.[42] Especially the fashion and entertainment journals, with their numbers mushrooming toward the end of the eighteenth century, served to "reduce the information gap between city and country, between metropolis and province."[43] The journal became the "key medium of bourgeois society."[44]

In the 1798 *Journal of Luxury and Fashions* (*Journal des Luxus und der Moden*), an anonymous author offered the following observation about the preceding 1797 season at the spa of Pyrmont: "Our German Fashion Journal is rightfully held in some public libraries. Because in later centuries, when perhaps our nation will have melted into the chaos of the commonality of a universal nation, it may still be a welcome find for many a historian to draw from it the customs, fashions, and practices of the present world."[45] This study takes the author at his or her word, examining as one of the two main types of primary sources the printed material that earned the spa its increasingly strong media presence over the course of the second half of the eighteenth century.

Regarding censorship, historians have long agreed that the "opposing institutions and interests of the eighteenth century . . . led to 'inefficiency,' and, from another perspective, to freedom of action."[46] In fact, censorship was largely a *quantité négligeable* during the early modern period and the eighteenth century, which were marked by movements like the Reformation and the Enlightenment that sparked unprecedented expansions of print media. When publications making similar arguments appeared on a mass scale and in different German territories, authorities could not effectively censor them.[47] This changed, however, in the 1820s and the 1830s: "In the German Confederation, the old traditional censorship with the censor in action was revived, but it was now institutionalized throughout Germany much more systematically than in the Old Empire.

The foundation was laid by the so-called Karlsbad Decrees of 1819, which provided for general censorship of print material."[48] As we will see later, these developments also had a profound impact on the way spas were discussed in the print media.

This study focuses on the role of the eighteenth-century German spa as a multiplier of cultural and social ideas rather than the development of one or more individual spas. The representation of spas in eighteenth-century German-language print media functions as an indicator to determine which spas contemporaries encountered in their reading materials and would therefore have considered fashionable. The spas included in this study were thus chosen because at least a regional, if not a supra-regional, German-speaking audience had access to and shared information about them. A secondary, geographical criterion was applied to the sample of spas, focusing on what contemporaries defined as "German" (*teutsche*) spas. In this way, about 80 spas and seaside resorts were identified that made up the map of fashionable German spas in the long eighteenth century.

Roughly 40 spas were represented in the print media for an extended period of time over the course of the eighteenth and early nineteenth centuries. They were at least of regional significance and sought to establish themselves among spa visitors through supra-regional publicity. These spas constituted a small minority among the broad spectrum of healing springs in the early modern period and the long eighteenth century, which included numerous springs that sold their mineral waters but did not function as spas and many spas that attracted only local visitors. These 40 spas cover an area stretching from Aachen in the West to Bohemia in the East, and from Freienwalde in Brandenburg in the North to the Black Forest in the South. In addition, roughly another 40 spas, some newly founded, garnered supra-regional publicity at the beginning of the nineteenth century. These included rural spas in areas such as the Giant Mountains (*Riesengebirge*) in Silesia, Saxon Switzerland (*Sächsische Schweiz*), and the Renchtal in the Black Forest, as well as seaside resorts on the Baltic and North Sea coasts.[49]

Overall, this study covers the period between 1680 and 1830 as the "long eighteenth century." The analysis of primary sources focuses on the period between the mid-1700s and 1820 – a period when the representation of spas in the print media intensified considerably and the spa functioned as a multiplier of new cultural and social ideas. This "watershed period" (*Sattelzeit*)[50] between early modernity and modernity was, as Reinhart Koselleck put it, a "transitional period . . . in which it becomes more and more difficult to mediate between the handed-down traditions and necessary innovations."[51] This study supports the proposition of the watershed period as a formative era of change between the early modern and the modern period, while at the same time drawing attention to the slow and meandering nature of that change. In contrast to periodizations like "Enlightenment," "Counter-Enlightenment" or "Anti-Enlightenment" (*Gegenaufklärung*), "Romanticism," and so forth that evoke specific intellectual and literary movements,[52] the notion of a watershed period facilitates the perception of the decades between 1750 and 1820 as a unity. This, however, in no way negates the Enlightenment as an intellectual and social movement. Rather, as will be shown later, the spa functioned as a multiplier of Enlightenment ideas during the watershed period.

The first main group of primary sources analyzed in this study consists of printed texts from a wide variety of authors and genres, from spa guides and travelogues to plays and didactic poems. The titles of all these works bear witness to the fact that they deal with one or more spas beyond a purely chemical or medical-balneological analysis.[53] These texts describe the spa as a place of social encounter and recreation, thus explicitly addressing spa visitors. Articles and reviews in journals are also included as sources, especially the "Spa Chronicle" ("Badechronik") in the *Journal of Luxury and Fashions* (*Journal des Luxus und der Moden*).[54] These were published regularly after the annual spa season and provide a clear indication of how closely the reading public followed the news about spas. All publications offer a wide range of information about the spa, from travel arrangements, the landscape surrounding the spa, accommodations, amusements, and services to health benefits – with a different degree of coverage in each publication.

Spa guides often contained engravings depicting the interior spaces or the surrounding landscape of the spas or maps of spa regions. Images of spas can also be found as paintings or as single-leaf prints used for advertising purposes. Susanne Müller's statement about the *Baedeker* guidebooks of the later nineteenth century is also true for the spa guides of the late eighteenth and early nineteenth centuries: "Printed tourist guides . . . are . . . in constant interplay with other visual media."[55] This study aims to show the interplay of textual and pictorial sources but does not aspire to provide an art historical analysis. As will be shown later, intermediality[56] was an important factor in persuading readers of spa guides to trust an author's claims about the interior spaces and the surrounding landscape of a spa.

Analyzing printed material *en masse* yields broad insight into how the reading public viewed the phenomenon of the spa, insight that cannot be obtained by doing research on only one or several spas. The spa publications examined here formed a "spa discourse," describing the spa in a largely uniform manner. The method of historical discourse analysis employed in this study is inspired by Michel Foucault. It is based on the idea that not everything that could theoretically be put into words is actually "sayable," and that societies always limit what can legitimately be said in any given context or period.[57] In other words, in view of the infinite number of possible statements a language offers, discourse analysis asks which statements actually appear and thus constitute a discourse.[58] A statement is "the atom of discourse,"[59] and the possibilities of making a statement are – in comparison to the infinite possibilities of language – historically limited, even "scarce."[60]

Foucault speaks of a discourse or a "discursive formation" when statements occur with a certain regularity, when series of statements emerge and certain relationships between statements and their "rules of formation" can be identified.[61] Discourses are "contexts of speech . . . with rules of expression and of truth that are historically situated, i.e. they have a beginning and an end as well as a specific social (and . . . cultural) place."[62] Thus, the rules of formation can be made visible in a specific historical context because discourses are "practices that systematically form the objects of which they speak."[63] The bibliography at the end of this book provides a list of publications that form the backbone of the spa discourse analyzed in this study. In Parts II and III, quotations from these publications illustrate various types of discursive statement about the spa as a multiplier of cultural and social ideas. These quotations were chosen because they are typical examples of such statements, but they are only the tip of the iceberg. There are multiple further examples of similar discursive statements in the printed primary sources that could not be included in the text.[64]

Adapting Foucault's rejection of categories such as book, work, and also author,[65] this study does not classify and analyze works according to genre or author but seeks to understand the discourse that arises anonymously and beyond the individual author. An objection often raised against Foucault, namely that he depersonalizes discourse, turns into an advantage because many of the texts examined here, especially journal articles, were published anonymously.[66] Nevertheless, "power" is expressed through the spa discourse – not in its traditional sense with regard to the state or authorities – but in terms of the production and dissemination of discursive formations that "structured the thinking and acting of the many."[67] A critical exploration of the published spa discourse requires careful attention to the specific interests and biases expressed, above all in promotional works and advertising materials. Nevertheless, it will be shown later that the range of statements in the spa discourse transcended authors and genres, as well as fictional and nonfictional texts.

The second main group of primary sources analyzed here encompasses personal narratives – diaries, letters, and autobiographies – in order to compare the experiences of individual spa visitors to the published discourse. Finding letters, diaries, and autobiographies describing spa visits comes with its own challenges. In particular, editions often do not have indices, and their titles or tables of contents do not indicate whether spa visits are mentioned in the text. In many ways, finding personal narratives recounting spa visits resembles searching for the proverbial needle in the haystack. In comparison to the printed sources that form an almost

continuous chronological sequence – and in which statements about the
social and cultural role of the spas are repeated over and over – the personal narratives of spa visits are far fewer in number. In addition, personal
narratives do not cover the same broad geographical area as the published
discourse, in terms of either the spas visited or the areas from which the
authors originated. Overall, however, the corpus of personal narratives
examined here is large enough to compare the experiences of spa visitors
and to identify similarities and contrasts between spa visitors' experiences
and the published discourse.

Authors from northern and central Germany are most prominent,
including writers from the outer regions of the German lands such as
the Danish-German writer Jens Baggesen (1764–1826), Johann Schopenhauer (1766–1838) from Danzig (today Gdańsk in Poland), as well
as Elisa von der Recke (1754–1833) and Sophie Becker (later Schwarz,
1754–1789), the latter two from Courland. With regard to social status,
most of the personal narratives were written by members of the upper
middle class and the nobility, including ruling princes. The personal narratives from the "lowest" social ranks are those of 24-year-old Johann
Christian Kestner (1741–1800), offspring of a family of Hanoverian state
officials and the husband-to-be of Charlotte Buff, the inspiration for Lotte
in Goethe's novel *The Sorrows of Young Werther* (*Die Leiden des Jungen
Werther*);[68] of Ludwig Friedrich Christoph Schmid (1736–1798), a bailiff
and councillor in the town of Uffenheim in Ansbach;[69] of the aforementioned Sophie Becker, daughter of a Lutheran pastor; and of Goethe's
partner Christiane Vulpius (1765–1816), daughter of a poor princely
official in Weimar. Male and female authors are roughly equal in number.
Pyrmont, Karlsbad, and Lauchstädt are the most prominent among the
spa towns visited by these authors.[70]

The usual interval of years or even decades between an actual event
and its narration in an autobiography not only results in a streamlined
narrative, which focuses on a select number of events and experiences in
a person's life, but also leads to more reflection and potentially the benefit
of hindsight. In contrast, diaries and letters are often written closer to the
events and experiences and provide more detailed narratives. This does
not entail, however, that diaries and letters present experiences in a more
direct or immediate way. There is simply no way to commit an experience[71] directly to paper – it must be put into words and concepts that
emerge from the social environment of the writer. And letters need to meet
the expectations of their recipients, including narrative conventions.[72]

As Fulbrook and Rublack point out, "The purpose of reading personal
narratives, then, is not to recover a more authentic non-discursive voice
of subjects, but to use personal narratives to see as far as possible how
people worked their way through dimensions of norms and relationships,
through conflicting demands, ambivalent fears and other emotions, how
men and women gave these meaning, what narrative forms this took and

what this means in a particular context."[73] While personal narratives were embedded in contemporary discourses, they nevertheless offer the historian insights that printed sources cannot. In contrast to the often anonymous discourse, personal narratives allow us to access the perceptions of individuals whose social status and previous life experiences influenced how they responded to what they witnessed during spa visits.

The question of the relationship between the published discourse and individual experiences is therefore fundamental to this study. Both the personal narratives and the printed sources address perceptions of the natural and built environment, of social interactions, of conflicts over spaces and values. This study assumes a circle or circuit of communication embedding both the personal narratives and the printed sources. In other words, I argue that personal narratives are integrated into the discursive structures of a society. In order to communicate their experiences at spas, people had to use the established communicative patterns about spas, including those found in the published discourse. At the same time, the spa discourse could only gain credibility in society because its statements were regarded as plausible by contemporaries. The claims made and narratives told about spas in various genres of writing had to echo the expectations and experiences of readers to be persuasive.

Historians working on spas, seaside resorts, and other leisure spaces like summer retreats between the late eighteenth and the twentieth centuries have used a variety of terms to describe these spaces: "spaces of freedom,"[74] "liminoid spaces,"[75] "counter-worlds," and "safe spaces."[76] All of these terms seek to encapsulate the nature of a space situated outside the everyday world but at the same time closely connected to it. Contemporaries considered the spa to be full of ambiguities and tensions. While the spa was separated from everyday life, the published discourse and the personal narratives of spa visitors revolved around questions about the relationship between everyday spaces and the spa as a "separate world."

I argue that Michel Foucault's concept of "heterotopia"[77] aptly describes spas and their function in late eighteenth- and early nineteenth-century society. According to Foucault, heterotopias are places in a society constructed as "mirrors" to everyday spaces. They are "real places – places that do exist . . . – which are something like counter-sites, a kind of effectively enacted utopia in which the real sites, all the other real sites that can be found within the culture, are simultaneously represented, contested, and inverted."[78] These "places . . . outside all places,"[79] which are nevertheless not utopias but actual spaces, are connected to all other spaces in society but at the same time contradict them.[80] Foucault emphasizes that there are different forms of heterotopias in every society and that every society creates its own heterotopias or can change the function of existing heterotopias. Thus, heterotopias are historically variable.[81]

Contemporaries recognized and defined this specific "intermediate position" of the eighteenth-century spa as a heterotopia. The spa was outside the world, and yet it reflected the world. On the one hand, the spa was characterized as "paradise," "arcadia," "Elysium,"[82] or even "an enchanted island."[83] On the other hand, it was described as "the world in miniature."[84] As a space outside of everyday life, it was at the same time integrated into the everyday world through various communication processes.[85] During the late eighteenth century, the spa became a "heterotopia of compensation"[86] by multiplying cultural and social ideas of the Enlightenment. The spa thus offered an alternative space that, at least at first glance, seemed to be better than social reality. This defined space was also associated with a defined period of time: "The heterotopia begins to function at full capacity when men [*sic*] arrive at a sort of absolute break with their traditional time."[87] For the spa guests, this "heterochrony"[88] was the time they spent at a spa. For the spas, this heterochrony was the so-called season, the busy summer months. The spa existed as a heterotopia only in the summer; during the rest of the year it was a small town, a village, or even just a vacant facility in the open countryside.

As a heterotopia of compensation, the spa was separated from the everyday world, but everyday life also protruded into the heterotopia and was reflected, disputed, or confronted with an ideal. This is why contemporaries perceived the spa to be full of contradictions – between health and disease, between leisure and work, between social integration and social ruptures. The political and military upheavals of the late eighteenth and early nineteenth centuries are another case in point. Given the importance of these political changes – and the fact that the spa often served as a place for (secret) diplomatic meetings – the relatively small number of statements in the published spa discourse that refer to these events is striking. In contrast, we know from personal narratives that the spa was a hotbed of political conversations and people were always eager for news.[89] But, as a heterotopia, the spa was supposed to offer a better life, separated from the upheavals of the time.[90] As a result, the spa discourse rarely discusses the political disruptions that marked the late eighteenth and early nineteenth centuries.

It is therefore significant when statements about political events break into the spa discourse. The French Revolution is a case in point. It became a topic in the published discourse after the revolution had entered a phase of extreme violence. In 1793, after King Louis XVI had been executed in January, the French Revolution was on everyone's lips in Karlsbad. An article in the *German Magazine* (*Deutsches Magazin*) reported, "It absorbs all objects of conversation, and nothing else is spoken of but it."[91] Similarly, in the summer of 1815, Napoleon's final battles against the Coalition armies and the conclusion of the Congress of Vienna, which reordered the European political landscape after the Napoleonic Wars, were discussed in spa publications. The *Journal of Luxury and Fashions* (*Journal des Luxus und der Moden*) commented that spa guests in Karlsbad had been eager for news about these momentous events.[92]

As a *spatial heterotopia*, the spa served as a multiplier of new perceptions of the natural and built environment that laid the foundation for
modern tourist experiences. "Nature" and "the landscape" are decidedly
cultural categories. They are created in people's minds through widely
shared experiences and discourses. At the spas, an early modern paradigm
of urbanity was slowly replaced by a paradigm of rurality. By the turn of
the nineteenth century, new ways of perceiving mountains and the seaside were propagated and then gradually consolidated, leaving a marked
imprint on the "tourist gaze" until today.[93] This modified perception of
nature brought about new individual and collective practices, namely outings into the surrounding countryside, enabling spa visitors not only to
see the landscape in a new way but also to experience it.

As a *social heterotopia*, the spa was characterized by a "system of
opening and closing,"[94] which Foucault defines as typical of a heterotopia.
There are seemingly open heterotopias that, in fact, hide exclusions: "One
thinks one has entered and, by the sole fact of entering, one is excluded."[95]
The German spa in the long eighteenth century was just such a place,
where all social groups were allowed to enter, but the interior spaces of the
spa were, in fact, marked by numerous processes of exclusion.[96] Against
this background, the spa served as both an actual space for encounters
between the nobility and the upper middle class, and a "projection surface" for the bourgeois media discourse.

In analogy to salons, Masonic lodges, and other institutions of Enlightenment sociability in the eighteenth century,[97] the spa was defined as
a meeting place of the nobility and the bourgeoisie where they could
practice new forms of communication and interaction. Therefore, the spa
was separated from everyday social life in terms of both space and time.
Enlightenment ideas were projected onto the spa, and this led contemporaries to associate the spa with expectations for the future of society.
In the bourgeois discourse, the forms of communication and interaction
practiced at the spa were expected to transfer into society and fundamentally change the course of history.

Overall, the German spa served both as a discursive multiplier and as
a setting for cultural and social processes of transformation during the
watershed period between the early modern and modern eras. The spas
analyzed here were visited by members of the nobility and upper middle
class, who traveled at least regionally, and sometimes "nationally" and
"internationally," for the annual spa season. As a result, the spas were
multifunctional spaces for these social elites, while at the same time spa
visitors and the published spa discourse perceived the spas as special
places where different social rules were supposed to apply. At the spas
– both in actual spaces and in the published discourse – questions about
society's relationship to the natural world, about the interaction between
the nobility and the middle class, and about a new bourgeois self-image
were discussed and negotiated.

In light of the dearth of research on the German spa in the early modern period and the long eighteenth century, Part I provides foundational background information. Chapter 1, "Spas from the Late Middle Ages to the Eighteenth Century," gives an overview of the development of central European spas between the late fifteenth and the eighteenth centuries and provides a hierarchy of spas derived from two categories decisive for their success: support by their owners and the social composition of the spa-goers. Chapter 2, "Spas as Centers of Communication: Face-to-Face Interactions and Print Culture," discusses the spa as a center of communication networks, which extended from one-on-one interactions to a spa discourse that became part of the Enlightenment public sphere.

Part II deals with the rise of the spa as a multiplier of new ideas about nature and the creation of a daily "vacation" routine at the spa, concepts that have fundamentally influenced modern tourism. This part is based on both textual and visual sources. Chapter 3, "Reinventing the Eighteenth-Century Spa as a Leisure Space," explores the gradual transformation of the urban ideal of the early modern spa into a new ideal, now combining urban amenities and leisure activities with "rural" landscape gardens. Chapter 4, "Spas and Seaside Resorts on the Cusp of Modern Tourism: New Perceptions of Nature and a Daily Routine," traces how the spa of the late eighteenth and early nineteenth centuries functioned as a multiplier of a modern perception of nature that valued rugged mountains and the seaside over townscapes. This chapter also analyzes how spas developed a specific daily routine.

Part III examines the social function of the late eighteenth- and early nineteenth-century spa as a meeting place for the nobility and the rising bourgeoisie. Contemporaries regarded spas as analogous to Masonic lodges, salons, and other institutions of Enlightenment sociability. Each of these spaces was supposed to allow the nobility and the bourgeoisie to meet on an equal footing and, over time, create a new social order. Chapter 5, "The Spa in the Eighteenth Century: From Social Hierarchy to New Demands for Equality," traces the development from social separation at the spa during the early modern period to the outspoken demands for social equality that characterized the spa discourse of the late eighteenth century. Chapter 6, " Nobility and Bourgeoisie at the Spa: Creating Unity and Maintaining Differences," analyzes in detail the different ways in which contemporaries conceptualized the relationship and interactions between the nobility and the middle class at the spa – both in a lively Enlightenment debate and in practice. This chapter also explores the limitations of the spa as a social heterotopia.

Notes

1. Hufeland, *Praktische Uebersicht der vorzüglichsten Heilquellen Teutschlands*, 1815, 94: "Da es einer der besuchtesten, und zwar von den höhern und reichsten Klassen besuchtesten, Bäder ist, so ist natürlicher Weise die

Lebensart geräuschvoll, luxuriös, kostbar und vornehm, daher auch oft gezwungen und drückend für geringere Stände. Es läßt sich jedoch hoffen, daß sich dies immer mehr verlieren, und man endlich zu der Einsicht kommen werde, daß ein Hauptreiz solcher Anstalten der ist und seyn soll, aus den gewöhnlichen Verhältnissen und steifen Einengungen des bürgerlichen Lebens herauszutreten, sich einmal in freier Luft auch der Freiheit des Lebens zu erfreuen, und die reine Natur mit ihren Gaben auch natürlich zu genießen."

2. See Bergdolt, *Wellbeing*, 261; Lempa, *Beyond the Gymnasium*, 47–63. For a broad chronological European overview, see Porter, *Medical History of Waters and Spas*; Boisseuil, Wulfram, *Renaissance der Heilquellen*.

3. See Rosseaux, *Städte in der Frühen Neuzeit*, 45–46, 144.

4. See Rosseaux, *Freiräume*, 211–224; Steward, "Role of Inland Spas"; Wurst, *Fabricating Pleasure*, 255–261.

5. See Bitz, *Badewesen*; Eßer, Fuchs, *Bäder und Kuren in der Aufklärung*; Fuhs, *Mondäne Orte*; Kaufmann, *Gesellschaft im Bad*; Loleit, *Wahrheit, Lüge, Fiktion*; Kuhnert, *Urbanität*; Ziegler, *Deutsche Kurstädte*.

6. See, e.g., Wood, *Health and Hazard*; Geisthövel, "Promenadenmischungen"; Sommer, *Zur Kur nach Ems*; Fuhs, *Mondäne Orte*; Triendl-Zadoff, *Nächstes Jahr in Marienbad*, translated as Zadoff, *Next Year in Marienbad*. For the seaside resorts, see, e.g., Bresgott, *Ostseeküste*; Kolbe, "Viel versprechende Strandwelten"; Kolbe, "Strandurlaub."

7. Daniel, *Kompendium Kulturgeschichte*, 11: "kollektiven Sinnstiftungen."

8. See Introduction to Part III.

9. See Introduction to Part II.

10. See Porter, *Kunst des Heilens*, 246–306.

11. Even in 1831, Hufeland declared, "I come back to this again and again, as I have often said, that mineral waters represent a class of their own as products of nature and as agents, and that our chemistry is still far from being able to decide about their compounds, their value or worthlessness." ("Ich komme immer wieder darauf zurück, was ich schon öfter gesagt habe, daß die Mineralwasser eine große, ganz eigene Klasse von Naturprodukten und Agentien darstellen, und daß unsere Chemie noch lange nicht im Stande ist, über ihre Mischung, Werth oder Unwerth, zu entscheiden.") Hufeland, *Praktische Uebersicht der vorzüglichsten Heilquellen Teutschlands*, 1831, 6. See also Lotz-Heumann, "Repräsentationen."

12. See Trampel, *Beschreibung des Bades zu Meinberg*, 1770, for an example of comparative advertising of Meinberg and Pyrmont.

13. See Eulner, "Kur- und Badebetrieb," 129–130; Kuhnert, *Urbanität*, 60.

14. See, e.g., Mosch, *Bäder und Heilbrunnen*, 1819; Reichard, *Passagier auf der Reise*, 1801.

15. Scheidemantel, *Anleitung zum vernünftigen Gebrauch*, 1792, V: "So ist der Grund, warum sie ein gewisses Wasser vor andern auslesen, keiner weiter, als der, daß sie Freunden versprochen haben, in deren Gesellschaft an diesem Orte eine Brunnen- oder Badecur zu halten."

16. Frankenau, *Pyrmont*, 1799, 122: "Diejenigen, welche Drang fühlen, das eine oder andere Bad zu besuchen, besonders Damen, sollten nicht schwazsüchtige Freundinnen zu einer Theeassemblee einladen, um bey der Gelegenheit, unter unzähligen O! und A! eine Stimmensammlung anzustellen, welches Bad die gnädige Frau mit der Gegenwart ihrer hohen Person beehren mag."

17. Paul, *Dr. Katzenbergers Badereise*.

18. [Möser], *Schreiben des Verfassers*, 1746, 26: "der Richter zu Lüda."

19. Scheidemantel, *Anleitung zum vernünftigen Gebrauch*, 1792, Vorbericht, 2: "von sehr vielen Menschen, vorzüglich von deren höhern oder mittlern Classe in jedem Sommer gebraucht."

20. Schopenhauer, *Im Wechsel der Zeiten*, 194: "Überhaupt gab es bei sehr mangelhafter Einrichtung der Brunnenorte damals in Deutschland derselben nur wenige; jetzt würde es schwerfallen, mehr als zehn Meilen zurückzulegen, ohne auf eine größere oder kleinere, dem menschlichen Erfindungsgeist oder der Natur entspringende Heilquelle zu stoßen. Vor fünfzig oder sechzig Jahren waren viele der jetzt besuchtesten teils noch unbekannt, teils nur von in der Nähe derselben Wohnenden spärlich benutzt und ärmlich ausgestattet; an die zweckmäßige Einrichtung von Seebädern wurde aber noch gar nicht gedacht."

21. See Kuhnert, *Urbanität*, 34.

22. See Bahlcke, Eberhard, Polívka, *Handbuch der historischen Stätten: Böhmen und Mähren*, article "Karlsbad," 250.

23. See Martin, *Deutsches Badewesen*, 330–331.

24. On social differentiation within the German *Bürgertum*, see Introduction to Part III.

25. See Behringer, *Im Zeichen des Merkur*, 436–485; Bödeker, "Reisebeschreibungen," 283.

26. "Badechronik," *JLM* (October 1805), 677: "Das Beispiel der Großen und Reichen wirkt hier wie überall im Gebiet des Luxus und der Mode unvermerkt in absteigender Linie. Daher die Manie, auch der mittleren Stände, ohne krank zu seyn, blos der lieben Mode wegen, eine Badreise zu machen."

27. "Badechronik," *JLM* (June 1800), 296: "So wie es an keinem Bedürfnisse, weder für Kranke noch für Gesunde, weder zur Nothwendigkeit noch zum Vergnügen fehlt."

28. Willebrand, *Carlsbader Brunnenreise*, 1780, 52: "Aber gedenken Sie, mein Liebster! ja nicht, daß alle Menschen, die hier auftreten, wirklich Kranke und Brunnengäste sind. Neine – dafür behüte der Himmel! – Sehr viele reisen hierher, um die Langeweile zu verkürzen – cum privilegio etliche Wochen müßig zu gehen, und sich ihrer Amtssorgen zu entschlagen – den Hausfrieden hier zu suchen – die Leber abzuspülen, um zu neuen Schmausereyen sich geschickt zu machen. Viele sind hier, um ihre Pferde, Stallknechte in modernen Livereyen – auch ihre Läufer u.s.f. bewundern, und ihre neuen Ritterorden beschauen, beneiden oder sich baronisiren zu lassen." See also [Schulz], *Reise eines Lief-länders*, 1795, 76–77.

29. On eighteenth-century consumer society in Germany, see North, "*Material Delight.*"

30. "Ueber den Luxus des Badereisens," *JLM* (July 1798), 320: "Zu unsrer Zeit werden sie als Plaisirörter von den Meisten betrachtet und besucht; bey solchen ist also das Badewesen bloßer Luxus. Der größte Theil der Brunnen- und Badegäste trinkt kein Wasser und badet nicht; ihre Absicht ist lediglich, eine Lustreise zu machen, Freunde kennen zu lernen, zu tanzen, zu spielen, sich zu zerstreuen u.s.w." See also Reichard, *Passagier auf der Reise*, 1801, 351–352.

31. Möser, *Briefwechsel*, letter from Möser to Nicolai, 17 April 1789, 699: "Am 4. Juli abends um Glock 9 werde ich g[eliebts] G[ott] in Pyrmont seyn; und das Vergnügen, Sie dort zu sehen, wird auf meine Gesundheit besser wirken als Bad und Brunnen, deren ich keins gebrauche."

32. See Marcard, *Beschreibung von Pyrmont*, vol. 1, 1784, 43–44.

33. Deneken, "Bemerkungen bey dem Rehburger Gesundbrunnen," 1796, 193: "Jeder will hier seine Geschäfte vergessen und den Geist erheitern. Alle, welche sonst in ganz verschiedenen Verhältnissen leben, haben sich die Beförderung des wechselseitigen Vergnügens hier zum gemeinschaftlichen Berufe gemacht. – Dem Grabe entgegenwankende – Leichenähnliche Kranke sind zu Rehburg seltene Erscheinungen. Viele kommen blos hierher, um sich zu ergötzen."

34. Hoser, *Beschreibung von Franzensbrunn*, 1799, 115: "Nicht minder weit weg von sich verscheucht ein Brunnenort, dem es an Vergnügungen fehlt, jeden Gesunden der für sein Geld nur Zerstreuung sucht, und der . . . eigentlich die Seele der Unterhaltung und des freien heitern Tons in solchen Oertern ist."

35. Ketelhodt, *Tagebuch einer Reise*, 300: "ist doch dieses Bad um deswillen sehr belebt und lustig, weil nur sehr wenige Personen zur Wiederherstellung ihrer Gesundheit, die meisten aber für ihr Vergnügen hier sind."

36. [Möser], *Schreiben des Verfassers*, 1746, 25: "Wer hier krank ist, der ist im Paradiese verloren."

37. "Badechronik," *JLM* (October 1805), 677: "Wir leben in einem Zeitalter der Widersprüche. Selbst da, wo der Leidende für Gebrechen seines Körpers Linderung und Heilung sucht, selbst da baut der Sibarit sich Tempel der Freude und des Wohlbehagens, und die Heilquellen, welche die Natur zur Labung des Siechen rinnen ließ, schafft der Genuß dürstende nie zu sättigende Weltmann, zu Quellen der feinsten, nicht immer lautersten Vergnügungen um."

38. See Melton, *Rise of the Public*.

39. See Faulstich, *Medien*; Faulstich, *Die bürgerliche Mediengesellschaft*; Würgler, *Medien*, 63.

40. See Wehler, *Deutsche Gesellschaftsgeschichte*, 310; Fischer, Haefs, Mix, *Von Almanach*, 20; Gestrich, *Absolutismus*, 185; Maurer, *Biographie des Bürgers*, 57.

41. See Faulstich, *Die bürgerliche Mediengesellschaft*.

42. See Fischer, Haefs, Mix, *Von Almanach*.

43. Cilleßen, "Modezeitschriften," 211: "das Informationsgefälle zwischen Stadt und Land, zwischen Metropole und Provinz zu verringern." See Faulstich, *Die bürgerliche Mediengesellschaft*, 242–250. See also the assessment by Wehler, *Deutsche Gesellschaftsgeschichte*, 309: "More than one third (742) of the journals between 1765 and 1790 were limited to entertainment, while the other two thirds were dominated by literature, politics, and science." ("Mehr als ein Drittel [742] der Zeitschriften zwischen 1765 und 1790 beschränkte sich auf Unterhaltung, aber die anderen zwei Drittel wurden von Literatur, Politik und Wissenschaft beherrscht.")

44. Faulstich, *Die bürgerliche Mediengesellschaft*, 225: "Schlüsselmedium der bürgerlichen Gesellschaft." See also 250.

45. "Badechronik," *JLM* (September 1798), 497–498: "Unser deutsches Moden-Journal wird mit Recht auf einigen öffentlichen Bibliotheken gehalten. Denn nach Jahrhunderten, wenn vielleicht unsere Nation in das Chaos der Allgemeinheit einer Universalnation geschmolzen seyn wird, kann es noch manchem Geschichtsschreiber ein willkommener Fund seyn, um die Sitten, Moden und Gebräuche der Jetztwelt daraus zu schöpfen."

46. Haefs, "Zensur," 415: "gegenläufigen Institutionen und Interessen im 18. Jahrhundert . . . zu 'Ineffizienz', aus anderer Perspektive zu Freiräumen führten." See also Müller, *Aufklärung*, 35–36.

47. See the 1814 statement by Perthes, quoted in Kiesel, Münch, *Gesellschaft*, 118: "Germany always had the most complete freedom of the press, . . . because what was not allowed to be printed in Prussia was allowed in Württemberg, what was not allowed in Hamburg, [was allowed to be printed] ten steps away in Altona. No book remained unprinted, no book uncirculated." ("Deutschland hatte immer die vollständigste Preßfreiheit, . . . denn was in Preußen nicht gedruckt werden durfte, das durfte es in Württemberg, was in Hamburg nicht, zehn Schritte davon in Altona. Kein Buch blieb ungedruckt, keines unverbreitet.")

48. Siemann, "Zensur," 366: "Im Deutschen Bund wurde die alte traditionelle Zensur mit dem Zensor in Aktion wieder belebt, aber nun deutschlandweit

und erheblich systematischer institutionalisiert als noch im Alten Reich. Das Fundament bildeten die sogenannten Karlsbader Beschlüsse von 1819, welche die generelle Zensur des Schrifttums vorsahen."

49. See Chapter 4 and the map at the end of this book.

50. See Koselleck, "Einleitung"; Koselleck, "Das achtzehnte Jahrhundert."

51. Koselleck, "Das achtzehnte Jahrhundert," 280–281: "Übergangszeit . . . in der es immer schwerer wird, die überkommenen Traditionen mit den notwendigen Neuerungen zu vermitteln."

52. See, e.g., Raymond, *Von der Landschaft*; Trepp, *Sanfte Männlichkeit*; Borgstedt, *Zeitalter der Aufklärung*, 5–9; Müller, *Aufklärung*, 10–12, 100–108.

53. The works excluded here are medical dissertations and treatises on the chemical composition and analysis of healing waters as well as treatises on the application and therapeutic effects of one or more healing waters primarily targeting physicians. Libraries often group such works together with the spa literature examined here in a category labeled "balneology." This study also does not take into account works that were part of the growing late eighteenth-century discourse on the use of water for the purposes of hygiene and health maintenance, covering topics such as regular washing with water, swimming in rivers, municipal baths, and the production of artificial mineral waters. See Frey, *Der reinliche Bürger*; Cilleßen, *Exotismus*.

54. The *Journal des Luxus und der Moden* changed its title slightly several times over the decades of its publication history. See the note in the bibliography. For more details, see Borchert, Dressel, *Journal des Luxus und der Moden*, 9–10. For an analytical bibliography of the *Journal*, see Kuhles, Standke, *Journal des Luxus und der Moden*.

55. Müller, *Welt des Baedeker*, 275: "Reiseführer . . . befinden . . . sich im ständigen Wechselspiel mit anderen visuellen Medien."

56. See Emich, "Bildlichkeit und Intermedialität."

57. See Baberowski, *Sinn der Geschichte*, 196–197: "A discourse is everything that can be said, and it is the set of rules that determines what and how something can be said. Foucault is not interested in the question of how language functions, he is interested in the regimes of sayability." ("Ein Diskurs ist alles das, was gesagt werden kann, und es ist das Regelwerk, das darüber bestimmt, was und wie etwas gesagt werden kann. Foucault interessiert sich nicht für die Frage, wie Sprache funktioniert, ihn interessieren die Sagbarkeitsregime.")

58. See Foucault, *Archaeology*, 42–44; Sarasin, "Diskurstheorie," 61.

59. Foucault, *Archaeology*, 80.

60. Sarasin, *Geschichtswissenschaft und Diskursanalyse*, 34: "Knappheit."

61. Foucault, *Archaeology*, 49.

62. Sarasin, "Diskurstheorie," 61: "Redezusammenhänge . . . mit Aussage- und Wahrheitsregeln, die historisch situiert sind, das heißt einen Anfang und ein Ende sowie einen bestimmten sozialen (und . . . kulturellen) Ort haben."

63. Foucault, *Archaeology*, 74. See also Daniel, *Kompendium Kulturgeschichte*, 171.

64. Beyond the primary sources analyzed for this study, there are many others that could not be covered here. The *Verzeichnis der im deutschen Sprachraum erschienenen Drucke des 18. Jahrhunderts* (*VD 18*, www.vd18.de) is incomplete. In addition, numerous reviews of spa publications as well as accidental finds in the *Zeitung für die elegante Welt*, which has not yet been indexed, and in regional intelligencers (*Intelligenzblätter*), which have also not yet been systematically indexed, show that the spa discourse of the late eighteenth and early nineteenth centuries reached a broad reading public.

65. See Foucault, *Archaeology*, 22–25.

66. See Foucault, *Archaeology*, 122; Landwehr, *Geschichte des Sagbaren*, 80.
67. Sarasin, "Subjekte," 145: "das Denken und Handeln der Vielen strukturierten." See also Haslinger, "Diskurs," 33.
68. See Kestner, *Die wahre Brunnenfreiheit*; Lampe, *Aristokratie*.
69. See Schmid, *"Wer an seinem Schöpfer sündiget . . .".*
70. For a detailed description of the hierarchy of early modern and eighteenth-century spas, see Chapter 1.
71. On the complexity of applying the category "experience," see Münch, *"Erfahrung"*.
72. See Günther, "'And Now for Something Completely Different'," 51.
73. Fulbrook, Rublack, "In Relation," 271. See also Jancke, Ulbrich, *Vom Individuum*, 26; Stolberg, *Homo patiens*, 30–31. Sarasin argues more forcefully, "Most of what appears in so-called ego-documents as the 'experience' of the speaking subject simply refers back to the discursive conditions that formed this experience." ("Das meiste, das in so genannten Ego-Dokumenten als 'Erfahrung' des sprechenden Subjekts erscheint, verweist schlicht zurück auf die diskursiven Bedingungen, die diese Erfahrung formten.") Sarasin, *Geschichtswissenschaft und Diskursanalyse*, 120.
74. Rosseaux, *Freiräume*; Mai, "Touristische Räume," 13: "Freiräume."
75. Kolbe, "Strandurlaub," 188–189: "liminoide[r] Raum."
76. Triendl-Zadoff, *Nächstes Jahr in Marienbad*, 18–19, 39, 76–77, 133, 210, 215 and passim: "Gegenwelten" – "Schutzräume." Triendl-Zadoff also uses the concept of "heterotopia." See also Zadoff, *Next Year in Marienbad*.
77. See Foucault, "Of Other Spaces"; Foucault, "Of Other Spaces: Utopias and Heterotopias"; Foucault, "Des espaces autres."
78. Foucault, "Of Other Spaces," 24. See also Foucault, "Des espaces autres," 755; Foucault, "Of Other Spaces: Utopias and Heterotopias," 352.
79. Foucault, "Of Other Spaces," 24. See also Foucault, "Des espaces autres," 755.
80. See Foucault, "Of Other Spaces," 24; Foucault, "Des espaces autres," 755.
81. See Foucault, "Of Other Spaces," 24–25; Foucault, "Des espaces autres," 756–758.
82. See, e.g., "Badechronik," *JLM* (October 1799), 490.
83. Pauline zur Lippe and Herzog Friedrich Christian von Augustenburg, *Briefe*, 17 August 1790: "bezauberten Insul" (i.e., Pyrmont).
84. See, e.g., [Grundig], *Beschreibung seiner, im Jahr 1751 in das Käyser Carls-Bad gethanen Reise*, 1754, 80–81; "Teutsche Badechronik," *JLM* (November 1796), 558.
85. See Chapter 2.
86. Foucault, "Of Other Spaces," 27.
87. Foucault, "Of Other Spaces," 26. See also Foucault, "Des espaces autres," 759.
88. Foucault, "Of Other Spaces," 26. See also Foucault, "Des espaces autres," 759.
89. For example, in 1793, Lavater described in his travel diary how the spa guests in Pyrmont discussed the news of the surrender of the city of Mainz on 22 July. The city had been occupied by the French army during the War of the First Coalition. See Lavater, *Reisetagebücher*, 290. See also Luise von Preussen, *Fünfundvierzig Jahre aus meinem Leben*, 295, about the War of the Sixth Coalition (*Befreiungskriege*) against Napoleon in 1813.
90. See Grattenauer, *Über Neutralität, Erhaltung und Sicherheit der Bäder*.
91. [Giseke], "Fortsetzung der Briefe über Carlsbad," 1793, 824: "Alle Gegenstände der Unterredung absorbiert sie, und es wird von sonst nichts gesprochen als von ihr."
92. "Bade-Chronik," *JLM* (November 1815), 658–659.

93. Urry, Larsen, *Tourist Gaze.*
94. Foucault, "Of Other Spaces," 26.
95. Foucault, "Of Other Spaces: Utopias and Heterotopias," 355. See also Foucault, "Des espaces autres," 760.
96. See Chapter 6.
97. See Hardtwig, *Genossenschaft,* 285–320.

Part I
Foundations

1 Spas from the Late Middle Ages to the Eighteenth Century

The Development of Spas and Health Practices Between the Late Middle Ages and the Eighteenth Century

The Romans started the long tradition of central European spas. Among others, Aachen, Baden-Baden, and Wiesbaden were Roman baths. With the collapse of the Roman Empire a long period of decline began, and it was only in the thirteenth and fourteenth centuries that people used these hot springs again.[1] By the late fourteenth century a "new pattern of bathing behavior" had emerged: people increasingly went on "bathing trips" to existing or newly discovered hot springs.[2] New spas like Wildbad in Württemberg or Karlsbad in Bohemia were mostly situated in the open countryside. Without protective walls, spas could be dangerous places for guests. In 1367, for example, Count Eberhard II of Württemberg and his son Ulrich were attacked in Wildbad by the counts of Eberstein. Count Eberhard and his family escaped with their lives because a peasant warned them of the impending attack.[3]

In the fifteenth century, due to the increasing popularity of bathing trips, many spas underwent major transformations. These were usually initiated by their princely owners. Bathing ordinances were issued, spas were fortified with walls and declared independent legal districts, and bathing pools and spa hostels were built.[4] The architectural ensembles of Plombières (or Plummers) in Lorraine (Figure 1.1) and Bagno Vignoni in Tuscany, with centrally located bathing pools surrounded by hostels, were typical of the late Middle Ages and the early sixteenth century. As a result, the material culture of these spas conveyed a sense of urbanity. The lower social orders usually bathed in open-air or partially covered pools. For the higher social classes separate baths were provided, and enclosed bath-houses became more common. Before the early modern period, however, baths continued to be used primarily in groups.[5] Physicians recommended that spa-goers bathe for a very long time – four to ten hours a day – with the purpose of causing a so-called bathing rash (*Badeausschlag*). Based on the contemporary idea of the permeability of the skin,[6] the bathing rash was considered a sign of inner cleansing and thus the beginning of healing.[7]

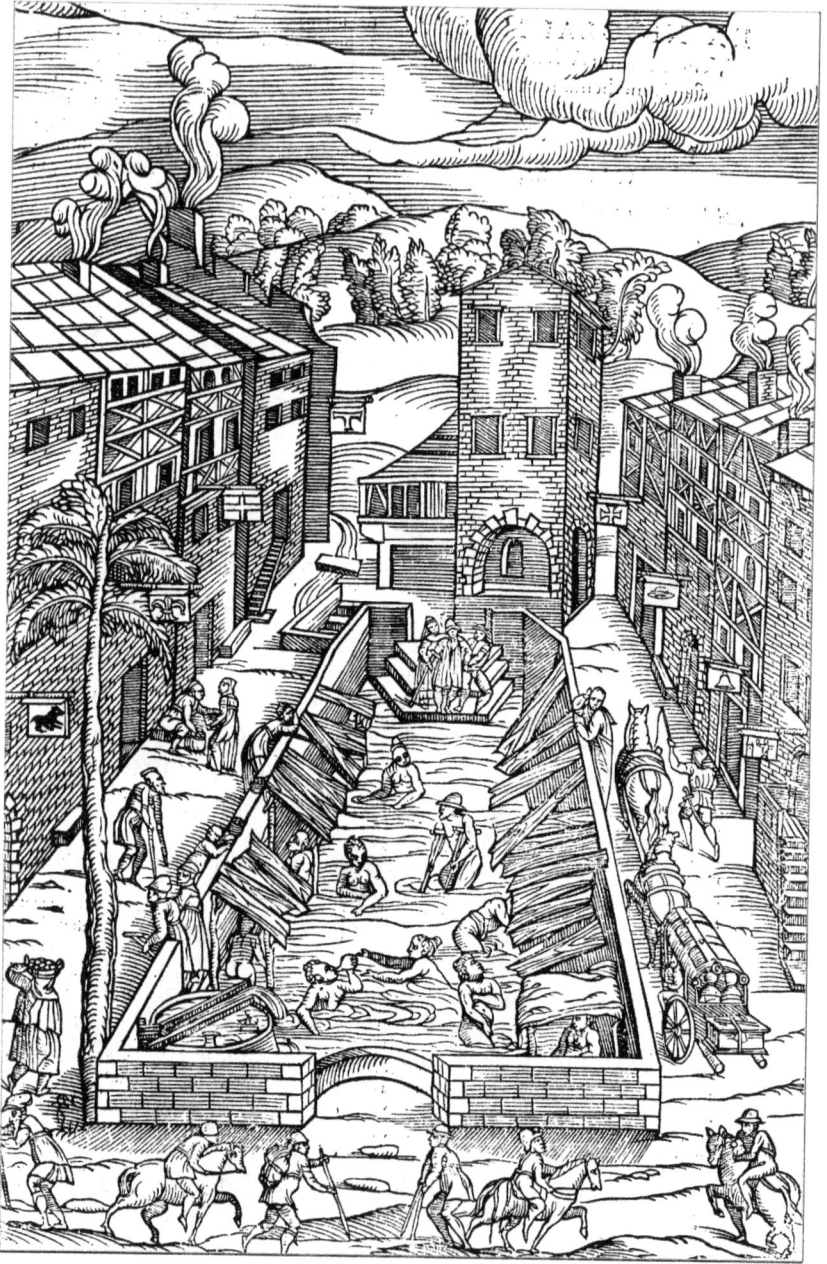

Figure 1.1 Plombières or Plummers in Lorraine, engraving, 1553. ("Balneum
Plummers." In *De balneis omnia quae extant*, 299. Venice: Iuntas,
1553. Staats- und Stadtbibliothek Augsburg, shelf mark 2 Med 19.)

This is illustrated by the diary of the Augsburg merchant Lucas Rem, who traveled to Pfäfers in Switzerland and to Wildbad in the Black Forest in the early sixteenth century.[8] During his visit to Pfäfers from 20 May to 9 June 1511, Rem extended his daily bathing time from four to eleven hours before shortening it again. On 30 May, his bathing rash broke out. He reported that he also made use of cupping therapy. Rem followed the same basic pattern while staying at Wildbad in the years 1521, 1525, 1530, 1535, 1536, and 1540, usually in August/September. He regularly extended his bathing times from three or four hours to seven or eight. In addition to cupping, he also used sweat baths.

During the second half of the sixteenth and the early seventeenth centuries, two fundamental changes in the usage of healing waters impacted the history of spas. First, in addition to hot springs, acidulous and other cold mineral waters, the so-called health springs (*Gesundbrunnen*),[9] became more popular and led to a sharp increase in the number of springs available for healing purposes. Second, as supplements to bathing, the drinking cure and the shower (*Dusche*), namely a jet of water aimed directly at the head or another part of the body, were introduced (Figure 1.2).[10] The

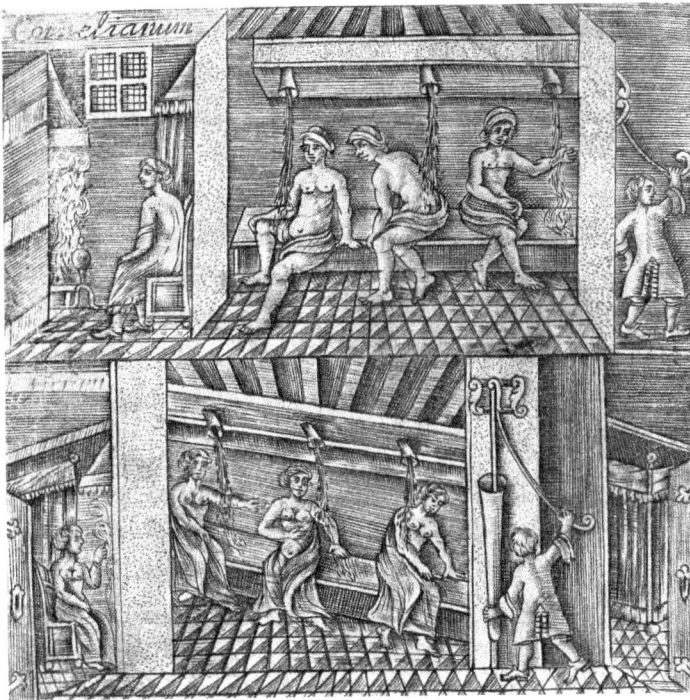

Figure 1.2 Aachen, therapeutic showers, engraving, 1688. (In Blondel, François. *Außfürliche Erklärung vnd Augenscheinliche Wunderwirckung Deren Heylsamen Badt- und Trinckwässern zu Aach*, 85. Aachen: Clemens, 1688. SLUB Dresden/Deutsche Fotothek/DDZ.)

introduction of the drinking cure led to the construction of stone wells that provided comfortable access for spa guests (Figure 1.3). Servants were at hand to scoop the healing water. (See the picture-in-the-picture depicting the Wine Spring [*Weinbrunnen*] in Schwalbach in the bottom

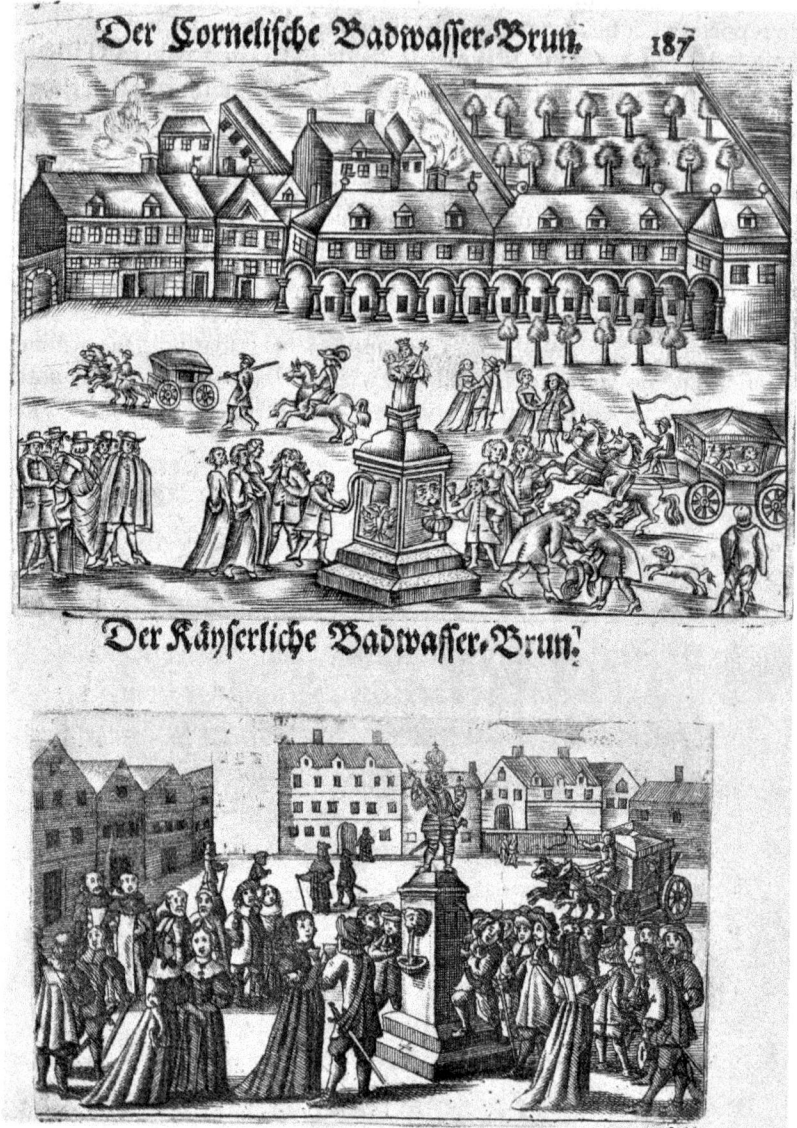

Figure 1.3 Aachen, drinking wells, engraving, 1688. ("Der Cornelische Badwas-ser-Brun. Der Kayserliche Badwasser-Brun." In Blondel, François. *Außfürliche Erklärung vnd Augenscheinliche Wunderwirckung Deren Heylsamen Badt- und Trinckwässern zu Aach*, 187. Aachen: Clemens, 1688. SLUB Dresden/Deutsche Fotothek/DDZ.)

left corner of Figure 3.4.) Over the course of the seventeenth century, the drinking cure became the most popular therapy at the spas, even at those with hot springs like Aachen and Karlsbad, but bathing cures continued to be used as well. In fact, bathing, albeit with shortened bathing times, remained an integral part of the therapies offered at spas. This is confirmed by personal narratives from spa visitors[11] and by the fact that even newly built spas in the eighteenth century had bathhouses.[12]

The spread of these new spa practices from the second half of the sixteenth century onward is illustrated by the travel diary of the French nobleman Michel de Montaigne, famous for his *Essais*, and the letters of the Nuremberg merchant Balthasar Paumgartner. Montaigne visited Plombières in Lorraine and Baden in Switzerland in 1580–1581, as well as Bagni di Lucca and other Tuscan baths, to seek a cure for his bladder stones.[13] Paumgartner traveled to Bagni di Lucca in 1584 and 1594, to Karlsbad in 1591, and to (Langen-)Schwalbach in the Taunus mountains in 1596.[14] Both Montaigne and Paumgartner used the drinking cure and the shower. Their bathing times were limited to between half an hour and two hours.[15] The contrast between Lucas Rem at the beginning of the sixteenth century and Balthasar Paumgartner at the end is particularly striking: while Rem sat in the water for long hours during his visit to Wildbad, Paumgartner traveled to Schwalbach primarily for a drinking cure.

The transformed spa map of central Europe reflects this shift in spa treatments over the course of the sixteenth century. Hot springs like Aachen, Baden-Baden, Ems, Wiesbaden, and Wildbad were leading spas in the Holy Roman Empire at the beginning of the early modern period. In addition, other European spas with hot springs like Bagni di Lucca and Plombières (Figure 1.1), and spas in Switzerland such as Baden, Leuck, and Pfäfers (Figure 3.1), were established names in the perception of central European spa visitors. With the growing popularity of cold mineral waters and the drinking cure, Schwalbach quickly turned into a highly successful spa. While Schwalbach was on the rise at the end of the sixteenth century, the popularity of Wildbad declined.[16] In the long run, Pyrmont and Karlsbad, which Balthasar Paumgartner still considered "a very rough hot spring" in 1591,[17] gained in importance. Pyrmont and Karlsbad became two of the leading spas of the empire in the late seventeenth and eighteenth centuries.

The Thirty Years' War resulted in a general decline of the spas; nevertheless, the spa tradition of the early modern empire continued after the war. Between the late seventeenth and the early nineteenth centuries, spas expanded almost without interruption. The Seven Years' War and the Napoleonic Wars left their mark on different spa regions at different times. For example, the success story of Aachen came to an abrupt end with the French occupation from 1792/1794 onward, while the spas in the central and eastern parts of the empire were negatively affected by the military operations of the early nineteenth century.[18] Overall, however, long-term processes profoundly contributed to the establishment of spa travel as a regular summer activity for the middle classes and the nobility by the second half of the eighteenth century. The network of roads in the empire was vastly improved by the construction of causeways.[19] The "regular passenger transport" of the postal service and the *Extrapost* became integral elements of traveling.[20] In addition, the countryside was generally safer in the eighteenth century than in preceding times, so that traveling to and staying at a spa became far less risky.

The rise of the spas in the eighteenth century found expression in the architectural redesign of existing spas, among others Pyrmont and Lauch-städt. This development reached its peak in the late eighteenth and early nineteenth centuries, with new spas emerging at mineral springs that had previously been neglected or were newly discovered, such as Wilhelms-bad, Hofgeismar, and Berka. Therefore, the spa hierarchy and spa map of the long eighteenth century look very different when compared to those of the late sixteenth and early seventeenth centuries. Most of these new spas were located in or near towns or villages and depended on continuous support from the local prince.

Spas and Their Patrons in the Long Eighteenth Century

In the 1669 novel *Simplicius Simplicissimus*, Hans Jacob Christoph von Grimmelshausen describes the importance of sustained support and promotion by the spa owner for a spa's development. The novel's protagonist Simplicissimus receives a stone from the prince of the Mummel Lake (*Mummelsee*) that supposedly causes a healing spring to appear upon touching the ground. Simplicissimus imagines how the healing well would prove beneficial to him:

> I already had ideas about the impressive structure I would build there so that the guests could be put up in style, and about all the money I would earn by renting lodgings, I was already thinking about how much I would have to bribe the doctors to persuade them to recommend my marvelous mineral springs over others, even the ones in Schwalbach, so that I'd have a bunch of rich guests. I was already grading whole mountains so that those who came and went wouldn't complain about the road. I was even hiring crafty houseboys, miserly cooks, careful maids, vigilant stable boys and orderly bath and water supervisors. I even thought of a place near my farm where I could plant a beautiful, level pleasure garden on the side of the wild mountain. There I would raise all kinds of rare plants, and my gentlemen guests and their ladies could go walking there, the sick could refresh themselves and the healthy could philander or amuse themselves with all sorts of entertaining games. The doctors would have to compose a fabulous testimonial about my springs and its [*sic*] qualities – for a

price, of course – which I would have printed along with an engraving
of my farm; then any patient who hadn't yet been there could work
up his hopes by reading himself half-well.[21]

Not without irony, Grimmelshausen gives the reader a detailed view
of how to create and promote a spa in the long eighteenth century. A
spa furthered its owner's social advancement by drawing "gentlemen
guests and their ladies" to a place that is, in effect, described as a country
farm. At the same time, the spa is a source of (hoped-for) financial profit.
Later on in the chapter, Simplicissimus states that he wants to "make a
gentlemanly business" out of the "precious springs on my farm."[22] Grimmelshausen touches upon the various aspects of promoting and sustaining
a spa in order to make it a success with spa visitors, whether they were
sick or healthy. Convenient access roads, gardens, and various forms of
entertainment were particularly important.

At the same time, Grimmelshausen emphasizes that the spa of the long
eighteenth century was a creation of the media. His character Simplicissimus explicitly discusses the role of the spa discourse for the success of a
spa in attracting visitors. In order to ensure a spa's presence and visibility
in the published discourse, spa owners commissioned advertising material like spa guides and engravings. Often, comparative advertising was
the method of choice; Simplicissimus compares his spa with Schwalbach,
the most famous spa at the time. Spa owners hired spa physicians (*Brunnenärzte*) not only to care for spa visitors but also to write spa treatises,
thus propagating the spa in the published discourse. Grimmelshausen
is brutally honest with his readers about the fact that the healing qualities of a water spring were largely constructed through persuasion and
social consensus. While Grimmelshausen discusses all of this with irony,
he refers to lived experience. For instance, Count Wilhelm IX of Hanau
commissioned the fictional *Letters of a Swiss* (*Briefe eines Schweizers*) as
well as copperplate engravings to establish the spa of Wilhelmsbad in the
late eighteenth-century spa discourse.[23]

For eighteenth-century Germany, three main categories of spa patrons
can be identified: princes, urban magistrates, and private entrepreneurs.
Whereas in England private initiatives and private investors played a central role in the development of spas,[24] the vast majority of central European spas were princely spas, including Alexandersbad, Baden-Baden,
Berka, Bertrich, Bocklet, Boll, Brückenau, Freienwalde, Godesberg, Hofgeismar, Lauchstädt, Liebenstein, Meinberg, Nenndorf, Pyrmont, Teinach, Teplitz (today Teplice in the Czech Republic), Wilhelmsbad, as well
as many others.

The number of urban and private entrepreneurial German spas was
small. Two of the most important spas of the long eighteenth century, the
imperial city of Aachen and the royal town (*königliche Stadt*) of Karlsbad,
were supported by urban magistrates.[25] The spa district of Aachen was

actively promoted by the imperial city council until the French conquest in 1792/1794, while the spa of Karlsbad was neither systematically promoted by its overlords, the German and then Austrian emperors, nor by its urban magistrates.[26] The success of Karlsbad as a spa was to a considerable degree due to the circumstance that the town burned down by chance twice, each time at a moment when its architecture threatened to be perceived as unfashionable. The medieval town burned to the ground in 1604 and was replaced by new, uniform half-timbered structures. In 1759, the town burned down again and was rebuilt with stone houses in a uniform style.[27] As cynical as it may sound, these events contributed to Karlsbad's long-term success. In addition, as we shall see in Chapters 3 and 4, the change in landscape perception also secured the spa's success.

Other spas maintained by a municipality were Überkingen,[28] which belonged to the imperial city of Ulm, and especially Franzensbad in Bohemia (today Františkovy Lázně in the Czech Republic), founded in 1793.[29] Franzensbad (or Franzensbrunn) was owned and supported by the nearby town of Eger (today Cheb in the Czech Republic) and was accordingly often called "Eger" or "Egerbrunn" in contemporary sources. Exclusively private entrepreneurial initiatives were rare in the empire. Only Driburg, which was leased by the Braunschweig court hunt master (*Hofjägermeister*) and chamberlain Caspar Heinrich von Sierstorpff in 1782 and located in the territory of the prince-bishops of Paderborn, can be considered a success story.[30]

In contrast to Grimmelshausen's fictional spa owner Simplicissimus, who is described as a private entrepreneur, in most cases a spa depended on the sustained support of a territorial ruler to be successful. Princely support ranged from the construction of spa facilities and the creation of avenues and gardens at existing spas to the founding of new spas after the (re)discovery of water springs considered to have healing qualities. Contemporaries already noticed the essential role of territorial princes in spa development. In his diary about Duke Karl Eugen of Württemberg's "journeys to the countryside" (*Land-Reisen*), Baron von Buwinghausen-Wallmerode reported, "The 5th of July 1770. Teinach. After the duke had resolved to improve the reputation and acceptance of the Teinach mineral spring, it was decided to go to Teinach this year instead of making the annual journey to Graveneck."[31] And in a fictional travelogue entitled *Letters from a Traveler to his Friend about his Visit to the Godesberg Spa (Briefe eines Reisenden an seinen Freund Ueber den Aufenthalte beim Godesberger Gesundbrunnen)* published in 1793, the narrator commented on the former spa of Tönnisstein,[32] which had been promoted by Elector Clemens August of Cologne but fell into disrepair under his successors: "It is a pity, an eternal pity, that it is no longer what it used to be. The wildly overgrown avenues, the magnificent staircases and balustrades that are lying around broken everywhere, . . . all are evidence of its former glory. . . . Elector Clemens August treated this place very well.

He stayed there often, and he would have invested large sums of money for its glorification, if death had not prevented him from doing so. The most beautiful models of all that he planned to build are still on display there."[33]

On rare occasions, a ruler's support could result in the elevation of a village to the legal status of a town. Wildbad is an example from the Middle Ages. It was granted a town charter some time after the attack on Count Eberhard in 1367, potentially as an expression of gratitude by the counts of Württemberg.[34] In early modern times, the landgrave of Hesse-Darmstadt granted Schwalbach the freedom of the *Burgfrieden* in 1643, after it had risen to become one of the most popular spas in the empire.[35] And Pyrmont, built as a spa located near two villages and a castle, was elevated to the status of an excise town (*Akzisestadt*) in 1720. Nevertheless, Pyrmont's elevation was largely the result of an attempt by Prince Friedrich Anton Ulrich of Waldeck and Pyrmont to alleviate his financial difficulties.[36]

The day-to-day operation of a spa was entrusted to the territorial administration. This included issuing spa ordinances (*Brunnenordnungen*), the deployment of administrative officials and small military units, the organization of poor relief – either by establishing a bathhouse for the poor or by setting up a poor relief fund – and the granting of licenses to merchants, bankers, and casino operators.[37] The inhabitants of new spas often received tax concessions or building materials for the construction of lodging houses.[38] Inhabitants operating spa facilities undoubtedly profited from the establishment of a spa, but Grimmelshausen also stresses that others suffered when a prince decided to create a new spa. In his novel, Simplicissimus' stone touches the ground in the middle of a forest and causes a mineral well to spring forth. He then tries to convince the peasants in the vicinity that they will prosper if their lord decides to create a spa. They would be able to "sell . . . chickens, eggs, butter, livestock and so on for good prices."[39] But the peasants want none of it: "Our master will put an innkeeper there, and he'll be the one to get rich, while we'll have the short end of it by having to keep up the roads and paths."[40]

While most of the spas in the empire were supported by princes, the leading territorial rulers, including the electors, hardly engaged in spa development, if at all. The dukes and, from 1623, electors of Bavaria did not support a spa in any meaningful way during the early modern period and the eighteenth century. Strikingly, numerous spas in Franconian territories were advertised as "Bavarian spas" soon after these territories had fallen under Bavarian rule in the early nineteenth century.[41] Although the electors and, from 1701, kings of Brandenburg-Prussia supported Freienwalde north of Berlin, the spa was mostly frequented by the territory's nobility and remained small. The Silesian spas came under Prussian rule initially after the First Silesian War in 1742 and then permanently with the Treaty of Hubertusburg in 1763, but their rulers did not systematically support them. Nevertheless, the Silesian spas became popular with the change in landscape perception at the turn of the nineteenth century.[42] Although the electors of Hanover (and from 1714 kings of Great Britain) promoted Rehburg as a spa from the middle of the eighteenth century, Rehburg did not become one of the leading spas of the empire.[43]

Lauchstädt, one of the most prominent German spas, was situated in the electorate of Saxony. However, it was originally built and supported by the dukes of Saxe-Merseburg, and the electors of Saxony had inherited it. Dresden, the residence town of the electors of Saxony, was surrounded by a veritable ring of small spas at the end of the eighteenth and the beginning of the nineteenth centuries.[44] None of these spas, however, gained more than limited supra-regional significance. The three spiritual electors (of Mainz, Trier, and Cologne) were slightly more active in their support of spas than their secular colleagues. The electors of Mainz supported Schlangenbad, the electors of Trier promoted the small spa of Bertrich at the end of the eighteenth century, and the electors of Cologne developed Godesberg into a spa, after Tönisstein had been given up. However, none of these were among the leading spas of the empire.

Most spas during the long eighteenth century were supported by princes who ruled over medium-sized and small territories. These rulers viewed spas as a means of increasing their prestige among the princes of the German lands. The list of secular territorial rulers who supported existing spas or founded new spas is long. To name just a few: the counts and (from 1712) princes of Waldeck and Pyrmont with Pyrmont; the margraves, then grand dukes of Baden with Langensteinbach and Baden-Baden; the dukes of Sachse-Meiningen with Liebenstein; the princes and later dukes of Nassau with Wiesbaden; the princes of Hohenzollern-Sigmaringen with Imnau; the margraves of Ansbach-Bayreuth with Alexandersbad; the counts of Lippe with Meinberg; from 1810 Duke Alexius Friedrich Christian of Anhalt-Bernburg with Alexisbad; from 1812 Duke Carl August of Saxe-Weimar-Eisenach with Berka, which was to a large degree planned by Goethe.[45] Count Wilhelm of Hanau, from 1785 landgrave and from 1803 elector of Hesse-Kassel, built no less than three spas: Hofgeismar, Wilhelmsbad near Hanau, and Nenndorf.[46] Over the course of the early modern era and the eighteenth century, the dukes of Württemberg promoted the spas of Boll, Wildbad, and Teinach.[47] Ecclesiastical princes ruling over small and mid-sized territories were also actively involved in the foundation and development of spas. The prince-abbots and, from 1752, prince-bishops of Fulda developed the "spa (*Kurbrunnen*) near Brückenau."[48] The prince-bishops of Würzburg founded Bocklet. They also supported the spa of Kissingen, but to a lesser degree because the townspeople of Kissingen were rather ambivalent about their rulers' interventions.[49]

Within a territory, the ruler's support for individual spas helped them to rise above the rest, and, conversely, a lack or withdrawal of support led to a spa's decline. Bocklet and Kissingen are typical examples. In 1793, the dean of Würzburg cathedral, Baron von Zobel, reported a conversation with the publisher Friedrich Justin Bertuch in Kissingen: "While taking a walk together, we discussed the possibility of improving Kissingen, and Bertuch came up with several ideas about how to make this spa more popular in a short period of time. Zobel merely regretted that the prince favored *Bocklett,* and that there were no funds available for improvements in Kissingen."[50] Strikingly, in the same year, Kissingen was described in the *Journal of Luxury and Fashions (Journal des Luxus und der Moden),* which was published by Bertuch, as a "still too little known spa."[51] Other examples include the spas of Baden-Baden, Langensteinbach, and Badenweiler[52] in the Margraviate of Baden, their fate tied to the changing favors of the margraves. The same applies to the spas of Hofgeismar, Wilhelmsbad, and Nenndorf. Their rise and fall was directly connected to the support of Count Wilhelm IX of Hanau, later landgrave of Hesse-Kassel.

The competing goals and initiatives of rulers and townspeople often left their mark on the development of princely spas. These tensions between princes' ambitions and urban communities attempting to preserve their autonomy are part of the larger story of early modern towns. During the early modern period, princes increasingly solidified their power over the towns and cities in their territories.[53] Some spa towns paid a price for preserving their independence in the eighteenth century. The aforementioned case of Kissingen is a typical example. In the middle of the eighteenth century, Prince-Bishop Friedrich Karl von Schönborn equipped Kissingen with a spa garden and assembly rooms (*Kurhaus*). However, because of the recurring conflicts between the town and the prince-bishops, the latter began to actively promote and expand the spa of Bocklet instead from the 1780s onward.[54] Wiesbaden is another case in point. This spa's healing springs were mostly located in the lodging houses owned by urban middle-class families. Since the Nassau rulers lacked access to these springs, their attempts to modernize Wiesbaden were unsuccessful in the early modern period and during most of the eighteenth century. Toward the end of the century, and even more so in the early nineteenth century, the rulers' initiative dramatically changed the course of Wiesbaden's history. By creating a brand-new spa district outside the town proper, the Nassau rulers set up Wiesbaden to become one of the most popular spas of the nineteenth century.[55]

A limited number of spas received support through more than one source. Nevertheless, these cases confirm the broader picture of a German spa map dominated by princely spas. Ems and Schlangenbad, for instance, were divided between two territories. Ems belonged to Nassau and Hesse-Darmstadt,[56] while Schlangenbad lay on the border between Hesse-Kassel and the electorate of Mainz.[57] These spas were developed by a mixture of joint ventures and competition between their princely owners. In general, while not among the most successful, these spas prospered enough to remain popular throughout the early modern period and the long eighteenth century. In addition, mixed forms of state and private entrepreneurial support could occur, such as when a ruler sought private investments for the construction or operation of a spa through shareholding. This can be observed in Godesberg.[58] Nevertheless, the vast majority of such spas should still be considered princely because both major investments and decision-making authority remained firmly with the ruler. Kissingen is a case in point here. Bertuch submitted a plan to the prince-bishop of Würzburg for a private-public partnership. He proposed to increase the rent of the saltworks (he himself wanted to become the tenant) and to develop the spa, but – significantly – he was dependent on the attitude of the prince-bishop, without whose consent none of these ideas came to fruition.[59]

The majority of spas also served their rulers as summer residences. When a prince traveled to a spa in his territory in the summer, the members of his court gathered at the spa as well.[60] Among many others, Pyrmont,[61] Hofgeismar, and Teinach are examples of this practice. Spas thus became spaces of princely and noble representation. In some cases, a reduced form of the princely spa developed, one that was largely reserved for members of the court, after initial attempts to make the spa more widely known had faltered. An example of this type of spa residence is Auerbach, which was built between 1787 and 1795 by Landgrave Ludwig X of Hesse-Darmstadt.[62]

Recent research has looked at the way rulers of small and medium-sized territories – the princes who were also the most active in founding and supporting spas – perceived their role in the empire, expressed their political and cultural identity, and projected their princely status. In light of the rise of Brandenburg-Prussia and the deep rivalry between Austria and Prussia that defined the empire in the eighteenth century, this group of rulers was politically and militarily largely powerless. Accordingly, they were keen to represent their status in other ways. Contemporaries were aware that a popular spa and the presence of a prince's court at that spa fulfilled an important representational function. Upon learning during a stay in Pyrmont in 1719 that the king of England had gone for a walk alone, Duchess Elisabeth Charlotte of Orléans, better known as Liselotte von der Pfalz, commented, "The count [*graff*] of Waldeck, who is a completely new prince [*Fürst*], is quite right to walk around with the members of his court, for otherwise one might forget that he has become a prince. One cannot forget this about the king of England, it is too long that he has been a great prince."[63]

Princely representation in the eighteenth century always targeted two separate audiences: other princes and courts on the one hand and the ruler's own subjects on the other. Ute Daniel has defined a princely court "as a social, economic, political, and cultural phenomenon [that] constitutes a medium of communication for the respective male or female ruler 'outwards' – towards other courts – and 'downwards' – towards his or her own population."[64] Given this context, a spa was a princely creation, equivalent to a palace, with buildings, gardens, and courtly amusements expressing the ruler's intention to represent his status both internally and externally. For the second half of the eighteenth century, this self-representation focused on the image of the "enlightened prince."[65]

At the spa, a prince projected his status and self-image to his subjects, especially the noble and bourgeois elites of his own territory. The space was constructed as a stage for the prince's enlightened-absolutist self-representation and as a heterotopia of the ruler's making. In connection with the creation and promotion of spas, princes invoked the argument of *bonum commune*, of the prince acting for the common good. At the same time, the spa served to represent the prince to the outside world, for instance by enabling a prince to act as a host to other princes. At "his" spa, an inferior imperial ruler like the prince of Waldeck and Pyrmont could host the kings of England and Prussia. For example, in 1796, Prince Friedrich Karl August of Waldeck and Pyrmont made his palace available to King Frederick William II of Prussia for the duration of his visit to Pyrmont.[66] The spas thus functioned as spaces of princely representation for the less powerful territorial rulers in the empire and enabled them to project "the prestige of power to the outside world."[67]

The late seventeenth-century Bohemian spa of Kukus (today Kuks in the Czech Republic) is an extraordinary example of a spa that was built to project its owner's "prestige of power" but ultimately failed to fulfill this function. In 1692, Count Franz Anton von Sporck founded Kukus in his territory of Gradlitz. The count was the son of Johann von Sporck, himself the son of serfs and born in the principality of Paderborn around 1600. Johann von Sporck served in the Bavarian and then imperial army during the Thirty Years' War and rose to the rank of count. He eventually became the owner of both a considerable amount of land in Bohemia and a handsome fortune. His son Franz Anton von Sporck, born in 1662, enjoyed a Jesuit education, attended Prague University, and later went on the Grand Tour. Count von Sporck acted as a patron of the arts and editor of edifying treatises. He rose in imperial service to become one of the governors (*Statthalter*) in Bohemia and a privy councillor. In spite of holding high office, he did not succeed in marrying into the Bohemian aristocracy; his wife Franziska Apollonia came from a poor noble family in Silesia.[68]

Throughout his life, Count von Sporck devoted himself to the expansion of his estates, underpinning his noble lifestyle with the creation and promotion of Kukus. The spacious complex on both sides of the river Elbe encompassed a palace, a spa, and other facilities, including hunting grounds, a park with various sculptures, an avenue of linden trees, and a theater.[69] Kukus also had a stately church with a crypt as well as a zoo, a race track, and the so-called philosophical house, which contained a library. The architectural layout of the spa put the accommodations for noble guests next to the palace, while the bathhouse for the poor was placed on the edge of the complex.[70]

The amusements offered in Kukus were clearly aimed at a noble audience. Hunting and prize-shooting played a central role, and there were also tournaments (*Ringrennen*), billiards, pall-mall, and so forth. The library, theater and music performances, illuminations, balls, and banquets in the count's palace served the entertainment needs of the aristocratic spa guests.[71] These courtly amusements, the architectural layout of the spa – with the count and his family at the center – and the count's self-promotion as a philanthropist and patron of the arts clearly hint at Count von Sporck's intentions: the spa of Kukus served as a space where he could display his noble status to other nobles. Kukus was, in effect, a spa residence.

Count von Sporck's hope to attract higher-ranking nobles rested on the appeal of his estate as a spa – the spa thus served as a pretext for the count's aspirations. To this end, he commissioned extensive advertising for Kukus. For example, Gottfried Benjamin Hancke's treatise on Kukus, under the guise of describing the alleged curative powers of the healing water, attempted to increase the fame of Count von Sporck. Hancke wrote that the count "made the spa into a paradise" – a clear hint at the spa as a heterotopia – and substantiated this not only with a list of the numerous entertainments offered but also with references to Count von Sporck's Christian acts of poor relief. The treatise combined a detailed description of the spa facilities with information about the true nobility and "heroic blood" of the count's father Johann.[72] The spa thus served as a backdrop for the display of noble family tradition and the expression of noble status through architecture, landscape design, and aristocratic activities. Count von Sporck even went so far as to publish a fake article in the newspaper *Prager Post-Zeitungen* in 1723: "It is said" that the "king of England" will "make use of the so-called Kukus spa belonging to the Count von Sporck."[73]

Kukus was a highly complex spatial arrangement that served the count's purpose of representing his and his family's noble status in a space constructed as a spa, since only a spa made it possible for him to attract higher-ranking nobles to Kukus. His goal was to secure and expand his position in Bohemian and Habsburg aristocratic society. Significantly, the spatial construction of Kukus placed the noble guests as close to the host as possible. The spa of Kukus thus represents a specific early modern phenomenon, namely the attempt to secure a family's ascent into the nobility. Although Kukus did attract noble guests, neither the emperor nor the king of England visited the spa.[74] Count von Sporck ultimately did not reach his goal. This is clearly illustrated by the fate of his two daughters: the older daughter entered a convent, and the younger married a man from her mother's family.

Finally, the economic interests of territorial princes who created and supported spas merit a closer look. Did spas function as economic enterprises oriented toward making a profit? How did the representational function relate to the economic interests of these rulers? The emerging picture is highly ambivalent. It is important to recognize that for early modern and eighteenth-century contemporaries, the display of a ruler's status in and of itself, be it at a spa or at the princely court, justified the expense of large sums of money. Using Pierre Bourdieu's terms, economic capital was transformed into symbolic capital. It would therefore be a mistake to describe early modern and eighteenth-century spas as solely profit-oriented enterprises.[75] Even a successful spa like Pyrmont was not administered by its ruler with the single objective of profit maximization but rather with the intent of transforming economic into symbolic capital. A good part of the income from the spa went into covering the costs of the prince's annual summer residence there.[76]

Nevertheless, economic (and specifically mercantilistic) interests were important in the development and promotion of spas. By investing in a spa facility and in the often much more lucrative bottling and shipping of healing water,[77] princes sought to achieve mercantilistic objectives, such as creating work for local craftsmen and promoting trade, ensuring a positive trade balance, and deterring their subjects from visiting an extra-territorial spa and thus spending their money elsewhere. Accordingly, Göckingk observed about Lauchstädt, "Since, however, the large majority of those who stay here for a part of the summer do so mainly to amuse themselves, it is a reasonable policy to make the place more pleasant for them, and the government certainly manages to keep three times as much money in the country, or draws money in from outside, than it uses annually for the improvement of L[auchstädt]."[78] Count Wilhelm of Hanau provides another good example of this mercantilistic reasoning in the long eighteenth century. Wilhelm invested the payments he received for contributing troops to fight in the American Revolutionary War (subject to his subsidy treaties with England) into the development and expansion of his spas.[79] He thus expected long-term benefits through both additional income for his territories from spa guests and a gain in prestige for himself as ruler.

Spa Visitors and the Hierarchy of German Spas in the Long Eighteenth Century

The population and social structure of spas could fluctuate considerably over the course of each year. In extreme cases, a spa was a bustling space frequented by the upper social classes, including the ruling nobility, during the summer season, but turned into a sleepy village or small town for the rest of the year. Johanna Schopenhauer described this pattern for Schwalbach: "And in the middle of August Schwalbach sinks almost completely back into the loneliness in which it lies buried almost ten months of the year."[80] In order to reconstruct the hierarchy of German spas during the long eighteenth century, it is necessary to gain insight into the number of spa guests at individual spas and to gather basic information about spa guests, such as their social status and hometowns. This line of inquiry leads to the only quantifiable primary sources, the spa lists (*Brunnenlisten*) – guest lists that were assembled and distributed at eighteenth-century spas in either manuscript or printed form.[81]

Upon closer examination, however, the substantial limitations of these guest lists quickly become apparent. Above all, contrary to what one might expect, guest lists were not compiled to provide the territorial administration with data for statistical or fiscal purposes.[82] While in the eighteenth century the collection of population and other data by state bureaucracies generally increased, guest lists were created to fulfill the interests and needs of spa visitors, namely to learn who was staying at the spa with them.[83] As an "informal handout,"[84] the production of guest lists, handwritten or printed, depended on the interest of the public. Guest lists went from manuscript to print when the number of guests passed a certain threshold to ensure enough prospective buyers for the printed lists. For example, printed lists were first published in Pyrmont in 1735, while they were not available in Wiesbaden until 1774.[85] Their publication was discontinued when the number of spa guests decreased at the end of the season and printing them was no longer worthwhile.[86] Mosch remarked about Pyrmont, "When the number of spa guests becomes so small that the arrivals do not fill half a sheet, the lists are no longer printed."[87] Moreover, guest lists were not systematically collected before the nineteenth century.[88] As a result, even the lists in archival holdings of major spas such as Pyrmont and Karlsbad are incomplete.[89]

In addition to these issues, contemporaries already knew of further problems and described them in some detail. First, the lists were often manipulated in order to inflate the number of spa guests. For example, the *Journal of Luxury and Fashions* (*Journal des Luxus und der Moden*) reported about Pyrmont in 1801, "During this year's spa season, 6[00] to 800 visitors were often counted and entered on the guest list. However, there is also some ostentation involved here. The entire crew of Walter's theater company performing in Pyrmont, a considerable number, were entered as spa guests."[90] Second, different spas followed varying conventions in recording their guest lists, which makes it difficult to compare the lists. For example, Pyrmont counted individual persons, whereas Karlsbad listed parties.[91] In 1802, the *Journal of Luxury and Fashions* explained that a party registered in the Karlsbad guest lists consisted of at least three, but often five or more persons, not counting the servants.[92]

Third, contemporary sources constantly note that the guest lists are incomplete and unreliable because an unknown number of spa visitors were not listed at all. For instance, in 1799, the *Journal of Luxury and*

Fashions noted about Karlsbad, "The annual guest lists . . . do not give an exact indication of the actual number of spa guests, as many did not consent to be included in them, not only people from the insignificant social classes, but also from the fashionable classes."[93] Writing about the 1797 spa season in Karlsbad, another author in the *Journal* discussed the number of unrecorded guests and the potential reasons for these omissions: "The printed guest list contains 715 entries[94] up to 16 August, and one can assume with certainty that at least one sixth of spa guests did not have their names printed. Nearly all guests who came from what used to be Poland,[95] who perhaps had gathered for a common political purpose, refused to be included in the guest list."[96] In 1805, Marcard noted in his *Little Book about the Pyrmont Spa* (*Kleines Pyrmonter Brunnenbuch*), "Often, however, names of persons are omitted from the lists because they have their reasons to not want to see their names printed in public (perhaps because they are in Pyrmont without having asked for permission to take a vacation), and therefore object to being included."[97] It is not clear how many persons chose not to have their names included in the lists. Furthermore, we can only speculate about the reasons for such a decision, presumably ranging from the desire to avoid the costs of entry to the wish to remain unrecognized. Members of the high nobility often traveled to spas incognito.[98]

Thus, guest lists were regarded as problematic by eighteenth-century spa visitors, and they also create challenges for today's researchers. The author of a 1798 travelogue about Karlsbad summarized, "The names of the most common people and of servants are completely omitted from these lists. Also, many guests, either to save money or for other reasons, do not agree to be included in these lists. Consequently, one never quite knows exactly how many guests there are in Karlsbad, and thus the main purpose of this institution, namely, that one gets a complete overview of exactly who is present at the spa at the same time as oneself, is partially defeated."[99] While contemporaries lamented the extensive gaps in the spa lists because these omissions defied the lists' purpose, these gaps also render a statistical analysis of guest lists questionable.[100] Because of the richness of information contained in the published discourse, however, a close reading of this material allows us to extract sufficient information about the approximate number of spa guests at individual spas. Contemporaries not only were aware of the limits of guest lists but also paid close attention to any type of dramatic change in the numbers of guests, such as a decline in spa visitors due to conflict and war. This, in turn, enables us to make out a rough hierarchy of German (*teutsche*) spas during the long eighteenth century.

Spas exhibited a considerable range in terms of their number of annual visitors, correlating with the popularity of the spa and its position in the hierarchy of spas. Around 1800, an average of 600–700 parties visited Karlsbad annually, ranging from a mere 500 parties at the lower end and extending up to 1,000. According to contemporary estimates of the size of a party mentioned earlier, this corresponds to between 1,500 and 5,000 visitors.[101] The higher number, however, is probably unrealistic, considering that Karlsbad was effectively still a small town and that many of its visitors also brought along servants.[102] In Pyrmont the number of names recorded in the guest lists averaged between 1,000 and 1,200 in the same period but increased up to 1,500 visitors.[103]

Unlike prominent spas such as Karlsbad and Pyrmont, many other spas attracted only a small number of guests – in spite of their presence in the published discourse. Schandau in the electorate of Saxony, for instance, first appeared in the spa discourse at the beginning of the nineteenth century, advertising itself as the gateway to Saxon Switzerland.[104] In 1821, Schandau's guest list named only 50 parties, that is, between 150 and 250 guests, mainly coming from Saxony.[105] The spa of Rippoldsau in the Black Forest had 47 visitors in 1774. Even in 1830 only 86 guests were listed in spite of the spa's (limited) presence in the published discourse of the early nineteenth century.[106] In contrast, the list of spa guests in a mid-sized spa like Bertrich in the electorate of Trier counted 661 persons in 1790.[107] Alexisbad in Anhalt-Bernburg, a spa in the Harz Mountains, recorded 719 persons in its guest list of 1817.[108] Small and mid-sized spas clearly made an effort to register every single guest.

Overall, until the turn of the nineteenth century, a spa's ability to accommodate large numbers of guests was limited by the number of available lodgings. Therefore, on average, the large spas probably did not have much more than two to four times as many visitors as the medium-sized spas. This changed dramatically as the nineteenth century progressed. The leading spas of the nineteenth century, including Baden-Baden and Wiesbaden, recorded a massive increase in their number of guests, which quickly exceeded the dimensions of the early modern period and the eighteenth century. After a new spa district had been constructed, Wiesbaden saw a huge rise in the number of visitors. In 1813 it recorded 5,779 spa guests, and in 1817 already more than 10,000.[109] An even greater increase in the number of guests occurred in Baden-Baden, which saw a rise in popularity after the Second Congress of Rastatt (1797–1799).[110]

The number of visitors, however, is only one part of the story. The hierarchy of German (*teutsche*) spas in the perception of contemporary observers during the long eighteenth century was determined by a combination of different factors: the number of guests at a spa, their social status, the spa's catchment area, and the attention the spa garnered in the published discourse. In most cases, the social rank of the guests at a spa correlated with the spa's catchment area. The spas at the top of the hierarchy attracted guests from all German territories, even from all over Europe. Accordingly, many visitors belonged to the ruling aristocracy and the high nobility. These spas also drew significant attention in the published discourse. At the bottom of the hierarchy were spas with only a local catchment area, attracting visitors from the lower middle class and the peasantry. With rare exceptions, these spas did not draw the attention of the published discourse. However, the examples of Karlsbad and Pyrmont show that a Europe-wide or even international catchment area did not rule out the possibility of local and regional importance and the presence of guests from all walks of life.[111] This study focuses on spas that figured in the published discourse during the long eighteenth century, ranging from internationally known spas visited by the German and European ruling princes to regional spas that primarily attracted visitors from the lower nobility and the middle class.

Karlsbad was the most international spa of the long eighteenth century. It was a meeting place of the European aristocracy. King Frederick I of Prussia visited in 1708, Tsar Peter I in 1711, and the German and then Austrian emperors or their wives were frequent guests.[112] Many Russian nobles spent their summers here, as did exiled noblemen like the Scottish Earl of Findlater (1750–1811) and the Prince of Ligne (1735–1814).[113] Territorial princes from the empire were represented in large numbers – from the Anhaltine dynasty to the dukes of Württemberg, to name just two.[114] A broad spectrum of people from the lower nobility and the upper middle class made their way to Karlsbad; among them were Johann Wolfgang von Goethe, "Educator" (*Schulrath*) Joachim Heinrich Campe from Braunschweig (1746–1818), and "Mr. Z.W. Stevenson with his wife from New York in America."[115] Teplitz and Franzensbad were two spas in close proximity to Karlsbad, attracting many of the same visitors, especially because people moved between spas during the season. But these were considered less important than Karlsbad.

Also at the top of the hierarchy, the spa of Pyrmont ranked immediately behind Karlsbad, in terms of both the social status of its guests and its catchment area.[116] Peter the Great visited Pyrmont in 1716 and Frederick II of Prussia in 1744 and 1746.[117] It was a meeting place for the north and central German nobility and bourgeoisie, including members of the Brandenburg-Prussian dynasty and the court and aristocracy of the electorate of Hanover.[118] Pyrmont also attracted international nobility, not least from northern and western Europe, but to a lesser extent than Karlsbad.[119] At the end of the eighteenth century, members of the exiled French nobility arrived in Pyrmont in droves, an occurrence noted in the published discourse because German writers attributed a negative influence on the social environment in Pyrmont to these French exiles.[120] Although the proportion of spa guests from the middle and upper middle classes increased significantly at the end of the eighteenth century,[121] Pyrmont's social atmosphere was often criticized for noble pride, as will be shown in detail later.[122]

Ranking behind Karlsbad and Pyrmont, Schwalbach in the Taunus mountains, the imperial city of Aachen, and Lauchstädt in Saxony were the next three most prominent German spas of the long eighteenth century. They differ primarily in their individual development trajectories. As mentioned earlier, Schwalbach (Figure 3.4) began to rise as early as the middle of the sixteenth century, and it held the status of a leading spa of the empire in the period before and after the Thirty Years' War. Its ascent and heyday preceded Aachen's,[123] Karlsbad's, and Pyrmont's. Prominent visitors to Schwalbach included Elector August of Saxony in 1584[124] and the future Elector Georg Wilhelm of Brandenburg and his new wife Elisabeth Charlotte, the daughter of the Palatine elector, in 1616.[125] Protestant nobility from all parts of the empire as well as members of the higher clergy from the electorate of Mainz frequently stayed here. In particular, territorial princes and nobles of the Mainz and Hessian regions and of the Wetterau counties were regular visitors, as were the citizens of the nearby imperial city of Frankfurt.[126]

Toward the middle of the eighteenth century, Schwalbach experienced a gradual decline. The landgraves of Hesse largely stopped investing, leaving the spa's facilities out of date and even somewhat dilapidated.[127] In his autobiography, Johann Stephan Pütter looked back on his visit to Schwalbach in 1754: "The local circumstances, as far as avenues and other public amenities are concerned, I found in no comparison whatsoever with what I had seen in Pyrmont in 1749, much less how I got to know Pyrmont in later years (1770–1794)."[128] These conditions affected the social composition of Schwalbach's spa guests and its catchment area. By the early nineteenth century, Schwalbach was perceived as an outdated spa, visited mainly by Jewish spa guests from Frankfurt and Mainz and for the primary purpose of gambling.[129] In contrast to many other spas during the late eighteenth and early nineteenth centuries, Schwalbach failed to increase the number of its spa visitors, which remained at about 500 guests per season.[130]

The imperial city of Aachen compares to the royal town of Karlsbad in terms of the social composition of its spa society and its Europe-wide catchment area, although Karlsbad remained successful over a longer period of time. These two spas were located on the western and eastern edges of contemporaries' (mental) map of German fashionable spas. Aachen's rise began after the city fire of 1656 and the publication of a treatise by the spa physician Franz Blondel in 1688, which was translated into several languages.[131] The spa of Aachen competed with, but also benefited from, its proximity to Spa, the town just across the border in the prince-bishopric of Liège that lent its name to all watering places in the English language. The first preserved guest list for Aachen dating from 1768 names 391 persons, but the figure probably does not reflect the entire spa season.[132] Toward the end of the eighteenth century, Aachen counted roughly as many guests as Pyrmont, namely between 800 and 1,500 or more people.[133] Aachen attracted European rulers, German territorial princes, and the members of various German ruling houses: King Frederick IV of Denmark visited in 1724, King Frederick II of Prussia in 1742, and the Swedish King Gustav III in 1780.[134]

Aachen's catchment area stretched from England and the Netherlands in the West to Poland and Russia in the East, and it also drew guests from Italy and Sweden. Aachen's status as an imperial city and as a place of peace negotiations and treaties (notably the Treaty of Aachen in 1748 that ended the War of the Austrian Succession and the Congress of Aix-la-Chapelle between Austria, Great Britain, Prussia, Russia, and France after the Napoleonic Wars in 1818) contributed to its success as a spa. Members of the nobility and their entourages, who spent extended periods of time in the city for other reasons, also made use of the city's spa facilities. Toward the end of the eighteenth century, Aachen, like all German spas, attracted an increasing number of bourgeois visitors.[135]

Aachen's success came to an abrupt end with the invasion of French troops at the end of 1792 and again in 1794. In 1806, only 125 guests visited. Despite the French administration's intent to revive the spa, these plans were not implemented. A gradual process of revival started only after the end of French rule and the return of the spa facilities to the possession of the city in 1818.[136] Aachen therefore occupies a special place in the sample of spas analyzed here because its development was hampered for years by war and foreign policy factors. The city abruptly lost its position as one of the leading spas of the empire and was soon neglected in the published discourse.[137]

Besides Karlsbad, Pyrmont, and Aachen, the Saxon spa town of Lauchstädt near Halle played a leading role in Germany during the last third of the eighteenth century. In terms of the number of guests, Lauchstädt was not able to fully compete with these other spas. Its guest lists, which only listed parties, were never printed. Between 1751 and 1775, a range of between 100 and 200 parties were recorded annually. The number occasionally rose to 300 after 1775 but fell below 200 again starting in 1792.[138] Taking Karlsbad's ratio between party and persons as a guide, Lauchstädt had anywhere between 300 and 1,500 guests per season. Given the size of its spa district and the nearby town, Lauchstädt could have probably accommodated about as many guests as Pyrmont, but it most likely had fewer visitors than its more famous competitor.

In addition to the nobility from the various Saxon territories, nobles from Brandenburg-Prussia regularly visited Lauchstädt. Since the owners of the spa, the electors of Saxony, had intermittently been kings of Poland, the frequent visits of Polish nobles as well as members of the Russian nobility are not surprising. In addition to the nobility, spa guests from the middle and upper middle classes, mostly from cities and towns nearby, frequented Lauchstädt. Merchants from Leipzig joined professors from the universities of Halle and Leipzig.[139] The regular influx of students and inhabitants from Halle, a Brandenburg-Prussian university town close to the spa, was a special hallmark of Lauchstädt. The students came for day trips to attend the theater. The Lauchstädt theater was a significant attraction because Bellomo's company from Weimar played there from

1785 onward and, starting in 1791, the Weimar court theater under the direction of Goethe transferred to Lauchstädt for the summer months.[140] The residents of Halle mainly visited on weekends, a practice that was also common at other spas near cities or larger towns. This was the case in Wilhelmsbad, for example, which was situated close to Hanau and not far from the imperial city of Frankfurt.[141] Lauchstädt became more popular during the last quarter of the eighteenth century, resulting in the shortest heyday among the leading German spas. As mentioned earlier, its number of spa guests also lagged behind the other leading spas. However, Lauchstädt garnered considerable attention in the published discourse of the late eighteenth century. The relative preponderance of aristocratic visitors made the spa a primary target for bourgeois criticism of noble pride.

It is neither possible nor useful to order the many mid-sized and smaller spas of the long eighteenth century into a hierarchy based on the social composition of their visitors or their catchment area. All were represented in the published discourse, but these spas usually had a catchment area that only encompassed the territory in which they were situated and the surrounding region. As Bitz has shown for southwest Germany, most guests traveled about 100 kilometers to visit these spas.[142] This indicates that the territorial nobility and the upper middle and middling classes in most areas of Germany were able to travel to a regional spa. At the same time, knowledge about these spas was more widespread among the reading public than their catchment areas imply. The large number of small spas that did not leave a trace in the published discourse had only a local catchment area, and their visitors were predominantly from the lower middle class and the peasantry. However, their existence and their efforts to imitate the better-known spas in terms of their facilities and services point to the breadth of spa experiences in Germany in the long eighteenth century.[143]

Among the group of mid-sized and smaller spas, some stand out for the social composition of their visitors. Spas in prince-bishoprics, such as Bertrich and Brückenau, hosted an above-average number of clergy, from the lower clergy to the members of the cathedral chapter.[144] Spas such as Baden-Baden and Wiesbaden – before becoming world-famous in the nineteenth century – mainly attracted visitors from the urban middle and lower middle classes.[145] As previously mentioned, some spas functioned primarily as summer residences for territorial princes and their courts. The members of the princely courts and the territorial nobility were predominant in Auerbach, as was also the case to a lesser extent in Hofgeismar in Hesse-Kassel and Langensteinbach in Baden-Durlach.[146] Similarly, Freienwalde was mainly a spa of the Brandenburg nobility and also served as a residence for the widows of the ruling dynasty.[147] The correlation between the presence of noble visitors and a large European catchment area typical of the leading German spas did not apply to these small and mid-sized spas, where most noble guests came from the surrounding region. Still, the function of most spas as summer residences for their rulers must be emphasized again; the differences between princely spas existed in degree, not in kind.

In the spas that catered to the entire social spectrum from the aristocracy to the poor, all groups from the lower middle class downward were represented in large numbers. In addition to the servants of the elite spa guests, whose numbers cannot be determined, we find members of the lower urban middle class, peasants from the surrounding area, and beggars.[148] For example, in addition to its northern German and northern European spa guests from the nobility and upper middle class, Pyrmont also accommodated visitors from the middle and lower middle classes and peasants from the surrounding area. As was the custom at all spas, middle-class visitors were considered "proper" spa guests and entered in the guest lists if they so wished. In contrast, the number of peasants coming to Pyrmont was only estimated by the authorities and listed as a rough figure at the end of the guest lists. Nevertheless, the annual number of around 2,000 shows that peasants were an important factor (including in economic terms) for the spa of Pyrmont. Spatial separation played a significant role in the spa's attempt to accommodate all of these social groups.[149]

And finally, beggars were present in all spas but were not welcome in any of them. The authorities repeatedly took measures to discipline or remove beggars. Pyrmont and other spas attempted to restrict access to the spa and offer poor relief only to beggars who were regarded as sick and "deserving"[150] – similar to the way all towns and territories during this era sought to regulate beggars and the poor. Spa visitors from the middle classes upward were clearly concerned about whether a spa had its beggars "under control." The "Spa Chronicle" ("Badechronik") in the *Journal of Luxury and Fashions* (*Journal des Luxus und der Moden*) complained about Teinach in 1814: "Unfortunately, the enjoyment of the beautiful walking trails . . . is ruined by the sight of begging people."[151] Therefore, spa treatises regularly assured readers that no beggars would bother them. Deneken, for example, claimed that in Rehburg "good policing removes beggars from the walking trails, where they otherwise interrupt the lonely thinker in his meditations and friends in their confidential conversations in the most unpleasant way."[152] And Göckingk stated succinctly – and implausibly – about Brückenau: "Beggars are not present here at all."[153]

All eighteenth-century spas competed with one another, as the aforementioned cases of comparative advertising underscore. In some regions, however, spas in geographical proximity either entered into more direct competition or served different purposes in order to ensure their long-term survival. Regional "clusters"[154] of spas were obviously a result of geological conditions; clusters developed in areas with a preponderance of water springs. Despite a considerable increase in summer travel to spas across central Europe and the heavy investment by princes in their spas in the eighteenth century, the potential for all spas in one cluster to prosper was clearly limited unless each of them could draw a sufficiently large number of guests. As a result, many spas within a cluster differed both functionally by offering different spa treatments and socially by tailoring their offerings to different social groups. Examples of such spa clusters are the Bohemian spas of Karlsbad, Franzensbad, Teplitz, and later Marienbad;[155] the spas of Pyrmont, Driburg, Meinberg, and later Limmer;[156] the spas of Schwalbach, Wiesbaden, and Schlangenbad;[157] Brückenau, Bocklet, Kissingen, and later Wipfeld;[158] as well as spa clusters that entered the published discourse in the early nineteenth century like the Saxon spas surrounding Dresden (Augustusbad near Radeberg, Berggießhübel, Buschbad near Meißen, Schandau, and Tharand);[159] the Renchtal spas (Antogast, Freiersbach, Griesbach, Peterstal, and Sulzbach) and other spas in the Black Forest;[160] as well as the Silesian spas (Altwasser, Charlottenbrunn, Cudowa, Flinsberg, Landeck, Reinerz, Salzbrunn, and Warmbrunn).[161] Contemporaries already took note of these clusters. The published discourse clearly reveals this: when none of the spas in a cluster rose above the others in popularity, the individual spas were often subsumed under the name of the cluster.[162]

The Taunus spas formed both a socially and a functionally differentiated cluster in the early modern period. Before the rise of Wiesbaden in the nineteenth century, the leading spa was Schwalbach. By the Thirty Years' War it had risen to become a fashionable spa known for its diverse leisure facilities.[163] However, since Schwalbach lacked attractive bathing facilities, at the end of the seventeenth century Schlangenbad was established at a hot spring in the woods near Schwalbach. Initially, Schlangenbad was a kind of functional supplement for Schwalbach. "People who neither like to have an active social life nor enjoy too lively entertainments"[164] arranged for mineral water from Schwalbach to be brought to Schlangenbad. And guests staying in Schwalbach made short bathing trips to Schlangenbad. This functional symbiosis came to an end when Schlangenbad – by then also equipped with a theater, assembly rooms, and gardens – increasingly attracted noble visitors and began to compete with Schwalbach in the eighteenth century.[165]

In contrast, Wiesbaden, another spa in this cluster, mainly served spa guests from the middle classes, about half of them coming from the imperial city of Frankfurt.[166] As we saw earlier, Wiesbaden's small-town structure prevented it from expanding and building fashionable facilities. Accordingly, the spa's entertainment offerings, such as its theater performances, were also tailored to the needs of its spa guests.[167] As Martina Bleimehl-Eiler argues, "To simplify, Wiesbaden embodies the spa of the petty bourgeoisie, Langenschwalbach the spa of a wide spectrum of social classes, and Schlangenbad the princely spa."[168] This social differentiation within the Taunus spa cluster was further complemented by a functional differentiation. Wiesbaden became a place where the upper classes received their initial medical treatments (*Vorkur*), namely the unpleasant purging, before moving on to Schwalbach to enjoy everything a fashionable spa had to offer.[169]

The spas of Pyrmont, Meinberg, and Driburg near Paderborn formed an eighteenth-century cluster, but in contrast to the Taunus spas, their relationship was above all characterized by demarcation and rivalry. To differentiate itself from the neighboring spa of Pyrmont, advertising material for Driburg aggressively propagated the spa as a rural idyll for the middle class. This was even reflected in its buildings, which displayed a visible half-timbered construction, a style otherwise considered out of fashion in the late eighteenth century.[170] Meinberg, on the other hand, sought to make a name for itself primarily by advertising the quality of its healing water. The spa physician Johann Erhard Trampel aspired to attract guests by emphasizing the greater healing power of the Meinberg water compared to the Pyrmont water, while also extolling the spa's simple pleasures and natural surroundings.[171]

In sum, spas were such a widespread phenomenon in Germany in the early modern period and the long eighteenth century that all social groups, from the aristocracy to the peasantry, had opportunities to experience a spa. Accordingly, spa experiences were not of a singular nature but entailed a broad variety. For the poor, spas primarily remained places for the sick seeking water treatments to heal their ailments. For most other social groups, spas combined a healing and a recreational function. But for the upper social classes this relationship increasingly reversed, and spas became resorts where recreational activities and social interactions took center stage. With the number of spa guests from the bourgeoisie on the rise during the second half of the eighteenth century, spas became centers of communication for the upper middle class and the nobility.

Notes

1. See Steudel, "Geschichte," 2, 4; Studt, "Badenfahrt," 35–36; Kuhnert, *Urbanität*, 32–33.
2. Studt, "Badenfahrt," 33: "neues Muster des Badeverhaltens" – "Badenfahrt." See Busch, "Reisen," 484–486; Fürbeth, "Bedeutung des Bäderwesens," 463.
3. See Steudel, "Geschichte," 4; Studt, "Badenfahrt," 36–37; Biehn, Herzogenberg, *Große Welt reist ins Bad*, 11.
4. See Bitz, "Bäder und Sauerbrunnen," 183; Rumpel, "Einfluss der Obrigkeit," 78; Studt, "Badenfahrt," 36; Fürbeth, "Bedeutung des Bäderwesens," 470.
5. See Studt, "Badenfahrt," 35–40; Bitz, *Badewesen*, 39; Bitz, "Bäder und Sauerbrunnen," 84; Mehring, *Badenfahrt*, 28, 136–137.
6. See Stolberg, *Homo patiens*, 144–150. The underlying medical ideas cannot be discussed in detail here. The contemporary idea of the permeability of the skin – from the inside to the outside and vice versa – was based on

humoral pathology and was essential for how people used hot springs. It was assumed that the bathing rash indicated that the bad humors had left the body.

7. See Steudel, "Geschichte," 5; Studt, "Badenfahrt," 40; Busch, "Reisen," 481–483; Křížek, *Kulturgeschichte des Heilbades*, 79–80. The poor often tried to stay in the bathing pool for as many hours as possible to speed up the healing process while keeping the cost of their spa visit down. Many ate and slept in the water, which sometimes led to death by drowning.

8. See Rem, *Tagebuch*.

9. See Bitz, *Badewesen*, 64, 66.

10. See Bitz, *Badewesen*, 66; Martin, *Deutsches Badewesen*, 359.

11. See, e.g., the spa visits by Goethe and his partner and later wife Christiane: Göres, *"Was ich dort gelebt, genossen"*, 15.

12. See, e.g., Wegner, "Staatsbad Bocklet," 259; Wegner, "Staatsbad Brückenau," 267.

13. Montaigne's travel diary is written partly as a first-person narrative and partly as a third-person narrative by a servant, to whom Montaigne probably dictated. See Montaigne, *Tagebuch*, 331.

14. See Paumgartner's correspondence with his wife Magdalena: Paumgartner, *Briefwechsel*.

15. See Montaigne, *Tagebuch*, 35, 205, 228; Paumgartner, *Briefwechsel*, 46, 52, 115, 226, 247, 251, 264. See also Steudel, "Geschichte," 7.

16. See Föhl, "Wildbad," 475–476.

17. See Paumgartner, *Briefwechsel*, letter Balthasar to Magdalena, from Karlsbad, 5 June 1591, 113: "ein sehr spröhttes willdbad."

18. See Marcard, *Kleines Pyrmonter Brunnenbuch*, 1805; "Bade- und Reise-Epoque," *JLM* (September 1807).

19. See Maurer, "Reisen interdisziplinär," 297.

20. Behringer, *Im Zeichen des Merkur*, 436: "Personentransport im Linienverkehr." See 436–485, 512–549.

21. Grimmelshausen, *An Unabridged Translation of Simplicius Simplicissimus*, 424–425. See also Grimmelshausen, *Simplicissimus Teutsch*, 516–517.

22. Grimmelshausen, *An Unabridged Translation of Simplicius Simplicissimus*, 425. See also Grimmelshausen, *Simplicissimus Teutsch*, 517.

23. See [Schäfer], *Briefe eines Schweizers*. This work is usually ascribed to Andreas Schäfer, a privy councillor of Wilhelm IX. Bott has argued that Knigge was the author of these fictional letters, but in my view he cannot convincingly substantiate this. See Bott, *Briefe eines Schweizers*. See also Conert, *Wilhelmsbad*, 46–47.

24. See Borsay, "Health and Leisure Resorts," 791.

25. Karlsbad was elevated to the status of a royal town by Emperor Joseph I in 1707. See Biehn, Herzogenberg, *Große Welt reist ins Bad*, 217.

26. See Campe, *Reise von Braunschweig nach Karlsbad*, 1806, 160; *Reise nach den Badeörtern*, 1798, 153–154.

27. See *Festschrift zur 74. Versammlung*, 165–169, 183–197.

28. Überkingen is not on the map at the end of this book because it remained a spa with only local significance during the period covered in this study.

29. See Bahlcke, Eberhard, Polívka, *Handbuch der historischen Stätten: Böhmen und Mähren*, article "Franzensbad," 144.

30. See Bothe, "Bad Driburg," in: *Kurstädte*; Bothe, "Bad Driburg," in: *Privat-Heilbad*; Kaspar, *Das Gräfliche Bad Driburg*; Kaspar, "Bad Driburg."

31. Buwinghausen-Wallmerode, *Tagebuch*, 190: "Den 5. Julii 1770. Deinach. Nachdeme Sich der herzog vorgenommen hatte, den Deinacher Sauerbronnen

ein wenig in bessern Ruf und Aufnahme zu bringen, so wurde vor heuer beschlossen, statt der alljährl. Reysse nach Graveneck, heuer nach Deinach zu gehen."

32. Tönnisstein is not on the map at the end of this book because it remained a spa with only local significance during the period covered in this study.

33. *Briefe eines Reisenden an seinen Freund Ueber den Aufenthalte beim Godesberger Gesundbrunnen*, 1793, 65–66: "Schade, ewig Schade, dass der nicht mehr ist, was er ehedessen war; denn die wild verwachsenen Alleen, herrlichen Treppen und Balustraden, die zerbrochen allenthalben herumliegen, . . . zeigen alle von seiner ehemaligen Pracht. . . . Kurfürst Clemens August war diesem Ort sehr gut. Er hielt sich öfters da auf, und würde zu seiner Verherrlichung grosse Summen verwendet haben, wenn ihn nicht der Tod daran verhindert hätte; denn noch zeigt man die schönsten Modelle von allem dem vor, was da als hat sollen hingestellt werden."

34. See Keyser, *Württembergisches Städtebuch*, article "Wildbad," 483; Föhl, "Wildbad," 475.

35. See Keyser, *Hessisches Städtebuch*, article "Schwalbach," 390.

36. See Engel, "Die 'Akzisestadt' Pyrmont"; Kuhnert, *Urbanität*, 96–97.

37. See Mehring, *Badenfahrt*, 76–98.

38. See Kuhnert, *Urbanität*, 97.

39. Grimmelshausen, *An Unabridged Translation of Simplicius Simplicissimus*, 428. See also Grimmelshausen, *Simplicissimus Teutsch*, 521.

40. Grimmelshausen, *An Unabridged Translation of Simplicius Simplicissimus*, 428. See also Grimmelshausen, *Simplicissimus Teutsch*, 521–522.

41. See Wetzler, *Beschreibung der Gesundbrunnen und Bäder Wipfeld, Kissingen, Bocklet und Brückenau*; Wetzler, *Blicke auf Baierns Heilbrunnen und Bäder*; Wetzler, *Gesundbrunnen und Bäder im Obermainkreise des Königreichs Baiern*.

42. Altwasser, Charlottenbrunn, Cudowa, Flinsberg, Landeck, Reinerz, Salzbrunn, and Warmbrunn. See Mosch, *Heilquellen Schlesiens*, 1821.

43. See Droste, . . . *der Gesundtheyt wegen und des Vergnuehgens halber*.

44. See "Badechronik," *JLM* (September 1801); Rosseaux, *Freiräume*, 211–224.

45. See "Badechronik," *JLM* (March 1813); Gräf, *Goethe in Berka*; Michels, *Anhalt in alten Ansichten*.

46. See Putschky, "Wilhelmsbad, Hofgeismar und Nenndorf." Wilhelm's promotion of spas underlines that the health function of spas was based on attribution. Of the three spas supported by Wilhelm, the mineral waters of two – Wilhelmsbad and Hofgeismar – are not curative by today's standards, and these spas therefore declined in the nineteenth century. Their eighteenth-century buildings and gardens are largely preserved today. Nenndorf's healing spring, in contrast, is still considered curative today, and the spa has therefore undergone restructuring and building activities, making it more difficult to see the original eighteenth-century design today.

47. See Föhl, "Wildbad"; Günther, Jäckh, Lubkoll, *Bad Boll*; Gemeinde Bad Boll, *Bad Boll*; Greiner, "Zur Geschichte von Bad Teinach."

48. See Wegner, "Staatsbad Brückenau."

49. See Wegner, "Staatsbad Bocklet"; Winkler, "Bad Kissingen."

50. Böttiger, *Literarische Zustände*, 297: "Bei einem Spaziergang wurde über die Verbesserungsfähigkeit des Kissinger Bades gesprochen, und Bertuch rückte mit mehrern Ideen hervor, wie diesem Bad schnell emporgeholfen werden könne. Zobel bedauerte nur, daß der Fürst mehr für *Bocklett* wäre, u. zu den Verbesserungen in Kissingen kein Fonds auszumitteln sei." (Italics in the original.)

51. Bucholtz, "Etwas über den Kißinger Gesundbrunnen," *JLM* (May 1793), 241: "noch zu wenig bekannte[s] Baad."
52. Badenweiler is not on the map at the end of this book because it remained a spa with only local significance during the period covered in this study.
53. See Schilling, *Stadt*, 75–79.
54. See, e.g., Winkler, "Bad Kissingen," 363.
55. See "Die Einweihung des neuen Saales in Wißbaden," 1810; Bleymehl-Eiler, "'Das Paradies der Kurgäste'," 60–64; Fuchs, "'Dieses Wasser'," 101.
56. See *Dehio – Handbuch der deutschen Kunstdenkmäler: Rheinland-Pfalz*, article "Ems," 63.
57. See *Dehio – Handbuch der deutschen Kunstdenkmäler: Hessen*, article "Schlangenbad," 780.
58. See, e.g., Wiedemann, *Geschichte Godesbergs*, 514–517.
59. See Böttiger, *Literarische Zustände*, 297–298.
60. Personal narratives by princes and noble members of princely courts confirm this. See, e.g., Faber, "Beschreibung einer Bade- und Rheinreise," 64–70 (Ems 1632); Buwinghausen-Wallmerode, *Tagebuch*, 190–204 (Teinach 1770); Friedrich I. von Sachsen-Gotha und Altenburg, *Tagebücher 1667–1686*, vol. 1, 192–193, 457 (Schwalbach 1671), vol. 2, 216–218 (Wildungen 1682).
61. See Kuhnert, *Urbanität*, 100–105.
62. See [Lichtenberg], *Nachricht von dem Auerbacher mineralischen Wasser*, c. 1778. See also Gröschel, *Staatspark Fürstenlager*.
63. Elisabeth Charlotte von Orleans, *Aus den Briefen*, 141: "Der graff von Waldeck, der ein gantz neuer fürst ist, hat groß recht, in staat mit seinen Leuten zu spatziren, denn man mögte sonst vergeßen, daß er ein fürst geworden ist; das kan man bey dem König von Englandt nicht vergeßen, es ist zu lang, daß er ein großer fürst ist."
64. Daniel, *Hoftheater*, 27: "als soziales und wirtschaftliches, politisches und kulturelles Gesamtphänomen immer auch Medium der Kommunikation des jeweiligen Fürsten bzw. der jeweiligen Fürstin 'nach außen' – gegenüber anderen Höfen – und 'nach unten' – gegenüber der eigenen Bevölkerung – darstellt." See also Gestrich, *Absolutismus*.
65. See, e.g., Arndt, "'Monarch'"; Berger, "Repräsentationsstrategien"; Umbach, *Federalism*; Schmidt, "Überleben der 'Kleinen'"; Winterling, *Hof*, 164.
66. See Kuhnert, *Urbanität*, 116.
67. Kuhnert, *Urbanität*, 103: "Machtprestige nach außen."
68. See Benedikt, *Franz Anton Graf von Sporck*; Dorgerloh, "Franz Anton Graf von Sporck," 124; Lietzmann, "Des Reichsgrafen Franz Anton von Sporck Kukus-Bad," 138–142; *Allgemeine Deutsche Biographie*, vol. 35, article "Sporck, Johann Graf von," 264–267.
69. From an art-historical perspective, Kukus is famous for its Baroque sculptures. See Schiff, "Der Gründer von Kuks."
70. See Benedikt, *Franz Anton Graf von Sporck*, 319–320; Dorgerloh, "Franz Anton Graf von Sporck," 114–115, 120; Lietzmann, "Des Reichsgrafen Franz Anton von Sporck Kukus-Bad," 146, 150–155; Tausch, "Franz Anton von Sporcks 'Kuckus=Bad'," 127, 129, 147.
71. See Benedikt, *Franz Anton Graf von Sporck*, 314; Hancke, *Beschreibung*, c. 1720, D2v; Lietzmann, "Des Reichsgrafen Franz Anton von Sporck Kukus-Bad," 148, 155–160; Tausch, "Franz Anton von Sporcks 'Kuckus=Bad'," 132–133.
72. Hancke, *Beschreibung*, c. 1720, Bv: "zu einem Paradieß gemacht" – "Helden-Blut."

73. Quoted in Lietzmann, "Des Reichsgrafen Franz Anton von Sporck Kukus-Bad," 164–165: "Man sagt" – "König von Engelland" – "[sich] des dem Grafen von Sporck zugehörigen so genannten Cuckus-Baad bedienen werde."

74. See Benedikt, *Franz Anton Graf von Sporck*, 406, note 200; Lietzmann, "Des Reichsgrafen Franz Anton von Sporck Kukus-Bad," 164.

75. Therefore, Kaspar's thesis – based on Driburg, as a private-entrepreneurial spa – that spas were places "where a lot of money could be made" ("an denen sich viel Geld verdienen ließ") should be rephrased in a much more nuanced way. Kaspar, "Bad Driburg," 81.

76. See Kuhnert, *Urbanität*, 100–103.

77. See Kuhnert, *Urbanität*, 101–102.

78. [Göckingk], "Briefe eines Reisenden," 1778, 469: "Da indes die Zahl derer, welche sich hauptsächlich des Vergnügens wegen einen Theil des Sommers hier aufhalten, ohnstreitig die größte ist, so räth schon die Politik, ihnen den Ort angenehmer zu machen, und die Regierung behält gewiß dreimal so viel Geld im Lande, oder zieht es von auswärts hinein, als sie jährlich zur Verschönerung von L[auchstädt] verwendet."

79. See Clausmeyer-Ewers, Löw, *Staatspark Wilhelmsbad Hanau*, 11; Wilhelm I. von Hessen, *Wir Wilhelm*, XII.

80. Schopenhauer, *Ausflucht an den Rhein*, 1818, 67: "Und in der Mitte des Augusts sinkt Schwalbach fast ganz in die Einsamkeit zurück, in welcher es beinah zehn Monate im Jahre begraben liegt."

81. Bitz and Kuhnert, in addition to their research on spa architecture and communication structures respectively, focused their attention on these spa lists and, for Pyrmont, additionally on the so-called *Schlüsselgeldbücher* (literally books of fees for keys), a list of fees for lending out the keys to the privies close to the main avenue in Pyrmont. See Kuhnert, *Urbanität*, 43. Kuhnert provides a statistical analysis of these lists for Pyrmont, and Bitz does the same for a number of southwestern German spas of varying size in order to draw conclusions about the composition of the spa audience in terms of their social and geographical origin. See Kuhnert, *Urbanität*, 44; Bitz, *Badewesen*, 25. The Pyrmont guest lists are available at https://owl.museum-digital.de/index.php?t=sammlung&instnr=13&gesusa=38 and the Karlsbad guest lists can be accessed at https://www.portafontium.eu/contents/kurliste/.

82. An exception among the spas was Lauchstädt. Its spa ordinance of 1780 instructed the owners of lodging houses to provide lists of their guests to the authorities. See *Reglement Wornach die Bürger und Hauß-auch Gast-Wirthe in der Stadt Lauchstädt sich zu achten haben*, 1780. Other exceptions were the aforementioned *Schlüsselgeldbücher* in Pyrmont and, in the case of some spas, account books the princely administration kept to record paid bills by spa guests. See Bitz, *Badewesen*, 31. However, these sources are only available for a select number of spas, and they only provided glimpses rather than complete sets of data.

83. See Frankenau, *Pyrmont*, 1799, 136; Marcard, *Beschreibung von Pyrmont*, vol. 1, 1784, 42; Kuhnert, *Urbanität*, 42; Engel, *Kulturgeschichtliche Streifzüge*, 261.

84. Kuhnert, *Urbanität*, 42: "informelle Handreichung."

85. See Kuhnert, *Urbanität*, 45; Bitz, *Badewesen*, 23.

86. See Frankenau, *Pyrmont*, 1799, 138; Kuhnert, *Urbanität*, 43.

87. Mosch, *Bäder und Heilbrunnen*, 1819, vol. 2, article "Pyrmont," [unpaginated]: "Wenn der Brunnengäste so wenig werden, daß die Zahl der Ankommenden keinen halben Bogen mehr füllt, druckt man die Listen nicht mehr."

88. See Kuhnert, *Urbanität*, 43. Johann Wolfgang von Goethe collected lists of spa guest, especially from the Bohemian spas. See Ruppert, *Goethes Bibliothek*.
89. See Kuhnert, *Urbanität*, 45, 124–125; Bitz, *Badewesen*, 461–463.
90. "Badechronik," *JLM* (September 1801), 492: "Man hat bei der heurigen Badezeit oft an 6[00] bis 800 Fremde gezählt und in die Badeliste eingetragen. Allein dabei ist denn freilich auch manche Ostentation im Spiele. Selbst das ganze nicht unbeträchtliche Personale der Walterschen Schauspielgeschaft, die in Pyrmont spielte, mußte sich als badend mit aufführen lassen."
91. See Frankenau, *Pyrmont*, 1799, 139; Kuhnert, *Urbanität*, 43.
92. "Badechronik," *JLM* (November 1802), 625. This obviously makes it difficult to estimate the size of groups composed of families, relatives, and potentially also friends visiting a spa together, let alone the number of accompanying servants beyond general observations such as the fact that rulers traveled with smaller courts by the end of the eighteenth century. See Kuhnert, *Urbanität*, 43–44; Bitz, *Badewesen*, 141.
93. "Badechronik," *JLM* (September 1799), 462: "Die jährlichen Badelisten . . . geben keinen genauen Aufschluß über die wirkliche Zahl der Kurgäste, indem sehr viele sich nicht darinn aufnehmen lassen, und zwar nicht nur aus den unbedeutenden, sondern auch aus den vornehmen Menschenklassen."
94. As explained later in this chapter, this refers to parties of several persons rather than individual spa guests.
95. This is a reference to the first partition of Poland in 1772, when the country was divided between Austria, Prussia, and Russia.
96. "Badechronik," *JLM* (November 1797), 544–545: "Die gedruckte Badeliste enthält 715 Nummern bis zum 16. Aug[ust] und man kann mit Gewißheit annehmen, daß zum wenigsten I[/]6 der Badegesellschaft die Einzeichnung ihrer Namen unterließ. Fast alle ehemaligen Pohlen, die vielleicht selbst ein gemeinschaftlicher politischer Zweck versammelt hatte, verbaten sich die Einrückung in die Badeliste."
97. Marcard, *Kleines Pyrmonter Brunnenbuch*, 1805, 163–164: "Oefters aber bleiben Namen von Personen aus den Listen weg, weil sie ihre Ursachen haben sie nicht öffentlich gedruckt zu sehen (vielleicht ohne Urlaub in Pyrmont sind), und die Einrückung daher verbitten." See also *Das Pyrmonter Brunnenarchiv*, 1782, 27.
98. See Lotz-Heumann, "Daheim und auf Reisen."
99. See *Reise nach den Badeörtern*, 1798, 122: "Die Namen ganz gemeiner Leute und Domestiken fallen daraus gänzlich hinweg; auch lassen sich viele Fremden, entweder aus Sparniß oder aus andern Absichten, gar nicht erst in diese Listen einzeichnen: folglich erfährt man nie ganz genau, wie groß die Anzahl der Fremden in Karlsbad sey, und so wird der Hauptzweck dieser Einrichtung, daß man nämlich vollständig übersehe, mit wem man sich zu gleicher Zeit hier in Gesellschaft befindet, zum Theil verfehlt."
100. Although Bitz attempts to establish a classification of spa guests by correlating title/occupation, hometown, and, if possible, lodging house, the problematic aspects of his approach are obvious. For example, he does not differentiate between old and new nobility and, moreover, from the late eighteenth century onward, puts "middle and lower nobility" ("mittleren und niederen Adel") together with leading territorial officials who could, however, also be of bourgeois background. German territorial rulers and foreign aristocracy are grouped together in one category, although it is precisely a distinction between these two groups that would allow one to answer questions about the international popularity of a spa. See Bitz, *Badewesen*, 26–29. Overall, a statistical analysis of the guest lists for the

purpose of a quantitative social history of spas could only hope to be meaningful if intensive additional research were carried out for each spa. This
would not only entail a very detailed classification system but also require
research on every single listed guest to determine his or her precise social
and geographical origin. Such a study would have to focus on one or at most
two spas and could, in light of the known gaps in the guest lists, still not be
certain in producing meaningful results.

101. Reichard writes that about 700 parties of spa guests visited Karlsbad each
year in 1799 and 1800. He estimates that this amounted to 4,000 spa guests
annually. See Reichard, *Passagier auf der Reise*, 1801, 353.

102. On the problem of reliably gauging the number of persons in a party, see
Stöhr, *Kaiser Karlsbad*, 1810; Stöhr, *Kaiser Karlsbad*, 1817; Karell, *Karlsbad*, 118; *Festschrift zur 74. Versammlung*, 593–594.

103. See Frankenau, *Pyrmont*, 1799, 139; Marcard, *Kleines Pyrmonter Brunnenbuch*, 1805, 166–167; Kuhnert, *Urbanität*, 45–47.

104. See, e.g., "Badechronik," *JLM* (August 1804), 402–403; "Von Schandau";
Schandau, seine Quellen und reizende Umgebungen, c. 1804.

105. See Johne, *Bad Schandau*, 17.

106. See Bitz, *Badewesen*, 251, 315.

107. See "Gästeliste Bertrich 1790."

108. See *Verzeichnis der im Sommer 1817 im Alexisbade angekommenen Badegäste und Fremden*.

109. See Fuchs, "'Dieses Wasser'," 101; Struck, *Wiesbaden*, 61.

110. See Bitz, *Badewesen*, 312.

111. See [Schulz], *Reise eines Liefländers*, 1795, 78; Kuhnert, *Urbanität*,
128–130.

112. See Stöhr, *Kaiser Karlsbad*, 1812, 81.

113. See Stöhr, *Kaiser Karlsbad*, 1810, 259 (de Ligne), 262 (Findlater).

114. See Stöhr, *Kaiser Karlsbad*, 1812, 285 (duke of Württemberg); 284–286
(members of the Anhaltine dynasty).

115. Stöhr, *Kaiser Karlsbad*, 1810, 260 (Campe and Stevenson): "Herr Z.W. Stevenson mit Gemahlin aus Neuyork in Amerika."

116. I disagree with Kuhnert, who sees Pyrmont and Karlsbad as equals in the
spa hierarchy of the eighteenth century and argues that Karlsbad only rose
above Pyrmont around 1800. See Kuhnert, *Urbanität*, 53–54.

117. See *Das Pyrmonter Brunnenarchiv*, 1782, 15–16.

118. See "Badechronik," *JLM* (November 1797), 555; Frankenau, *Pyrmont*,
1799, 141–142; *Das Pyrmonter Brunnenarchiv*, 1782, 16–40; Kuhnert,
Urbanität, 86–87.

119. See Frankenau, *Pyrmont*, 1799, 141; Kuhnert, *Urbanität*, 50–51.

120. See Kuhnert, *Urbanität*, 52; "Ueber Pyrmont," 1800, 505.

121. See Kuhnert, *Urbanität*, 124–125.

122. See Chapter 6.

123. Schwalbach and Aachen were the first spas in the empire with German-
language spa publications concentrating on amusements. This clearly indicates their importance in the late seventeenth and early eighteenth centuries.
See Chapter 2.

124. See Rossel, "Kurfürst August von Sachsens Badereise."

125. See Scultetus, *Selbstbiographie*, 73.

126. See Genth, *Kulturgeschichte*, 37–43; Genth, *Nachtrag*, 16–17.

127. See Bleymehl-Eiler, "'Das Paradies der Kurgäste'," 70–71.

128. Pütter, *Selbstbiographie*, vol. 1, 297–298: "Die Localumstände, was Alleen
und andere öffentliche Anstalten betrifft, fand ich in gar keiner Vergleichung
mit dem, was ich (1749.) zu Pyrmont gesehen hatte, viel weniger, wie ich

Pyrmont in späteren Jahren (1770–1794.) habe kennen gelernt." Bleymehl-Eiler, "'Das Paradies der Kurgäste'," 66, classifies Schwalbach together with Pyrmont, Aachen, Spa, and Bath as among the "famous fashionable spas of the time" ("berühmten Modebäder der Zeit"), but she disregards the necessary chronological differentiation.

129. See "Badechronik," *JLM* (December 1805); "Badechronik," *JLM* (September 1808).

130. See Bitz, *Badewesen*, 164–165, 312; Genth, *Nachtrag*, 16–17.

131. See Bernhard, "Bad Aachen," 129.

132. See Richel, "Aachener Fremdenliste von 1768."

133. See Erdmann, *Aachen im Jahre 1812*, 95.

134. See Richel, "Aachener Fremdenliste von 1768"; Bousack, *Heiße Quellen*, 75–76; Biehn, Herzogenberg, *Große Welt reist ins Bad*, 67.

135. See Bousack, *Heiße Quellen*, 76.

136. See Bernhard, "Bad Aachen," 138–139; Bousack, *Heiße Quellen*, 77–79.

137. Considering the urban character of Aachen's spa district, it remains a distinct possibility, however, that Aachen could have fallen behind anyway, independent of its occupation by the French. Aachen lacked features that catered to a changing spatial perception, and it is significant that from 1802 onward the French administration took measures to add rural aspects to the urban character of the spa, for example by laying out promenades and footpaths. See Bernhard, "Bad Aachen," 138. On the development of spatial perception at the spas, see Chapters 3 and 4.

138. See Reinhold, *Bad Lauchstädt*, 31. Ketelhodt, *Tagebuch einer Reise*, 300, writes that Lauchstädt rarely had more than 120 or 130 visitors, but it is not clear whether he meant parties or persons, and whether he actually consulted the spa lists or was just estimating. It is also possible that he was talking about the number of guests in Lauchstädt at any given time, rather than for the entire season.

139. See *Lauchstädt, ein kleines Gemählde*, 1787, 32; Reinhold, *Bad Lauchstädt*, 31.

140. See Heimühle, *Historische Kuranlagen*, 6–7, 22–23.

141. See Reinhold, *Bad Lauchstädt*, 34–35; Heimühle, *Historische Kuranlagen*, 23.

142. See Bitz, *Badewesen*, e.g. 126, 165, 235, 252, 314.

143. See in detail Kaspar, *Brunnenkur*.

144. See "Gästeliste Bertrich 1790"; Göckingk, "Von dem Kurbrunnen bei Brückenau," 1782.

145. See Bleymehl-Eiler, "Das Paradies der Kurgäste," 59–60; Bitz, *Badewesen*, 236, 277.

146. See Schneider-Strittmatter, *Langensteinbach*.

147. See *Dehio – Handbuch der deutschen Kunstdenkmäler: Brandenburg*, article "Freienwalde," 30–33.

148. See Kuhnert, *Urbanität*, 135, 138–140.

149. See Chapter 6.

150. See Kuhnert, *Urbanität*, 138–140.

151. "Bade-Chronik des Jahres 1814," *JLM* (September 1814), 583: "Schade, daß durch den Anblick eines bettelhaften Volkes . . . der Genuß auf den schönen Spaziergängen verdorben wird."

152. Deneken, "Bemerkungen bey dem Rehburger Gesundbrunnen," 1796, 198: "Durch gute Policey-Anstalten werden die Bettler aus den Spaziergängen entfernt, wo sie sonst den einsamen Denker in seinen Meditationen und Freunde in ihren vertraulichen Gesprächen auf die unangenehmste Weise unterbrechen." See also 195.

153. Quoted in Renner, "Dichter auf Badereise," 611: "Bettler finden hier gar nicht statt." See also [Gieseke], "Neue Briefe über Carlsbad, vom Jahre 1792, Zweiter Brief," 1793, 414.
154. Bitz, *Badewesen*, 21.
155. Marienbad (today Mariánské Lázně in the Czech Republic) joined this spa cluster in the 1820s.
156. Limmer joined this cluster at the beginning of the nineteenth century.
157. At the beginning of the nineteenth century Soden joined this cluster. Soden is not on the map at the end of this book because it remained a spa with only local significance during the period covered in this study.
158. Wipfeld joined this cluster at the beginning of the nineteenth century.
159. Augustusbad near Radeberg, Berggießhübel, Buschbad near Meißen, Schandau, and Tharand. See "Badechronik," *JLM* (September 1801); Rosseaux, *Freiräume*, 211–224. A little further away also in Saxon Switzerland were Wiesenbad and Wolkenstein. See "Bade-Chronik," *JLM* (September 1813); Heinsse, *Beschreibung des Wolkensteiner Bades*, 1808.
160. See Zentner, *Renchthal*, 1827. Rippoldsau is close by in the Wolftal. Other spas like Wildbad, Baden-Baden, Teinach, Huber Bad, and Langensteinbach are also in the Black Forest.
161. These spas are today located in Poland: Altwasser/Stary Zdrój, Charlottenbrunn/Jedlina-Zdrój, Cudowa/Kudowa-Zdrój, Flinsberg/Świeradów-Zdrój, Landeck/Lądek-Zdrój, Reinerz/Duszniki-Zdrój, Salzbrunn/Szczawno-Zdrój, and Warmbrunn/Cieplice Śląskie-Zdrój. In the early nineteenth century Langenau, today Długopole-Zdrój in Poland, joined this cluster. Langenau is not on the map at the end of this book because it remained a spa with only local significance during the period covered in this study. See Morgenbesser, *Nachricht an das Publikum*, 1777; Mosch, *Heilquellen Schlesiens*, 1821.
162. See Neubeck, *Gesundbrunnen*, 1798, 60; Gerning, *Heilquellen am Taunus*, 1814.
163. See Günzel, *Bäder-Residenzen*, 110; Bitz, *Badewesen*, 149; Bleymehl-Eiler, "'Das Paradies der Kurgäste'," 64–74.
164. [Merveilleux], *Amusemens des eaux de Schwalbach*, 1739, 37: "Personen, die weder eine starke Gesellschaft noch gar zu lebhafte Ergötzlichkeiten lieben."
165. See Bleymehl-Eiler, "'Das Paradies der Kurgäste'," 78–79.
166. See Chun, *Reise der Chunischen Zöglinge*, 1791, 40; Bleymehl-Eiler, "'Das Paradies der Kurgäste'," 59–64.
167. See Bleymehl-Eiler, "'Das Paradies der Kurgäste'," 62.
168. Bleymehl-Eiler, "'Das Paradies der Kurgäste'," 79: "Wiesbaden verkörpert stark vereinfacht gesagt das Kleinbürgerbad, Langenschwalbach das multiständische Modebad und Schlangenbad das Fürstenbad." – I would argue, however, that the term "Fürstenbad" ("princely spa") is misleading and that "noble spa" would be a more appropriate term.
169. See Bleymehl-Eiler, "'Das Paradies der Kurgäste'," 60.
170. See Bothe, "Bad Driburg," in: *Kurstädte*, 305–306. See also Chapter 6.
171. See Nohl, *Berichte vom Meinberger Brunnen*, 25–30; Trampel, *Beschreibung des Bades zu Meinberg*, 1770; Trampel, *Wie muß der Kranke*, 1806.

2 Spas as Centers of Communication
Face-to-Face Interactions and Print Culture

The spa as an eighteenth-century heterotopia – together with its inherent tensions, like those between its function as an aristocratic space of political and social representation and the bourgeois demand for equality – was created through a multitiered communication system. This communication system can also be described as a set of overlapping circles of communication with the spa at the center. In this chapter, I explore the two fundamental tiers of this communication system, namely interpersonal communication at the spa and the published discourse.

The direct face-to-face interaction of two spa guests formed the innermost circle of communication, spreading out to various overlapping communication circles between groups of spa visitors. Meetings in circles of friends in and around the spa extended this communication system. Letters written by guests to family and friends tied the spa into an even wider communication network. During the eighteenth century, spas became communication centers for Freemasons, and some spas even established their own Masonic lodges. Moreover, secret political negotiations were often conducted at spas. In addition to these interactions, inherently defined as private and confidential, the communication structure of the spa was characterized by diverse interactions in the public spaces of the spa, especially along the main avenue, in assembly rooms, and in coffeehouses. These different types of communication – from confidential to public – often mixed, either intentionally or unintentionally. At the spa, an extraordinarily high degree of social interaction and networking took place in a small, one might even say dense, space during a condensed period of time, the annual spa season.[1] This situation sometimes created severe tensions between expectations of confidentiality and the disclosure of supposed secrets to the public. Contemporaries were keenly aware of this and described the various facets of the spa as a center of communication both in personal narratives and in the published discourse.

Beyond these forms of interpersonal communication, the concept of the spa as a heterotopia was conveyed to the reading public through the various formats and genres of writing that constituted the published discourse. In the sixteenth and seventeenth centuries, spa publications centered around health and disease. A gradual change occurred in the late seventeenth century and accelerated during the eighteenth century. From the 1770s onward, the published discourse diversified dramatically. The reading public learned about life at the spa through a variety of functional and fictional genres, including advertising materials in textual and visual form, travelogues, novels, plays, poems, and journal articles. Tourist spa guides emerged, advertising the spa as a place of leisure and social interaction. During the late eighteenth and early nineteenth centuries, spa publications reached a wider audience and allowed readers to keep abreast of updates on individual spas as well as debates in the spa discourse. By the early nineteenth century, knowledge about spas had become so widespread in contemporary society that authors could use spa references to generate satire.

Interpersonal Communication at the Spa

In his 1798 autobiography, Johann Stephan Pütter (1725–1807), professor of law at the University of Göttingen, recounts his friendship with the lawyer and Hanoverian privy councillor Julius Melchior Strube (1725–1777). In this context, Pütter reveals Pyrmont's importance as a center of interpersonal communication and the spa's function as a social heterotopia. Pütter begins by explaining the limits of his intense, almost daily contact by letter with Strube: "Confidential information or other topics that we could not discuss in letters, we reserved for face-to-face meetings."[2] These meetings took place once a year in Pyrmont: "In the summer of 1771, he [Strube] suggested to me that we might both travel to Pyrmont at the same time. We soon agreed to arrive there on the same day and stay in the same lodging house. . . . we continued in this way during the following years as long as Strube was alive."[3]

Strube convinced Pütter that an annual visit to Pyrmont was of use to him beyond health and friendship: "In your profession, he said, you will end up sitting in your study and looking at everything from only one perspective and often in a distorted way if you don't continue to talk to businessmen and take a look at people of quality. Pyrmont will be the most appropriate place for you to achieve both these purposes."[4] Pütter concludes with satisfaction that "the experience soon taught me that my friend was right" and emphasizes the synergy created by "three weeks of continued confidential conversation with such a friend," "social interactions with so many other people," and "so many opportunities to make experiences and observations to broaden one's knowledge of human nature."[5] While at Pyrmont, Pütter recommended the University of Göttingen to other spa guests for their children or wards, he made a variety of acquaintances, among others the famous Osnabrück statesman Justus Möser (1720–1794), and he was able to deepen these contacts during his annual trips to the spa.[6] Pütter clearly recognized the advantages of the spa as a heterotopia – a place outside of everyday life – when he states that, although one can visit meritorious men in their hometowns, "this cannot be compared to the casual way in which one can talk to this or that person for a longer or shorter time in such a place as Pyrmont, without worrying about keeping the other person from their professional duties."[7]

In his autobiography, Pütter not only addresses the advantages of interpersonal communication at the spa but also directs our attention to the intimate connection between spa trips and letter-writing. Friends arranged to meet at a spa through letters exchanged in advance, and spa visitors reported to friends and family about their experiences at the spa. For example, Justus Möser wrote to his friend, the author, publisher, and bookseller Christoph Friedrich Nicolai (1733–1811), in May 1787, "If I am not to lose a minute of your pleasant company in Pyrmont, you must be at the center staircase in front of Niemeyer's lodging house at 10 o'clock in the evening of 30 June, and then I will rush to embrace you."[8] Nicolai's letter to Möser of March 1791 reveals the two interrelated functions contemporaries valued about the spa – the spa as a space of social interaction (rather than healing) and the opportunity for confidential face-to-face conversations: "As far as I am concerned, I think I will be in Pyrmont this year on 1 July, not to use the [healing] water, but to see my good friends. . . . Whether you will also come there is my question today, and it is my wish that you may answer with an audible yes! . . . and everything else I would like to say to you, [I ask you] to listen to in Pyrmont."[9]

Sometimes, arrangements for a spa visit did not work out as planned, so letters functioned as an information system in that regard as well. In 1766, for instance, Justus Möser wrote to his friend Thomas Abbt (1738–1766), the writer and mathematician, "I am just beginning to recover from an annoying indisposition, which I had contracted due to a cold. I have therefore canceled my trip to Aachen, . . . Meanwhile, my wife and sister left yesterday, and so I am now an abandoned grass widower. But I think I will travel to Pyrmont around 1 July."[10] During the season, guests staying at different spas also communicated by letter with each other. Möser's daughter, the writer Jenny von Voigts (1749–1814), for years hoped in vain for a meeting with Duchess Luise of Anhalt-Dessau (1750–1811) in Pyrmont, only to find herself writing letters instead when Luise stayed in Ems or Karlsbad: "How I envy all those who see you in Karlsbad, who can be with you."[11] And Adele Schopenhauer remarked in her diary on 16 July 1816 during her stay in Schwalbach, "No news from Pyrmont."[12]

Pütter also referred to the importance of meetings with friends and acquaintances in the vicinity of the spa: "Finally [there were] pleasant opportunities at times to make and renew valuable acquaintances in places close to Pyrmont."[13] One example was the so-called Pyrmont-Ohsen circle of friends, which regularly met at the estate of Eberhard (1743–1813) and Marie (1756–1849) von Grävemeyer in Ohsen in the 1780s.[14] The Pyrmont-Ohsen circle included the two spa physicians Johann Georg

Zimmermann (1728–1795) and Heinrich Matthias Marcard (1747–1817) and their wives, Justus Möser and his daughter Jenny von Voigts, as well as Christoph Friedrich Nicolai.[15] The ancestral castle of Baron vom Stein in Nassau near Ems served a similar function.[16] The house of the Gräve-meyers and Nassau castle were stopovers to and from the spas, allowing for frequent trips between the spas and these estates.

The aforementioned personal narratives reveal that leading figures of the German Enlightenment regularly met at the spas and looked forward to their conversations during these meetings. However, these narratives rarely inform us of the modes and content of these conversations. This is not surprising, considering how much contemporaries valued the spa as a space for confidential face-to-face interactions. In that regard, fictional treatments can be valuable to the historian because, while not document-ing actual, lived experiences, they provide a sense of what contempo-raries perceived as plausible depictions of these experiences. In his *Ernst and Falk: Conversations for Freemasons* (*Ernst und Falk: Gespräche für Freimaurer*), first published in 1778, the Enlightenment philosopher and dramatist Gotthold Ephraim Lessing (1729–1781) used sparse but highly pointed references to the spa of Pyrmont as the scene of a confidential conversation between two friends about Freemasonry.[17]

Although some researchers doubt that the first three conversations of Ernst and Falk are actually set in Pyrmont, this nevertheless becomes obvi-ous by taking into account contemporaries' knowledge about a typical day at the spa.[18] Reading *Ernst and Falk* (*Ernst und Falk*) in light of this knowledge, which was widespread among the eighteenth-century reading public, reveals that Lessing describes both the daily routine in Pyrmont, especially the spa's morning ritual, and typical communication situations between spa guests. Marcard writes about the morning ritual in Pyrmont:

> Already before six o'clock the genteel world [*feine Welt*] begins to appear in the avenue and hurries to the spring. . . . So many people who walk around without any constraint . . . , all of them in a casual morning suit, . . . without any further ceremony, except bidding each other a good morning while walking by; . . . Everyone participates in this pleasant scene in the way he likes best while drinking his spring water; he talks to whomever he wants, and no longer than it suits him, . . . At nine o'clock you can see small groups of people sitting down to have breakfast together . . . at the top of the avenue.[19]

A day in Pyrmont began by drinking the healing water and walking along the main avenue where the first two conversations between Ernst and Falk take place, interrupted by Falk's fascination with a butterfly.[20] "Intoxicated by the Pyrmont water,"[21] as Lessing refers to the morning activity of drinking spring water, Ernst and Falk have a confidential face-to-face conversation about Freemasonry. This exchange, however, takes

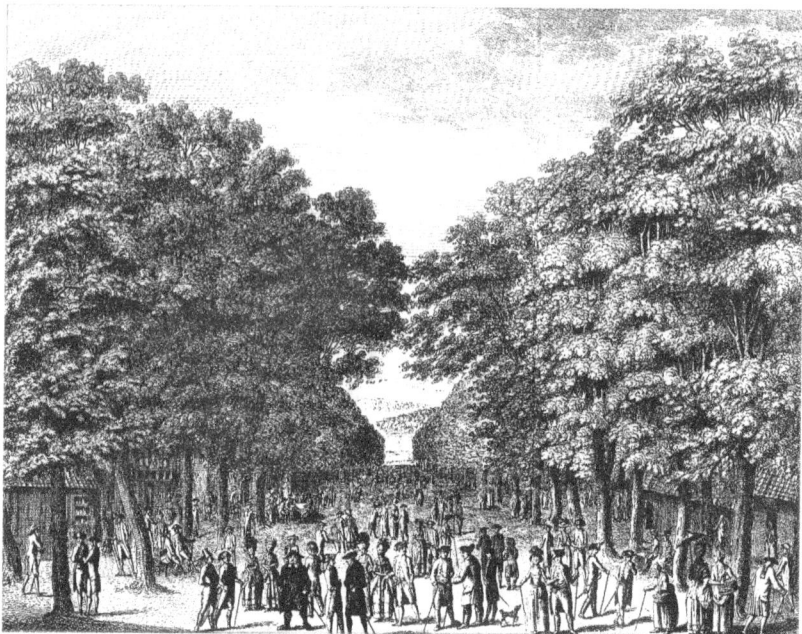

Figure 2.1 Pyrmont, main avenue, engraving by C.G. Geyser after a drawing
   by J.F. Weitsch, 1784. ("Marcard. Pyrmont. I." In Marcard, Henrich
   Matthias. *Beschreibung von Pyrmont.* Vol. 1, after 324. Leipzig: Weidmanns Erben and Reich, 1784. Bayerische Staatsbibliothek München,
   shelf mark M.med. 611–1/BHS II C 126–1.)

place in the midst of the crowd on the main avenue (Figure 2.1). Falk
concludes their second conversation by asking Ernst to seek the company
of other spa guests at breakfast: "There they wave to us for breakfast.
Come! . . . There in the larger company we will soon find topics for a
more suitable conversation."[22] Falk thus intentionally expands the circle
of communication, making it impossible to continue their private discussion. Falk keeps to this pattern of behavior throughout the day; he avoids
Ernst "in the jostling crowds" at the spa.[23] Ernst then tries to resume the
conversation with Falk in the evening by paying Falk a visit in his room.[24]
In his description of Pyrmont, Marcard clarifies that this was an expression of friendship, because "it is not at all customary in Pyrmont to visit
people in their rooms, only close acquaintances visit each other in their
rooms."[25] At the end of the third conversation, Ernst leaves his friend at
the spa to become a Freemason in "the city."[26]
   In this way, Lessing depicted different communication situations at the
spa. On the one hand, two people could successfully isolate their face-
to-face communication to such an extent that a confidential conversation

was possible – either in their rooms or even in the middle of the crowd of spa guests on the main avenue in Pyrmont. On the other hand, spa visitors could completely immerse themselves in the larger communication circles of the spa. As Pütter's aforementioned visits to Pyrmont and his annual meetings with Strube show, contemporaries deeply appreciated the opportunities offered by the spa, both for confidential conversations with friends and for mingling with strangers. Interpersonal communication about delicate topics could take place without "having to face . . . the dangers of a written record,"[27] and, moreover, the spa functioned as a communication hub that brought together people who may have otherwise not met.

Lessing's depictions in *Ernst and Falk* (*Ernst und Falk*) rang true for contemporaries because they had experienced similar situations, or because they had read about spas as gathering places for Freemasons. Lessing himself discussed Freemasonry with Möser in Pyrmont in 1766[28] – these conversations may very well have inspired him to use the spa as a setting for *Ernst and Falk* (*Ernst und Falk*). In fact, in the eighteenth-century published discourse, "art" and "life" often blended together. The function of the spa as a place for discussions of Freemasonry comes up in travelogues, for example. In Willebrand's *News from a Spa Visit to Karlsbad* (*Nachrichten von einer Carlsbader Brunnenreise*), the narrator talks to a Carmelite monk in Karlsbad about Freemasonry and about the attacks on Freemasons by townspeople in Aachen in 1779–1780.[29]

Even a short list of prominent men who were both Freemasons and spa guests in Pyrmont during the long eighteenth century shows that one cannot overestimate the importance of Pyrmont as a communication center for Freemasons. The list includes the publisher Friedrich Justin Bertuch (1747–1822), the educator and writer Joachim Heinrich Campe (1746–1818), Duke Carl August of Sachse-Weimar-Eisenach (1757–1828), the poet Matthias Claudius (1740–1815), Prince Frederick, duke of York and Albany and prince-bishop of Osnabrück (1763–1827), the writer and Prussian official Leopold Friedrich Günther von Göckingk (1748–1828), the writer and privy councillor Johann Wolfgang von Goethe (1749–1832), the philosopher Johann Gottfried Herder (1744–1803), the physician Christoph Wilhelm Hufeland (1762–1836), the writer Adolph Baron (*Freiherr*) Knigge (1752–1796), the writer August von Kotzebue (1761–1819), the writer, publisher, and bookseller Christoph Friedrich Nicolai (1733–1811), and the aforementioned law professor Johann Stephan Pütter (1725–1807).[30]

As early as 1746, Justus Möser, a regular Pyrmont visitor, advertised the spa's status among Freemasons to the reading public – or at least to those among the reading public with some insider knowledge about Freemasonry. In his anonymous work *Letter by the Author to His Sister About the Pleasant Stay in Pyrmont* (*Schreiben des Verfassers an seine Schwester über den angenehmen Aufenthalt zu Pyrmont*) he wrote,

"Here, as in paradise, one finds all kinds of nations and religions, from the judge from Lüda to the prince of Libanus."[31] The "prince of Libanus" (*Prinz vom Libanon*) constitutes the 22nd degree of the Scottish Rite of Freemasonry.[32]

The options for Freemasons to communicate at Pyrmont were expanded in 1776 with the foundation of the Masonic lodge named "Frederick at the Three Springs" (*Friedrich zu den drei Quellen*), which joined the Order of Strict Observance, the dominant Masonic system in Germany at the time.[33] The name of the lodge derived from the ruling Prince Friedrich Karl August of Waldeck and Pyrmont (1743–1812) and from the three main healing springs in Pyrmont.[34] Prince Friedrich also became the lodge's Protector. The Masonic Protector of the lodge was Prince Karl (also Carl, from 1794 Duke Karl II) Ludwig Friedrich of Mecklenburg-Strelitz (1741–1816), a frequent guest in Pyrmont.[35] Georg Friedrich Papen (or Pape), the prince's personal physician and "regular physician at the healing spring in Pyrmont," became the first Master of the lodge.[36] The lodge counted among its members numerous officials responsible for the operation of the spa as well as merchants in Pyrmont.[37] The Pyrmont lodge mainly served Freemasons visiting the spa, thus helping to maintain and consolidate the success of Pyrmont. In fact, the number of visiting Freemasons regularly surpassed the number of local members.[38]

The presence of a Masonic lodge at a spa created a heterotopia *within* a heterotopia, forming another space of "social extraterritoriality"[39] inside the larger social heterotopia of the spa. In addition to the various communication circles described earlier, the lodge added a space of "institutionalized intimacy"[40] to the spa where bourgeois and noble Freemasons were able to interact freely and overcome social boundaries. Freemasons visiting a lodge at a spa thus entered an exclusive circle of communication and interaction closed off to other guests. At the same time, the presence of a Masonic lodge at a spa implied that female spa guests and male spa guests who were not Freemasons were excluded from one of the communication circles of the spa.

In spite of their secret nature, however, eighteenth-century Masonic lodges were heterotopias with a "system of opening and closing,"[41] admitting people from the outside at certain intervals and following specific social rules. In her diary, Sophie Becker described a typical situation during a 1785 visit to Brückenau where she and Elisa von der Recke were invited to a banquet lunch at the "Freemason's club."[42] Becker commented, "I will not spend time on a description of the ceremonies performed at such banquets because everyone who has attended them knows them. The women all dressed in blue and white, something the gentlemen enjoyed very much."[43] As Becker's observations reveal, women, although excluded from membership in the lodges, were familiar with the rituals of the Masonic banquets where female guests were regularly admitted. Becker's experience as a woman entering the space of the Masonic lodge on a special occasion thus speaks to the functioning of Masonic lodges both in eighteenth-century society in general and at the spa in particular.

Unsurprisingly, given the spa's role as a multipurpose meeting place in eighteenth-century society, spas also served as neutral spaces for meetings and sometimes for secret negotiations of princes and their emissaries. Spas offered rulers and/or their representatives opportunities to meet outside their residence towns, and, as a result, strict diplomatic and court protocols could be relaxed.[44] Here, "politics could be conducted, as it were, in advance of official cabinet activities."[45] The heterotopia of the spa, with its various forms of social interaction, allowed for confidential interpersonal communication and for political agreements to be reached informally before negotiations became public knowledge.

During the so-called Pyrmont Summer of Princes (*Pyrmonter Fürstensommer*) of 1681, the northern German and European princes attempted to reach common ground in opposition to Louis XIV's Reunion policy while at the spa.[46] King Frederick II of Prussia revived his alliance with France against Austria in preparation for the Second Silesian War in Pyrmont in 1744, meeting with the French military representative Count Montaigne during a walk in the nearby woods.[47] In 1783, Prince Franz of Anhalt-Dessau[48] and Margrave Karl Friedrich of Baden met at the spa of Langensteinbach, located in the Margraviate of Baden, to initiate the League of Princes (*Fürstenbund*), a movement by the smaller German territories to counter Prussia and Austria, later taken over by Frederick II of Prussia.[49] In his travel diary, Franz von Waldersee, the illegitimate son of Prince Franz, hinted at the secrecy and intensity of these negotiations by commenting that the prince and the margrave "were always alone together."[50]

The representatives of the electors of Mainz, Cologne, and Trier, and of the archbishop of Salzburg met at the Congress of Ems in 1786 to oppose papal interference in their exercise of ecclesiastical authority. During the Napoleonic Wars and the gradual dissolution of the empire at the end of the eighteenth and beginning of the nineteenth centuries, Pyrmont again was the stage for political talks, especially on the occasion of the spa visits of King Frederick William II of Prussia in 1796 and 1797.[51] Yet another example is found in the Karlsbad Decrees of 1819, which were intended to push back on revolutionary tendencies in Germany by instituting censorship, among other measures. The role of the spa as a place for (secret) political negotiations was so much a part of the perception of contemporaries that journalists suspected diplomatic activities even when they did not take place. The presence of the Austrian "negotiator" Count Ludwig von Cobenzl and the former Russian envoy Count von Buxhöwden – both high-ranking diplomats – in Karlsbad in 1800 led to false newspaper reports about their "alleged congress."[52]

This incident leads us to further explore the tension at the spa between confidentiality or *arcanum* on the one hand and the public sphere on the other. In his 1746 *Letter by the Author to His Sister* (*Schreiben des Verfassers an seine Schwester*), Justus Möser emphasized the ambivalent nature of the communication system of the spa. With a good dose of sarcasm, he remarked, "I would like to ask all scholars who want to write biographies to come here because nowhere else are more secret messages whispered in your ear than here, and I hereby offer the most generous publisher *Memoires Aneckdotes* in twelve parts."[53] Kuhnert observes that "the confidentiality of the conversation, made possible by the setting of the spa, should not obscure the ambivalent character of a place that simultaneously functioned as a forum for increased publicity."[54] Two events in Wilhelmsbad and Pyrmont – the Masonic Congress of Wilhelmsbad in 1782 and the "scandal" in the early 1790s of the so-called Bahrdt pasquinade, a satirical pamphlet attacking various members of Pyrmont's spa society – provide examples of how confidential information was communicated to the larger spa society, or even further to the Enlightenment reading public.

From 16 July to 1 September 1782, Duke Ferdinand of Brunswick-Lüneburg-Wolfenbüttel, the Grand Master (*Magnus Superior Ordinis*) of the Order of Strict Observance, and his Deputy Prince Karl of Hesse-Kassel convened the so-called Masonic Congress of Wilhelmsbad at Wilhelmsbad near Hanau.[55] Count Wilhelm IX of Hanau, the owner of the spa, was Prince Karl's brother. The Congress was embedded in a longer-term controversy about the future of the prevailing Masonic system of Strict Observance, and the purpose of the convention was to reform the Strict Observance.[56] Due to the controversial nature of the negotiations, the organizers' major concern was to keep the deliberations secret. Therefore, Wilhelmsbad was chosen as the venue rather than the imperial city of Frankfurt, as had originally been planned.[57] The organizers of the Congress also wanted to prevent information about the negotiations from becoming known prematurely, even within the circle of Freemasons. They thus stipulated that "every delegate should take a pledge to tell his appointers [the lodges they represent] nothing about what is going on before the Congress ends."[58]

Duke Ferdinand and Prince Karl entirely overestimated their ability to keep information about the Congress from leaking, even in a small and newly established spa like Wilhelmsbad. The Congress started negotiations in mid-July, at the height of the spa season. As a result, Wilhelmsbad struggled to accommodate the delegates with their families and servants – a circumstance that necessarily caused the Congress to receive a certain amount of attention.[59] Furthermore, the spatial density of the spa led to a breach of the very confidentiality to which the organizers of the Congress had aspired. While spa guests like the aforementioned Pütter and Strube were usually able to convene confidential meetings apart from the rest of the spa society, the deep divisions among the delegates provoked them to spill out Masonic secrets into the wider public of the spa. The Masonic community eroded, resulting in a breakdown of trust and communication among the delegates, who started to speak openly to the other spa guests – not only in a clear breach of their pledges, but also of their Masonic oaths.

Franz Dietrich von Ditfurth, dissatisfied with the course of the Congress, reported that confidentiality could not be maintained at the spa. Ditfurth related that Count J. Gamba della Perosa (whom Ditfurth calls "Perouse") was "very upset about the Congress, so that he could not hide it from the Profane [non-Masons]."[60] Ditfurth, who stayed with his uncle in Hanau during the Congress,[61] clashed with Duke Ferdinand and Prince Karl during the 11th session. He remained in Wilhelmsbad after the end of the session on 30 July to vent his anger, also in the presence of non-Masons. Unable to successfully negotiate the tension between required secrecy and the opportunity to engage with the public sphere of the larger spa society, he reflected on the communication situation he found himself in by employing ironic exaggeration: "Then I told others: You people, I don't know anything to talk to you about, I don't know whether you are all Profane, but at least there are quite a lot of Profane in the Congress, and how can one deliberate in the presence of such people? Let us rather deliberate among the well-servants, the coachmen, and the retinue!"[62] It comes as no surprise that Count Wilhelm, who was not a Freemason but stayed at his castle in Wilhelmsbad over the summer, was well informed about the progress of the Masonic Congress.[63]

The reforms agreed upon at the Masonic Congress of Wilhelmsbad proved to be a Pyrrhic victory; they could not halt the erosion of the Strict Observance.[64] The Pyrmont lodge, which remained in the Strict Observance, gradually disintegrated.[65] The widespread system of Masonic lodges and secret societies that had been a hallmark of the age of Enlightenment in the empire began to splinter.[66] The Masonic systems of the Grand Landlodge (*Große Landesloge*) founded by the Prussian army physician Johann Wilhelm Kellner von Zinnendorf (1731–1782) and the new Eclectic League (*Ekklektischer Bund*) initiated in Wetzlar and Frankfurt, as well as the secret societies of the Illuminati and the German Union (*Deutsche Union*) of the radical Protestant theologian Karl Friedrich Bahrdt (1741–1792),[67] were committed to defending the radical Enlightenment against the anti-Enlightenment Order of the Golden and Rosy Cross (*Gold- und Rosenkreuzer*).[68] These were manifestations of the "clash of the late Enlightenment and early conservatism," resulting in the "emergence of political currents in Germany."[69] With the publication of the Bahrdt pasquinade in 1790, Pyrmont became a center of these developments.[70]

The scandal of the Bahrdt pasquinade started in 1788, two years before the publication of the pamphlet. Johann Georg Ritter von Zimmermann (1728–1795), a physician who practiced in Pyrmont during the spa season,[71] attacked the Berlin Enlightenment in his *On Frederick the Great and My Conversation with Him Shortly Before his Death* (*Über Friedrich den Großen und meine Unterredung mit ihm kurz vor seinem Tode*). In 1790, Karl Friedrich Bahrdt published a refutation, which, according to August von Kotzebue, was "devoured by all spa guests, smiled upon by some with pleasure" in Pyrmont.[72] In turn, Kotzebue decided to write a play (*Schauspiel*) in defense of Zimmermann. The pasquinade *Doctor Bahrdt with the Iron Forehead, or The German Union against Zimmermann* (*Doctor Bahrdt mit der eisernen Stirn, oder Die deutsche Union gegen Zimmermann*) was quickly published, appearing in the same year, 1790.[73]

Adolph Baron (*Freiherr*) Knigge was listed as the author on the title page of the Bahrdt pasquinade in an effort to conceal Kotzebue's authorship. The pamphlet vilified leading representatives of the German Enlightenment, among others Knigge himself, Joachim Heinrich Campe, Christoph Friedrich Nicolai, and Jacob Mauvillon (1743–1794), professor in Brunswick. The enlightened thinkers attacked in the Bahrdt pasquinade were Pyrmont visitors and, in their majority, also Freemasons and/or members of the Illuminati.[74] It soon became known that the Pyrmont spa physician Heinrich Matthias Marcard was the source of the information and rumors that Kotzebue had used for his personal attacks on these prominent Enlightenment figures.[75] Like Zimmermann, Marcard had been a member of Pyrmont's enlightened communication circles for many years, before increasingly adopting an anti-Enlightenment stance in the 1780s. Marcard later wrote in self-defense that he had found out about these "various messages, remarks, and well-known anecdotes" while serving as spa physician in Pyrmont and, as he claimed in blatant contradiction to the alleged "publicity" of these pieces of information, had passed them on to Kotzebue "in confidence and with discretion."[76]

The scandal surrounding the Bahrdt pasquinade once again illuminates the specific communication structure of the spa, as conveyed by Möser in his *Letter by the Author to His Sister* (*Schreiben des Verfassers an seine Schwester*) and by Lessing in *Ernst and Falk* (*Ernst und Falk*). The noble and upper-middle-class visitors to the spa formed a circle of communication. Within this larger circle there were various smaller communication circles, including formal organizations like Masonic lodges, informal circles of friends, and face-to-face conversations between two spa visitors. The option of conversing in secret in the middle of the public sphere of the spa rested on a mutual relationship of trust between the participants. However, a breakdown of trust, as we have seen in the case of both the Masonic Congress of Wilhelmsbad and the Bahrdt pasquinade, enabled the spread of information that was supposed to be confidential to ever larger communication circles, from the spa society to the reading public.

In contrast to confidential interpersonal conversations and Masonic lodges, coffeehouses during the Enlightenment era were quintessential public spaces. The *Pyrmont Spa Archive* (*Pyrmonter Brunnen-Archiv*) included the following description of the coffeehouse in Pyrmont in 1782:

"It is not easy to find a place in the world where one can find more topics for conversations about the gallant world and about the vanities of
human beings than in front of the coffeehouse on the grand avenue in
Pyrmont. . . . Imagine a mixed company of people from distant provinces,
often even from different nations, among these some of good mind, thor-
ough knowledge, and much experience, each of whom, by virtue of the
traditional spa freedom,[77] communicates without restraint."[78]

This passage points toward two aspects of the spa as a space for communication. First, the reference to the "mixed company of people" and
their accumulated expertise reminds us of Strube and Pütter, who valued this as one of Pyrmont's major advantages. Second, the coffeehouse
symbolizes the public sphere at the spa, where news and information
of various kinds as well as rumors were exchanged openly. To prove
this point, the author of the *Pyrmont Spa Archive* described a conversation that allegedly took place in front of the coffeehouse in 1780. Two
anonymous persons are credited with a discussion about the conduct of
Renatus Leopold Christian Karl von Senckenberg (1751–1800) in the
context of the War of the Bavarian Succession (1778–1779). The Austrian
state chancellor Wenzel Anton von Kaunitz tried to secure the Austrian
claim to parts of Bavaria by means of an enfeoffment by Emperor Sigismund to Duke Albrecht of Austria dated from 1426. Senckenberg in 1778
produced a release document by Duke Albrecht, nullifying these claims.[79]
According to the *Pyrmont Spa Archive*, the two protagonists in front
of the coffeehouse discussed whether Senckenberg's actions should be
regarded as meritorious or not, thus openly taking sides in one of the most
momentous political disputes in the empire at the time.[80]

Compared to other Enlightenment societies and associations, spas
served an important function as centers of interpersonal communication in eighteenth-century German society that has not yet been recognized sufficiently by historians. While Masonic lodges, reading societies,
salons, and coffeehouses primarily served local members and inhabitants
(with the exception of occasional outside visitors),[81] guests from a much
wider area came together during the season at the spas. As Kuhnert has
argued, spas helped to offset the lack of metropolises in the empire. Pyrmont, for example, served as a meeting place for the elites of the northern
German territories, a function that residence or university towns could
not fulfill.[82] Lucian Hölscher has argued that the literary public sphere
(*literarische Öffentlichkeit*) was a substitute for a capital city in Germany.[83] But the literary public sphere, however vibrant, still depended on
physical spaces for people to meet and engage in direct communication.
I argue that the spas met this need by bringing together different elite
groups to exchange information and to form and maintain relationships
during the long eighteenth century. At the same time, the spa was not
only a physical space but increasingly became a part of Enlightenment
print culture.

The Spa and Print Culture

In the long eighteenth century and even more so during the transitional period of the late eighteenth and the early nineteenth centuries, the presence of print culture at the spa and the presence of the spa in print culture were two sides of the same coin. On the one hand, a bookseller or bookshop and the availability of newspapers and journals were essential elements of cultural consumption at a spa. As early as 1706, Sigismund Beermann wrote about Pyrmont, "The scholars see there [in the main avenue] the bookshop on both sides, and an obsessive and insatiable bookworm, or whoever else is suffering from book sickness, can atone there for their passion."[84] In his poem *The Spa Guest* (*Der Brunnengast*) of 1744, Koromandel-Wedekind closely linked the two aspects of personal and printed communication:

> Whoever is a scholar,
> Enjoys books and reading journals,
> Will find opportunities at the linden trees in Pyrmont,
> Even find many a clever mind and good friend.[85]

Pütter in his autobiography dedicated an extensive footnote to the Pyrmont bookshop. It was operated "by . . . Helwing's bookstore [from Lemgo] carrying a large stock of books . . . and seldom [leaves] a request unanswered, or at least can easily provide advice in a short period of time."[86] And in 1796, Deneken announced in the *German Monthly* (*Deutsche Monatsschrift*) that an assembly hall would soon be built in Rehburg "that will be used for balls, for reading the newspapers and monthlies, and for other social entertainments."[87]

On the other hand, the expansion of the published discourse in the eighteenth and early nineteenth centuries gave spas an effective avenue to gain supra-regional attention and established the spa as a spatial and social heterotopia in contemporaries' minds. Until the end of the seventeenth century, spa publications focused on the treatment of illnesses. The science of balneology had developed in Italy since the thirteenth century,[88] but it was not until the second half of the fifteenth century that Italian balneological treatises became known north of the Alps. The turn of the fifteenth century, however, saw an increase in balneological works published in German, especially compendia[89] and "spa monographs,"[90] that is, balneological treatises on individual spas. While balneological treatises in Latin were aimed at physicians, spa publications in German addressed a lay audience and provided information about the range of available spas and healing waters as well as "instructions for self-medication."[91]

The balneological compendia and the spa monographs of the sixteenth and seventeenth centuries display a largely uniform structure. Their initial chapters present an analysis of the water and the water's healing powers (often including a list of people and their illnesses that had allegedly been healed by the water) as well as instructions on the proper use of the water. Throughout the early modern period, these instructions were based on traditional dietetics, the basic rules for a regulated, balanced way of life to help maintain health or cure disease. First enunciated by Hippocrates, Galen systematized these ideas into the *sex res non naturales*: light and air, food and drink, work and rest, sleep and wakefulness, excretions and secretions, and states of mind. Physicians propagated the rules of dietetics during the late Middle Ages, the Renaissance, and the early modern period, and, as a result, they became common lay knowledge.[92]

Dietetics also deeply influenced balneology and the medical instructions for a successful spa regimen. Balneological dietetics combined general dietetics with the specifics of healing water treatments. Instructions included not only which foods to eat or avoid, and how to achieve a balanced state of mind, but also details like the length of bathing times and how many glasses of healing water to drink. Chapter titles in spa publications expressly referred to these regimens. "Of the diet during the cure with acidulous water"[93] or "what kind of order of life to lead during the cure with acidulous water" were typical headings.[94] Spa physicians warned that failing to follow these medical rules would ruin the success of the water treatment. While spa monographs always included information about a spa's amenities and entertainments, these topics were only addressed briefly in later chapters.

Toward the end of the seventeenth and in the first half of the eighteenth centuries, the published discourse entered a long phase of expansion, with a growing number of spa publications emphasizing the function of the spa as a space of social interaction and recreation. A process of differentiation and diversification within the published discourse began. Publications focusing either primarily or entirely on the leisure function of spas appeared alongside publications about their health function. These developments became even more pronounced from the 1770s onward, when balneological spa guides and tourist spa guides gradually separated into distinguishable genres. During the late eighteenth and early nineteenth centuries, spas were represented in a wide variety of genres. As a result, knowledge about spas became deeply ingrained in the reading public by the early nineteenth century.

During his visit to Rehburg in 1765, Johann Christian Kestner kept a spa diary for his sisters at home in Hanover. He begins with a playful comment: "I am to provide you with a diary, yes I am to write *amusemens des eaux de Rehburg*. A difficult demand, as I am not Baron von Pöllnitz and Rehburg is not Spa. Moreover, I'm supposed to write *amusemens*. For the time being, I will only be able to tailor *rêveries*."[95] While letters and travelogues – both actual and fictional ones – played an important role in the history of spas and of communication in general during the eighteenth century,[96] it is not immediately clear what Kestner's allusions to *amusemens* and Baron von Pöllnitz refer to. In fact, Kestner connects his spa diary to a new genre of spa writings that has not yet been considered in historiography but that was clearly on contemporaries' minds. Since the 1730s, publications entitled *Amusemens de . . .* emerged as a new genre that mixed features of a spa guide, elements of the pastoral novel or the gallant novel (*galanter Roman*), and a frame narrative modeled on Boccaccio's *Decameron* or Chaucer's *Canterbury Tales*.[97]

Karl Ludwig von Pöllnitz dedicated his first *Amusemens* work (in French) to Spa in 1734 – indicative of Spa's importance in Europe at the time. His publication was translated into Dutch, German, and English.[98] A series of *Amusemens* publications followed.[99] In 1737, an *Amusemens* work about Aachen, *Amusements at the Waters of Aix la Chapelle, or Pastimes at the Waters in Aachen* (*Amusemens des eaux d'Aix la Chapelle, oder Zeit-Vertreib bey den Wassern zu Achen*), also by Pöllnitz, appeared.[100] In 1739, David François de Merveilleux published *Amusements at the Waters of Schwalbach, or Pastimes at the Waters in Schwalbach, the Baths in Wiesbaden and in Schlangenbad* (*Amusemens des eaux de Schwalbach, oder Zeitvertreibe bey den Wassern zu Schwalbach, denen Bäder zu Wisbaden, und dem Schlangenbade*).[101] In addition, we find *Amusemens* publications about the Swiss spas of Baden, Schinznach, and Pfäfers and about Baden near Vienna[102] – spas that, by the first half of the eighteenth century, were regarded as separate from *teutsche* spas like Aachen and Schwalbach.

In 1748, Johann Heinrich Schütte, the spa physician in Kleve, realized that the *Amusemens* title had become a recognizable feature and published *Amusements at the Waters of Kleve, or Enjoyments and Delights at the Waters in Kleve* (*Amusemens des eaux de Cleve, oder Vergnügungen und Ergötzlichkeiten bey denen Wassern zu Cleve*) to advertise Kleve as a spa. Schütte's work, however, was written with the members of the German and Dutch urban middle classes in mind, and he significantly modified the genre and its content. He retained the element of the frame narrative but moved away from the earlier *Amusemens* works with nobles as protagonists. Rather, the narrator accompanies a group of middle-class spa guests in and around Kleve, switching between descriptions of the spa as well as castles and small towns in its surrounding area and conversations about religion and philosophy.[103] Schütte thus explicitly targeted a middle-class audience of spa visitors, an important new element in the published discourse. All in all, it is not surprising that Kestner used the term *Amusemens* as a kind of household name and general reference point in his spa diary.

The *Amusemens* publications were part of a fundamental change in the published discourse closely reflecting the changes in the hierarchy of German spas.[104] The most fashionable spas were also the first to be associated with publications focusing on the spa as a space of social interaction and entertainment rather than healing. Not surprisingly, Schwalbach had been first in line with *The Schwalbach Perpetuum Mobile Lasting All Summer* (*Das Schwalbacher Sommer-wehrende Perpetuum mobile*), a burlesque poem first published in 1690, reprinted in 1701, and reissued in 1737 at the height of the wave of *Amusemens* publications as *Antics Seen at the Well-Cure in Langen-Schwalbach* (*Aufgefangene Grillen bey der Brunnen-Cur zu Langen-Schwalbach*).[105] As mentioned earlier, Schwalbach as the leading spa in the Taunus cluster was also the setting of an *Amusemens* publication, as was Aachen.

As Pyrmont and Karlsbad rose to the top of the spa hierarchy during the first half of the eighteenth century, they were increasingly associated with this new form of spa publication. For example, in 1706, Sigismund Beermann published *Some Historical News and Notes about the County of Pyrmont and Its Famous Mineral Spring* (*Einige Historische Nachrichten und Anmerckungen Von der Graffschafft Pyrmont und Ihren berühmten Saur-Brunnen*), a work that, in spite of its title, actually provides ample information about amenities and interactions at the spa "for the information of spa guests and as their pastime."[106] In 1719, *Perpetuum Mobile Pyrmontanum* followed, a burlesque poem in German, clearly modeled after the aforementioned *Perpetuum Mobile* publication about Schwalbach.[107] In 1744, Koromandel-Wedekind focused on Pyrmont in his poem *The Spa Guest* (*Der Brunnengast*),[108] and just two years later, in 1746, Justus Möser anonymously published *Letter by the Author to His Sister* (*Schreiben des Verfassers an seine Schwester*), also about Pyrmont.[109] The years 1750 and 1752 saw the publication of Charlotte Wilhelmine Amalie von Donop's ballad entitled *The Beauties of Pyrmont* (*Die Schönheiten Pyrmonts*)[110] and a poem by an anonymous author, *The Old, German, Honest, and Delightful Pyrmont* (*Das alte teutsche ehrliche und liebliche Pyrmont*).[111]

Karlsbad attracted numerous authors as well. Covering all aspects of a spa visit, *Newly Improved and Augmented Memorable Imperial Karlsbad* (*Neu-verbessert- und vermehrtes denckwürdiges Kayser Carls-Baad*), a three-part work first published in 1734 and reprinted in 1736, was intended "for the pleasure and as a pastime for all curious people and high-ranking spa visitors respectively."[112] In the same year, a fictional travelogue entitled *Moral and Satirical News from Karlsbad* (*Moralische und Satyrische Nachrichten aus dem Carlsbade*)[113] appeared. More publications followed: in 1751, *Innocent Pastimes in Karlsbad* (*Unschuldiger Zeitvertreib im Carlsbad*), another spa publication modeled after a gallant novel;[114] in 1754, Christoph Gottlob Grundig's travelogue *Description of His . . . Journey to Imperial Karlsbad* (*Beschreibung seiner . . . in das Käyser Carls-Bad gethanen Reise*), published anonymously and presented in the form of an epistolary narrative;[115] in 1756, the physician Balthasar Ludwig Tralles' *Ode* to Karlsbad;[116] and in the same year, Johann Christian Tilling's comprehensive spa guide, *News from Karlsbad* (*Nachricht vom Carlsbade*), which included advice on traveling to Karlsbad and a list of lodging houses at the spa.[117] All these examples illustrate the change and diversification that occurred in the published spa discourse in the first half of the eighteenth century.

From the 1770s onward, the number of spa publications rose significantly. By the turn of the nineteenth century, authors felt the need to justify why they added yet another publication to the existing corpus. In his work about Pyrmont, Frankenau argued, "'Again a mite of little value [added] to the large number of travelogues filling many a bookstore in our age that is so fond of writing' – I hear one or the other critic murmuring – 'and this mite is all the more unexpected because Marcard, who is famous far and wide, has already described a long time ago the famous spa of Pyrmont as an earthly paradise, as a *non plus ultra*.' It is true! I will therefore not repeat this man's description, which is much too charming, but provide a sketch of this spa as it really is."[118]

Spa publications of the late eighteenth and early nineteenth centuries covered a wide range of genres. Functional writings like spa guides and travelogues made up the majority of spa publications. Spa guides of various lengths, from short pamphlets to full-fledged books, came in a handy octavo or even duodecimo format. They were often explicitly labeled as "pocketbooks" (*Taschenbuch*) in their titles and, in fact, were increasingly sold (paper-)bound. This made spa publications everyday objects that could be taken on a trip and read in various circumstances.[119] In addition, anthologies, that is, collections of spa descriptions,[120] and educational writings, often in the form of travelogues,[121] became part of the published discourse. The onset of reports about spas in Enlightenment journals in the 1780s further expanded the published discourse and introduced an element of topicality. In 1796, the *Journal of Luxury and Fashions* (*Journal des Luxus und der Moden*) started to publish its regular "Spa Chronicle" ("Badechronik"), sometimes also titled "German Spa Chronicle" ("Teutsche Badechronik"), thus providing the interested public with news about spas after every season. Other journals and from 1801 the *Newspaper for the Elegant World* (*Zeitung für die elegante Welt*) also published articles about spas. Finally, at least one engraving with a view of the spa became *de rigeur* in spa guides and anthologies toward the end of the eighteenth century.

Spas also featured in fictional works like novels, novellas, short stories, fictional travelogues, poems, didactic poems, and comedies. These works were intended not only to provide light entertainment but at the same time to educate and foster a social identity among the middle class.[122] They did not exhibit the sophisticated language and complex plots of the "highbrow" literature of the Enlightenment, Storm and Stress (*Sturm und Drang*), and Romantic eras,[123] but they were also not as short and easy to read as "popular," or "lowbrow," literature. For lack of a better term, they can be characterized as "middlebrow" literature. In addition, these works often included descriptions of spas, thus blurring the lines between fictional texts and functional writings (*Gebrauchsliteratur*) like spa guides.

The highbrow and lowbrow works of the late eighteenth and early nineteenth centuries are well-researched in both literary studies and historiography,[124] but there are very few studies on the types of middlebrow works – both fictional and functional – that I analyze here. Manuel Frey, in his research on the bourgeois light novel (*Trivialroman*) between 1780 and 1815, pointed out the stark contrast between this dearth of research and the significance such works had for contemporaries.[125] Frey has shown that the light novels of the late eighteenth and early nineteenth centuries were not "disposable literature, but [figured as] expensive status symbols for a numerically small social elite."[126] "The bourgeois light novel was a preferred means of communication for the social elites of this period," in which "the expectations of the readership are revealed to us unobscured by political or aesthetic obligations, because market-oriented authors had to . . . seamlessly link ideas about the reorganization of the social world to the everyday lives of their readership."[127] Since light fiction "is bound by social norms . . . the ideas represented there . . . must be the expression of the binding cultural values of the times."[128] Frey's conclusions about the role of the light novel in late eighteenth- and early nineteenth-century society can be applied to the spa publications of the same period.

Even though they were often commissioned by princes, spa guides and other spa publications were undoubtedly written for a market; in other words, they responded to a demand. As spa experiences were common among the eighteenth-century reading public, spa publications had to contain plausible content in order to be viable. Fictional works had to reflect contemporaries' experiences, including social norms and values, to be convincing, and spa guides had to strike a careful balance between claims that were made for advertising purposes and the presentation of a realistic picture of the spa. An advertising pamphlet for Rehburg argued, "Anyone who wants to visit a spa will gladly look around for a publication in which he [*sic*] can find details about the spa. Or someone who visited it [will be looking for a publication] that can give him a complete recollection of everything he found interesting there."[129] In fact, the establishment of a published spa discourse in which, as I will show subsequently, certain statements were repeated over and over speaks to the fact that these statements were plausible. It is highly unlikely that implausible statements in the published discourse would have been repeated *en masse*.

Goethe's personal library and books he borrowed from the princely library in Weimar show how widespread spa guides and other spa publications were among the educated elite in Germany in the long eighteenth century. Goethe's library contained many of the works analyzed in this study, especially a large number of travelogues.[130] In addition, given the expansion of literacy in the German lands around 1800, spa publications probably also reached a wider, more heterogeneous audience beyond the upper middle class and the nobility.[131] As we have seen previously, a broader swath of the middle class traveled to spas, and servants accompanied their employers. It is therefore plausible to assume that someone who had spent three weeks in Rehburg would have purchased a spa guide about Karlsbad for the purpose of comparison, even if Karlsbad was out of his or her reach. Notwithstanding the fact that most of the readers of the spa publications were former, current, or future spa guests, these works were probably read out of curiosity as well, in order to get a glimpse of a heterotopia that was fascinating but unreachable.

As a result, the published discourse affected its readership in manifold ways. Consulted in preparation for a spa visit, spa guides – from short advertising pamphlets to more detailed works – served to influence guests' perception of the spa. Spa guides, fictional works about spas, and reports on the past season in the *Journal of Luxury and Fashions* (*Journal des Luxus und der Moden*) could all reaffirm (but also potentially realign) the perceptions of actual spa guests as well as satisfy the curiosity of those readers who were not spa visitors. In addition, fictional and functional spa publications instigated curiosity for previously little-known spas. In the long run, a mental concept of the spa as a heterotopia emerged among the readers of these publications and was stabilized by constant repetition.[132] The published spa discourse thus acted as a multiplier for essential elements of cultural and social modernity, especially the new landscape perception and the goal of a more egalitarian social order.

During the late eighteenth and early nineteenth centuries, the process of differentiation that had begun with the *Amusemens* publications and similar works also produced two separate strands of spa guides. The "balneological" strand examined the chemical composition and medical applications of the healing waters.[133] In contrast, the "tourist" strand of spa publications, while not excluding balneological aspects, such as the use of healing waters for bathing and drinking cures, focused on a description of the spa's role as a spatial and social heterotopia.[134] In general, both balneological works and tourist spa guides were available for all spas of regional and supra-regional significance.[135]

The tourist spa guides developed into a standardized form of "all around descriptions." Despite variations in content – for example, spa physicians tended to pay more attention to balneological aspects than lay authors – these spa guides turned into a recognizable genre with largely uniform content. The balneologically oriented sections of tourist spa guides usually elaborated on a selection of the following items: a history of the discovery and development of the healing water and the spa; a chemical analysis of the water, often augmented by explanations of its geological origins and "geognostic" observations about the surrounding area; a description of the healing effects of the spring water (increasingly including contraindications); and instructions for the application of the water for bathing and drinking cures and for dietetics. However, dietetics received far less space in these spa guides than it did during the early modern period,[136] and the concept of dietetics also changed.

The ideas of dietetics retained their legitimacy well into the nineteenth century,[137] but in the eighteenth century a shift toward the "dietetics of the soul" took place.[138] In the balneological treatises of the sixteenth and seventeenth centuries, dietetic recommendations focused on food and drink. The dietetics of the soul, in contrast, emphasized work and rest, sleep and wakefulness, and especially states of mind. Spa visitors were advised to avoid work as much as possible, as well as overexertion or excitement, caused, for instance, by gambling.[139] Stressful emotions and impressions were thought to endanger the success of the cure: "During the spa visit [*Kur*], all efforts of the mind and the body, all worries and burdens of life, all tempestuous passions, all games of hazard [gambling], all bacchanalia, [and] all nocturnal debauchery must be diligently avoided, and, in contrast, one must try to support the healing powers of the healing spring as much as possible through joyful moods of the soul, through innocent, sociable pleasures, through the refreshing enjoyment of the charming nature, through music, through an entertaining book, and through the skillful choice of food and drink."[140] The dietetics of the soul thus became a part of the recreational and entertainment function of the spa as a heterotopia, recommending positive social interactions, cultural consumption (including music and reading), and enjoyment of the landscape.[141]

Accordingly, tourist spa guides offered detailed descriptions of the spaces and activities that contributed to the perception and experience of the spa as a spatial and social heterotopia. They depict the spa's buildings and its gardens and parks; the landscape surrounding the spa and places of interest for outings; the entertainments and services available at the spa, such as theater performances, concerts, balls, communal meals, illuminations, shops ("boutiques"), the bookstore, the lending library, the reading room, equipment for exercise and games, and so forth. Spa guides describe the daily routine and social interactions at the spa. Other sections or chapters in these guides deal with practical information such as lodging houses and their prices, the accessibility of the spa by roads and postal routes, and its distance from important cities. Finally, all of these topics were often rounded off by comparisons with other spas, especially those nearby.[142]

By the end of the eighteenth century, the long process of differentiation in the published discourse came to completion. Many travelogues and articles in the *Journal of Luxury and Fashions* (*Journal des Luxus und der Moden*) ceased to discuss the health aspect of the spa and instead focused exclusively on descriptions of the landscape, entertainments, and social interactions. This transferred seamlessly to the genre of guidebooks, the forerunners of the famous *Baedekers*, which became popular at the beginning of the nineteenth century. The tourist aspect of the spas received primary attention, while their health function was considered secondary. Aloys Schreiber's *Handbook for Travelers Along the River Rhine* (*Handbuch für Reisende am Rhein*) of 1822 provides an example. In the main part of his guidebook, Schreiber introduces the spas as tourist destinations, leaving their description as medical facilities mostly for the appendix.[143]

Kestner's reference to the *Amusemens* works in his spa diary and Lessing's *Ernst and Falk* (*Ernst und Falk*) provided us with a first glimpse of the firm foothold that knowledge about spas and the social and cultural conventions of spa visits had gained in society by the second half of the eighteenth century. At the same time, the *Amusemens* works also illustrate that references between different publications within the spa discourse were common, and that such references and allusions also extended to personal narratives. A close reading of the spa discourse reveals a system of references and referencing between spa publications that, in turn, not only indicates contemporaries' deep interest in information about spas but also shows how closely spas were associated with certain expectations and social customs.

In the following pages, I explore the presence of the spa in the perception of contemporaries through two case studies. First, I examine a series of spa guides and reviews that constituted a reference network about Pyrmont. Second, I explore the broad scope of spa references in both the middlebrow and highbrow literature of the early nineteenth century by analyzing two light novels by Georg Christian Sponagel and Jean Paul's novella *Dr. Katzenberger's Spa Trip* (*Dr. Katzenbergers Badereise*). In these works, the authors make use of their readers' knowledge about spas. Similar to Lessing, they invoke an entire tableau of spa experiences by subtly referencing a variety of conventions associated with spa visits. They also create satire by exploiting the gap between the knowledge of their readers and the apparently incongruous and absurd conduct of their protagonists.

First, Heinrich Matthias Marcard's two-volume spa guide, *Description of Pyrmont* (*Beschreibung von Pyrmont*), published in 1784 and 1785,[144] served both as a positive and a negative reference point in the published discourse far into the nineteenth century. In 1799, the Danish physician Rasmus Frankenau published a rebuttal, attacking Marcard and accusing him of fraud: "Everybody refers to the famous Marcard's testimony about the wonderful virtues of the Pyrmont healing water. I do not deny the merits of Mr. Marcard's book; it shows very well that this man looks deep into the gullible human heart, and the book has undoubtedly put many a shiny thaler into the pocket of the personal physician [Marcard] and the inhabitants of Pyrmont. My pen is not guided by selfishness, nor am I paid by any prince who is in debt."[145] Mirroring the diverse content of a spa guide, Frankenau criticizes almost every aspect of Marcard's description of Pyrmont, from its healing water to its main avenue and theater.

Frankenau's attack fueled a wave of responses. The *General Gazette for Literature* (*Allgemeine Literatur-Zeitung*) published a scathing review, while a review in the *New General German Library* (*Neue allgemeine deutsche Bibliothek*) partially agreed with Frankenau's criticism.[146] In 1800, Gottfried Käppel published another spa guide, *Pyrmont's Noteworthy Features: A Sketch for Travelers and Spa Guests* (*Pyrmonts Merkwürdigkeiten: Eine Skizze für Reisende und Kurgäste*), refuting Frankenau. The subtitle of the work, *With Reference to Frankenau's Book: Pyrmont and Its Healing Spring* (*Mit Hinsicht auf Frankenaus Buch: Pyrmont und sein Gesundbrunnen*), informed readers to keep in mind the ongoing debate about Pyrmont when reading this spa publication. The preface contains short praise for Marcard's work and a long criticism of Frankenau's "libel."[147]

The dispute continued with the 1801 publication of *Remarks on the Work by Doctor Frankenau Concerning Pyrmont* (*Bemerkungen über die Schrift des Herrn Doctor Frankenau Pyrmont betreffend*) by the Marburg apothecary Georg Heinrich Piepenbring.[148] Once again, the title page referenced the ongoing controversy. Authors and reviewers obviously assumed that the reading public was aware of the debate about Pyrmont and took an interest in it. The reviewer of Piepenbring's work in the *New General German Library* (*Neue allgemeine deutsche Bibliothek*) in 1802 was certainly convinced that people were still motivated to follow the debate. After noting that Piepenbring tried to refute Frankenau in order to save Pyrmont's reputation, the reviewer stated, "We cannot say more about this short work, which of course everyone must read for themselves and compare with that of Frankenau."[149]

In 1805, Marcard himself jumped back into the fray with his *Little Book about the Pyrmont Spa* (*Kleines Pyrmonter Brunnenbuch*).[150] Without mentioning Frankenau or others by name, Marcard confidently denounced his critics as unworthy of a response and instead referred to Pyrmont's continuing success with spa visitors. The controversy trailed off after that, not least because Pyrmont did indeed lose favor with spa guests in the ensuing years. The advertising pamphlet of the spa physician Menke, published in 1818, does not mention the debate but only refers back to Marcard's original *magnum opus* of 1784/1785.[151]

As to the second case study, in the early nineteenth century, Georg Christian Sponagel (1763–1830) published two light novels, both first-person narratives: *My Four-Day Sufferings in the Spa of Pyrmont: Reading Matter for the Spa* (*Meine viertägigen Leiden im Bade zu Pyrmont: Eine Brunnen-Lectüre*)[152] and *The Cousin's Military Campaign to the Seaside Resort of Doberan* (*Des Vetters Feldzug in die Seebäder von Doberan*).[153] The protagonists of these novels reveal that they are visiting a summer resort for the first time and have no knowledge of spa customs. Due to their ignorance, they constantly find themselves in embarrassing situations. The protagonist in *My Four-Day Sufferings in the Spa of Pyrmont*, for example, is unfamiliar with the system of allocating privies in Pyrmont by renting out keys, and he consequently picks a fight with his landlord.[154] The protagonist traveling to Doberan takes the spa guide literally. Having read the oft-repeated topos of friends and acquaintances meeting at the spa, he expects to encounter his own friends there. When he cannot find them, he blames the spa physician for making false claims: "'What the spa physician writes is not really the Gospels [the truth],' I murmured to myself after I had already been roaming around quite a bit and could find neither an old friend nor an acquaintance. 'Here old friends, countrymen, relatives, and acquaintances from all areas are supposed to meet, but in spite of all my searching I have found neither old nor young friends.'"[155] Sponagel thus highlights the gap between the knowledge of the readers, who are aware of spa customs, and the ignorance and misunderstandings of his protagonist. The reader feels superior to the protagonist and laughs at his lack of knowledge and resulting clumsiness.

In a narrative sleight of hand, Sponagel seeks to create distance as well as closeness between the reader and the protagonist. Both are described as escaping from the constraints of busy professional lives and – according to the new paradigm of the body and illness[156] – as nervous and hypochondriacal. While the protagonist finds little rest at the spa, readers addressed as "spa guests" may hope to experience "mental exhilaration"[157] by reading about the protagonist's misadventures at the spa:

> So may you not spurn
> The burlesque that strives to amuse,
> Recognize with kindness the spirit,
> Which animates me when writing,
> Which, unconcerned about criticism,
> Does not dwell on stiff rules,
> Playing with unbridled whimsy,
> Wantonly and restlessly rushes forward.
> If [my text] succeeds, in gloomy hours,
> When discontent creeps up on you darkly,
> To win a smile from you,
> Then the purpose of this farce has been attained.[158]

In contrast to the rather coarse jokes and the obvious discrepancies between the experiences of the protagonists and of normal spa guests invoked by Sponagel, the allusions to the spa in highbrow literature are – as we have already seen earlier in *Ernst and Falk* (*Ernst und Falk*) – more subtle. However, they were no less obvious to contemporaries in the late eighteenth and early nineteenth centuries. Jean Paul's novella *Dr. Katzenberger's Spa Trip* (*Dr. Katzenbergers Badereise*) provides a striking example.[159] Jean Paul (1763–1825)[160] gave his fictional spa the name of Maulbronn, a monastery in Württemberg. When the story was written in 1807/1808, Maulbronn was not yet an urban settlement,[161] allowing Paul to create a spa without having to choose an actual spa as the setting of his novella.[162]

Dr. Katzenberger travels to "the spa of Maulbronn" ("Bad Maulbronn") with his daughter Theoda "not to bathe himself – or her – or to enjoy himself there. . . . Instead of a pleasure trip, Katzenberger actually went on a business trip to the spa in order to thoroughly beat up his reviewer, and to attack his honor with insults."[163] As we have learned from the examples of Pütter and others, Katzenberger's visit to the spa for professional purposes was not unusual. But Paul adds an exaggerated and absurd twist to the story by revealing Katzenberger's intention to beat up his scientific competitor. In contrast, Katzenberger's daughter Theoda is depicted as a model spa guest behaving entirely in accordance with spa customs. Not only does she (secretly) arrange to meet the writer Theodobach in Maulbronn,[164] she also promises her friend at home "a daily report of her spa trip."[165] This pattern continues through the entire narrative: on the one hand, the figure of Katzenberger, whose nonconformist behavior, bordering on absurdity, satirizes the spa experience; on the other hand, the figure of Theoda, offering the reader a conventional interpretation of the spa as a meeting place.

Maulbronn is also the setting for a love story between Theoda and Theodobach that at first seems to end tragically but then – predictably – comes to a happy conclusion.[166] Sociological and historical research has shown that the semantics of modern love and the notion of marriage based on romantic love originated in the late eighteenth and early nineteenth centuries.[167] This development is reflected in *Dr. Katzenberger's Spa Trip* (*Dr. Katzenbergers Badereise*) and in the published discourse in general. While earlier spa publications often associated the spa with sexual permissiveness and prostitution,[168] these references became rare by the end of the eighteenth century.[169] Instead, the new romantic notion of marriage based on love developed into a central motif in the spa discourse. Novels such as Adolph Bühren's *Four Weeks in Pyrmont, or: Whoever's Lucky Leads the Bride Home* (*Vier Wochen in Pyrmont, oder: Wer's Glück hat führt die Braut heim*) of 1824[170] and numerous other stories about falling in love and finding the ideal marriage partner were set in spas, thus linking the spa as social heterotopia to romantic love as part of the emerging bourgeois culture. For example, in Johanna Schopenhauer's short story *The Spa Guests* (*Die Brunnengäste*), this new ideal is embodied by two young nobles in financial distress who defend their romantic love and the marriage they secretly contracted against pressure by the groom's uncle, a baron. The pair of poor young nobles is thereby construed as defending bourgeois values.[171] Like the uncle in Schopenhauer's story, Dr. Katzenberger is, at the end, reconciled to his daughter's marriage to Theodobach.

In addition to the contrast between Dr. Katzenberger and his daughter, Jean Paul plays with numerous allusions and references to the spa experience of the late eighteenth and early nineteenth centuries. Paul combines features of several spas to create his setting of Bad Maulbronn, but his readers could easily decipher these references. Maulbronn is reached via "wide, shaded, intersecting chaussées,"[172] similar to many actual spas after the improvement of the road network at the turn of the nineteenth century. Visitors descend "down the last mountain in the independent principality of Großpolei (by now no longer independent) . . . to Bad Maulbronn, which seemed to be a little town of rural houses."[173] In one sentence, Paul captured shared knowledge about the majority of spas in the early nineteenth century: they were located in small and medium-sized territories, many of these principalities had lost their independence with the Imperial Recess (*Reichsdeputationshauptschluss*) of 1803, and the interior space of the spa as a heterotopia was expected to represent town and countryside rolled into one.[174]

Paul emphasizes the presence of the ruling prince at the spa as part of its "tableau." The "princely lord of the spa" brought with him "the prospect of new *scènes à tiroir*,[175] of new spectacles and scene painters for this small stage, especially the prospect of illuminating the cave."[176] In addition to Theoda's love story and Katzenberger's professional business, Paul introduces yet another aspect of the spa's multiple functions to his description of Maulbronn: the spa is presented as a place of (secret) political activities. The prince's spies appear in Maulbronn and "could invisibly eavesdrop [on the spa visitors] from the dark of the leaves all around."[177] Paul also refers to the widespread rivalry between spa physicians in the long eighteenth century by elevating the conflict between Dr. Katzenberger, his reviewer (the spa physician Dr. Strykius), and the prince's personal physician (Dr. Semmelmann) to a prominent position in his plot.[178]

Finally, Paul incorporates into his narrative recognizable features of contemporary spas as well as allusions to the daily routine and typical customs at spas.[179] Upon her arrival in Maulbronn, Theoda first looks in vain for Theodobach's name in the list of spa guests,[180] but she then finds an announcement of his expected arrival in the "newspaper of Großpolei."[181] Paul also refers to the "public table" (*öffentliche Tafel*), namely communal meals, usually breakfasts, that were common in Pyrmont and many other spas and that functioned as a meeting place for the spa society (Figure 2.2).[182] In addition, Paul alludes to specific spas and their customs, relocating them to Maulbronn. He references the famous cave in Liebenstein, where illuminations regularly took place: "She [Theoda] had retained an indelible image of the hour when as a child her mother had carried her around in a large, lamp-lit magic cave of the spa [of Maulbronn], similar to the cave in the spa of Liebenstein" (Figure 2.3).[183] Paul also hints at the customary trumpet fanfares in Karlsbad that signaled the entry of visitors to the spa. The nobleman von Nieß wants to enter Maulbronn "during the day while having the spa serenade played" for him.[184] In sum, Paul

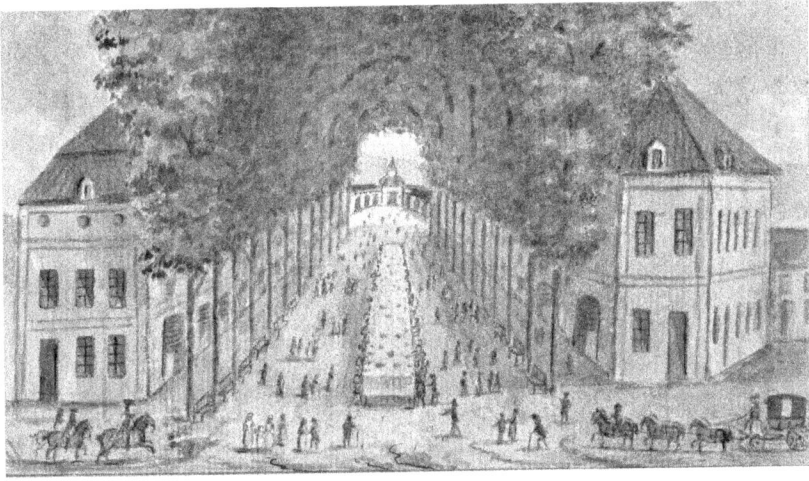

Figure 2.2 Pyrmont, communal breakfast, colored drawing by a French spa guest, 1795. (Museum im Schloss Bad Pyrmont, Inventarnummer: 1985/81.)

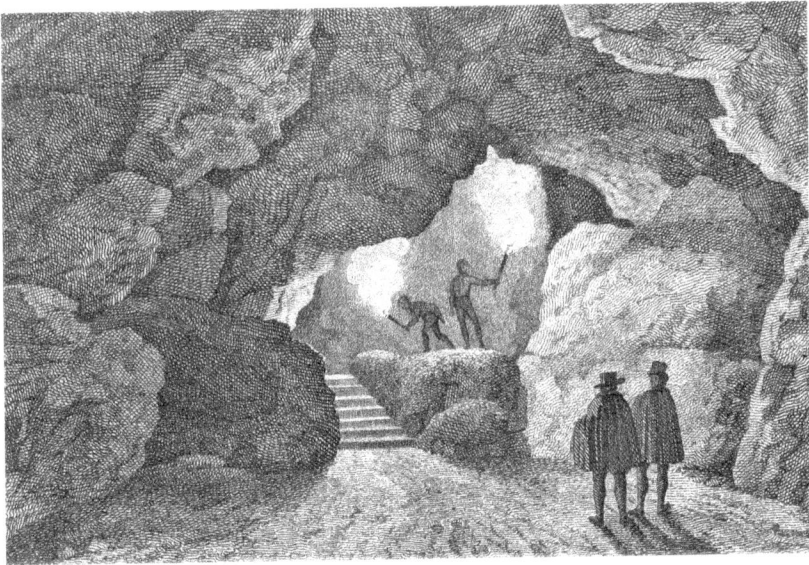

Figure 2.3 Liebenstein, cave, engraving by F. Rosmäsler junior, 1819. ("In der Liebensteiner Höhle." In Mosch, Carl Friedrich. *Die Bäder und Heilbrunnen Deutschlands und der Schweiz: Ein Taschenbuch für Brunnen- und Badereisende*. Vol. 2, unpaginated, in article "Liebenstein." Leipzig: Brockhaus, 1819. Collection of the author.)

characterizes the spas of the late eighteenth and early nineteenth centuries sarcastically, but also aptly, as spaces "of the fashionable morning drinking binge and the freedoms of the masquerades,[185] and the congress of wealth and education."[186]

The pervasiveness of knowledge about spas among the reading public of the early nineteenth century is evident in both middlebrow and highbrow literature. The novels by Sponagel operate through simple patterns, drawing on his readers' broad knowledge of contemporary spas to generate wit and laughter. Jean Paul, in contrast, offers his audience different views of the familiar spa experience via his two protagonists, Theoda and her father Dr. Katzenberger. On the one hand, readers can experience the spa as a social heterotopia by following Theoda's story. On the other, readers can question the social heterotopia constructed in the contemporary spa discourse by turning their attention to how Dr. Katzenberger ignores, or even actively renders absurd, the social and behavioral norms associated with spa visits. These literary treatments of the spa represent the end point of a long development beginning in the late seventeenth century. By the early nineteenth century, spas had been established in people's minds as recognizable spaces of recreation and social interaction with an associated repertoire of practices. As Susanne Müller has stated about the *Baedeker* handbooks, "Only a fully formed format, based on well-known standardizations, can become the subject of a satire."[187] The fact that authors were able to use spa conventions to create satire proves just how ingrained these spa conventions had become.

Notes

1. See Kuhnert, *Urbanität*, 17–18. Zaunstöck identifies this as a characteristic of Enlightenment societies. See Zaunstöck, "Die vernetzte Gesellschaft."
2. Pütter, *Selbstbiographie*, vol. 2, 547: "Was Briefen nicht wohl anvertraut, oder darin nicht ausgemacht werden konnte, verspahrten wir uns auf persönliche Zusammenkunft."
3. Pütter, *Selbstbiographie*, vol. 2, 548: "Im Sommer 1771 schlug er mir vor, ob wir nicht einmal beide zu gleicher Zeit eine Reise nach Pyrmont thun wollten. – Wir wurden bald darüber einig an einem Tage daselbst einzutreffen, und in einem Hause beysammen zu wohnen. Beides geschah. . . . daß wir auch die folgenden Jahre, so lange Strube am Leben blieb, auf gleiche Art fortfuhren."
4. Pütter, *Selbstbiographie*, vol. 2, 549: "Bey ihrem Berufe, sagte er, werden Sie in ihrer Studierstube zuletzt alles nur einseitig und oft schief ansehen, wenn Sie nicht zu Zeiten fortfahren, mit Geschäftsmännern sich zu unterhalten, und einen Blick in die große Welt zu thun. Beide Zwecke werden Sie zu Pyrmont am füglichsten erreichen können."
5. Pütter, *Selbstbiographie*, vol. 2, 549: "Die Erfahrung belehrte mich bald, wie richtig diese Vorstellung meines Freundes war" – "dreywöchentliche fortgesetzte vertrauliche Unterhaltung mit einem solchen Freunde" – "vergesellschaftet mit so vielerley anderem Umgange" – "so zahlreichen Gelegenheiten Erfahrungen und Beobachtungen zur Erweiterung der Menschenkenntnis zu machen."

6. See Pütter, *Selbstbiographie*, vol. 2, 555–556, 564.
7. Pütter, *Selbstbiographie*, vol. 2, 556: "So kömmt das doch in keiner Vergleichung mit der ungezwungenen Art, wie man an einem solchen Orte, wie zu Pyrmont, bald mit diesem, bald mit jenem sich länger oder kürzer unterhalten kann, ohne daß man besorgen darf, den andern von Berufsgeschäften abzuhalten."
8. Möser, *Briefwechsel*, letter from Möser to Nicolai, 23 May 1787, 680: "Wenn ich keine Minute von Ihrer angenehmen Gesellschaft zu Pyrmont verlieren soll, so müssen Sie den 30. Jun. abends um 10 Uhr bey der mittelsten Treppe vor dem Niemeyerschen Hause seyn, und dann fliege ich in Ihre Arme."
9. Möser, *Briefwechsel*, letter from Möser to Nicolai, 23 March 1791, 706: "Was mich anbelangen thut, so denke ich dieses Jahr am 1. Juli in Pyrmont zu seyn, nicht um das Wasser zu gebrauchen, sondern meine guten Freunde zu sehen . . . Ob Sie auch dahin kommen werden, ist heute meine Frage, und mein Wunsch, daß Sie diese mit einem vernehmlichen Ja! beantworten mögen. . . . und was ich Ihnen sonst noch zu sagen hätte, [bitte ich] von mir in Pyrmont anzuhören."
10. Möser, *Briefwechsel*, letter from Möser to Thomas Abbt, 18 June 1766, 406: "daß ich mich eben wieder von einer verdrieslichen Unpäßlichkeit, die ich mich durch eine Erkältung zugezogen hatte, zu erholen anfange. Ich habe meine Reise nach Aachen darüber eingestellet, . . . Indessen sind meine Frau und Schwester gestern abgereiset; und ich bin nun ein verlaßner Strohwittwer. Gegen d. 1. Juli denke ich aber doch nach Pirmont zu reisen." Note that Möser does not propose to travel to Aachen (or Pyrmont) to seek a cure for his "indisposition."
11. Voigts, *Im Geist der Empfindsamkeit*, letter from Voigts to Recke, 8 May 1790, 238: "Wie beneide ich alle, die Sie zu Carlsbad sehen, die bey Ihnen sein können."
12. Schopenhauer, *Tagebücher der Adele Schopenhauer*, vol. 1, 21: "Von Pyrmont keine Nachricht."
13. Pütter, *Selbstbiographie*, vol. 2, 565: "endlich [gab es] zu Zeiten angenehme Gelegenheit in den benachbarten Orten von Pyrmont schätzbare Bekanntschaften zu machen und zu erneuern." See 565–566.
14. See Erker, Siebers, "Justus Möser"; Erker, "'Brunnenfreiheit'," 81–83; Kuhnert, *Urbanität*, 171–177.
15. See Erker, Siebers, "Justus Möser"; Erker, "'Brunnenfreiheit'," 82, esp. footnote 122, which explains in detail the kinship and friendship relations within this circle; Kuhnert, *Urbanität*, 171–177.
16. See Duchhardt, *Stein*, 352–353.
17. In 1771 Lessing, privy councillor and librarian in Wolfenbüttel, was admitted to the Masonic lodge "Zu den drei Rosen" ("At the Three Roses") in Hamburg. Although Lessing was clearly unimpressed with Freemasonry and never entered a lodge again in his life, he was still very interested in Freemasonry, even after his disappointing experience. See Voges, *Aufklärung*, 148–149; Kelsch, "Freimaurer Lessing." As a result, Lessing wrote *Ernst und Falk: Gespräche für Freimaurer*. Lessing completed the text in 1777 and initially circulated it among his friends. See Lessing, *Ernst und Falk*, 93. He also sent the manuscript to Duke Ferdinand of Brunswick-Lüneburg-Wolfenbüttel, the Grand Master of the Masonic Order of Strict Observance and brother of the ruling prince Duke Karl I. See Kelsch, "Freimaurer Lessing," 111. The first three *Gespräche* were printed in 1778, while the last two were published in 1780. See Lessing, *Ernst und Falk*, 93–94. Lessing's texts subsequently became part of a media frenzy in the run-up to the

Masonic Congress of Wilhelmsbad in 1782, discussed later in this chapter. See Hammermayer, *Wilhelmsbader Freimaurer-Konvent*, 26–28.

18. See Voges, *Aufklärung*, 164; Appel, *Lessing als Freimaurer*, 19; Kelsch, "Freimaurer Lessing," 112. See also Kuhnert, *Urbanität*, 25, who does not apply his knowledge of everyday life in Pyrmont to this question and therefore does not recognize Pyrmont as the setting of *Ernst and Falk*. In 2015, Köhler followed my argument in "Pyrmont," 55–56.

19. Marcard, *Beschreibung von Pyrmont*, vol. 1, 1784, 55–58: "Schon vor sechs Uhr fängt die feine Welt an in der Allee zu erscheinen, und emsig zum Brunnen zu eilen. . . . So viele Menschen, die ohne allen Zwang durcheinander hingehn . . . ; alle im nachlässigen Morgenanzug, . . . ohne weitere Ceremonie, als daß sie sich im Vorbeygehn den guten Morgen wünschen; . . . An dieser angenehmen Scene nimmt ein jeder Theil, während er seinen Brunnen trinkt, auf welche Weise es ihm am besten gefällt; er spricht mit wem er will, und nicht länger als er Lust hat, . . . Um neun Uhr sieht man . . . oben in der Allee kleine Gesellschaften, die sich zusammen setzen, das Frühstück mit einander zu verzehren." See also Baggesen, *Labyrinth*, 163; Lavater, *Reisetagebücher*, 289.

20. See Lessing, *Ernst und Falk*, 10–28. In Lessing's story, the butterfly lured Falk "up to the brook" ("bis an den Bach"). A brook did indeed flow near the main avenue of Pyrmont, but not in its immediate vicinity, explaining why Ernst and Falk get lost. See Lessing, *Ernst und Falk*, 17. Marcard writes about the possibility of leaving the main avenue in the morning while drinking well water: "And [the spa visitor] sometimes leaves the colorful crowd in the large avenue to take a long walk through beautiful side gardens and have a different view." ("Und [der Kurgast] verläßt zuweilen auch die bunte Menge in der großen Allee, um einen längern Spaziergang durch schöne Seitenanlagen zu machen und die Gegenstände abzuwechseln.") Marcard, *Beschreibung von Pyrmont*, vol. 1, 1784, 58.

21. Lessing, *Ernst und Falk*, 29: "im Rausche des Pyrmonter."

22. Lessing, *Ernst und Falk*, 29: "Dort winkt man uns eben zum Frühstück. Komm! . . . Dort in der größern Gesellschaft werden wir bald Stoff zu einer tauglichern Unterredung finden."

23. Lessing, *Ernst und Falk*, 29: "im Gedränge der Gesellschaft."

24. See Lessing, *Ernst und Falk*, 29. Baggesen similarly describes the real-life experience of meeting his friend Adam von Moltke, whom he had believed to be dead, on the main avenue of Pyrmont: "Deep . . . in hazy thoughts, I strolled down the large avenue yesterday morning, without looking particularly to the right or left, when a long, pale, hollow-eyed figure came so close to me that it caught my attention . . . 'Baggesen! You!' – 'Moltke! You?' . . . Now he was standing, or more correctly: hanging in my arms – if not exactly healthy, then alive, and because of this encounter I forgot the avenue, all its water drinkers and the whole of Pyrmont. . . . Intoxicated we staggered arm in arm to his rooms in the bathhouse, where we rested for a few silent minutes recovering from our daze and then began to share our stories more calmly." ("In . . . nebelhaften Betrachtungen vertieft, schlenderte ich gestern morgen die große Allee hinunter, ohne sonderlich nach rechts und links zu sehen, als mir eine lange, totenbleiche, hohläugige Gestalt so nahe kam, daß sie meine Aufmerksamkeit erregte. . . . 'Baggesen! Du!' – 'Moltke! Du?' . . . Jetzt stand er, oder richtiger: hing er in meinen Armen – wenn nicht eben gesund, so doch lebendig, und ich vergaß über dieser Begegnung die Allee, alle ihre Wassertrinker und das ganze Pyrmont. . . . In diesem Rausch taumelten wir Arm in Arm zu seiner Wohnung im Badehaus, wo wir uns einige

stumme Minuten von unserer Betäubung ausruhten und dann ruhiger unsere Geschichten mitzuteilen begannen.") Baggesen, *Labyrinth*, 154–155.

25. Marcard, *Beschreibung von Pyrmont*, vol. 1, 1784, 64–65: "Visiten in den Wohnungen zu geben, ist in Pyrmont gar nicht gebräuchlich, nur besonders vertraute Bekannte besuchen sich einander auf ihren Zimmern." See also Lavater, *Reisetagebücher*, 287.

26. Lessing, *Ernst und Falk*, 35: "der Stadt." The last two *Gespräche für Freimaurer* are set in Falk's house in the countryside.

27. Kuhnert, *Urbanität*, 28: "man sich den Gefahren einer schriftlichen Fixierung . . . aussetzte." For further examples of letters that alluded to the possibility of speaking more openly during a personal meeting in Pyrmont, see Erker, "Friedrich Nicolai," 66.

28. This is confirmed by a letter from Möser to Abbt (see Kuhnert, *Urbanität*, 183) and by a diary entry by Georg Christoph Lichtenberg in 1772, to whom Möser had reported his conversations with Lessing (see Daunicht, *Lessing im Gespräch*, 207; see also Erker, *Justus Möser*, 9–10).

29. See Willebrand, *Carlsbader Brunnenreise*, 1780, 56–61.

30. See Erker, "'Brunnenfreiheit'," 86; Erker, *Justus Möser*, 10.

31. [Möser], *Schreiben des Verfassers*, 1746, 26: "Man findet hier wie im Paradiese allerley Nationen und Religionen, vom Richter zu Lüda an, bis zum Prinzen vom Libanon."

32. See Lennhoff, Posner, Binder, *Internationales Freimaurerlexikon*, article "Schottischer Ritus," 754.

33. See Trommsdorff, *Freimaurerei in Pyrmont*, 13.

34. See Zetzsche, *200 Jahre Freimaurerei*, 7.

35. See Trommsdorff, *Freimaurerei in Pyrmont*, 41–43; Erker, "Friedrich Nicolai," 58.

36. Trommsdorff, *Freimaurerei in Pyrmont*, 17: "ordentlichen Physikus bei dem Gesundbrunnen zu Pyrmont." See Zetzsche, *200 Jahre Freimaurerei*, 4.

37. See details about these social connections in Trommsdorff, *Freimaurerei in Pyrmont*.

38. For the years 1776–1780, the lodge recorded 56 members and 70 visiting Masons. See Trommsdorff, *Freimaurerei in Pyrmont*, 79–89.

39. Möller, *Fürstenstaat*, 480: "sozialen Exterritorialität."

40. Schneider, "Institution," 1670: "institutionalisierten Intimität."

41. Foucault, "Of Other Spaces," 26.

42. Becker, *Vor hundert Jahren*, 172: "Freimaurer-Klub."

43. Becker, *Vor hundert Jahren*, 172: "Ich halte mich nicht auf Beschreibung der Zeremonien ein, welche bei solchen Banketten gemacht werden, weil sie jeder kennt, der ihnen beigewohnt hat. Die Frauenzimmer hatten sich alle blau und weiß gekleidet, welche Aufmerksamkeit den Herren ganz wohlgefiel."

44. See Paulmann, *Pomp und Politik*, who discusses this phenomenon for the nineteenth century.

45. Kuhnert, *Urbanität*, 237: "Politik gleichsam im Vorfeld offizieller Kabinettsaktivitäten." See Luise, Königin von Preußen, *Briefe und Aufzeichnungen*, 277, 279.

46. See in detail Engel, "Pyrmonter Fürstensommer."

47. See Kuhnert, *Urbanität*, 235–237.

48. Leopold III Friedrich Franz, prince, then duke (from 1807) of Anhalt-Dessau (1740–1817), the founder of the Park of Wörlitz.

49. See Lotz-Heumann, "Daheim und auf Reisen," 114; on the League of Princes, see Umbach, "Politics of Sentimentality."

50. Schweinitz, *Fürst und Föderalist*, 63: "waren immer allein zusammen."
51. See Kuhnert, *Urbanität*, 237–239. Informers were also present in Pyrmont. See Kuhnert, *Urbanität*, 235–237.
52. "Badechronik," *JLM* (November 1800), 590: "Negociateurs" – "vermeintlichen Congreß." On the political situation in the summer of 1800, when Austrian diplomacy was virtually leaderless and "the whole world racked its brains over the reason for Austria's inactivity and suspected secret French-Austrian agreements" ("alle Welt sich über den Grund der österreichischen Untätigkeit den Kopf zerbrach und geheime französisch-österreichische Abmachungen argwöhnte"), see Aretin, *Das Alte Reich*, 473. Obviously, there were not only rumors about negotiations between Austria and France, but also about secret diplomacy between Austria and Russia, at that point still officially allied.
53. [Möser], *Schreiben des Verfassers*, 1746, 30: "Alle Gelehrten, die Lebensläufe schreiben wollen, will ich bitten hieher zu kommen, weil einem nirgend mehr heimliche Nachrichten ins Ohr gesaget werden als hier; und ich biete dem freygebigsten Verleger hiedurch zwölf Theile von Memoires Anecdotes an." (Italics by ULH.) See also the account of conversations one could allegedly listen to while strolling on the avenue in Pyrmont in "Pyrmonter Gemälde," 1800, 459–461.
54. Kuhnert, *Urbanität*, 28: "Die Vertraulichkeit des Gesprächs, die der Rahmen des Kurbades gewährte, darf . . . nicht über den ambivalenten Charakter eines Ortes hinwegtäuschen, der gleichzeitig als Forum gesteigerter Öffentlichkeit fungierte."
55. See Hammermayer, *Wilhelmsbader Freimauerer-Konvent*; Taute, *Wilhelmsbader Konvent*; Mensing, *Freimaurer-Konvent*; Mensing, "Illuminatismus"; Hessen, "Wilhelmsbader Freimaurerkonvent"; Hoede, "Wilhelmsbader Konvent"; Schüttler, "Wilhelmsbader Freimaurerkonvent." Count Wilhelm reports in his memoirs that Prince Karl had already met with other Freemasons in Wilhelmsbad in 1779. See Wilhelm I. von Hessen, *Wir Wilhelm*, 159.
56. Lessing's *Ernst und Falk* and the affair surrounding the Bahrdt pasquinade, which will be discussed later, also belong in this context.
57. The relative remoteness of Wilhelmsbad obviously led the organizers to believe that they would not only be able to separate the Congress from other spa visitors in Wilhelmsbad, but also from other Masons, especially from the Frankfurt Union Lodge, "the only German provincial lodge that had remained true to purely symbolic . . . Masonry" ("der einzigen deutschen Provinzialloge, die der reinen symbolischen . . . Maurerei treu geblieben war"). Hammermayer, *Wilhelmsbader Freimauerer-Konvent*, 42. See also Hoede, "Wilhelmsbader Konvent," 47.
58. Ditfurth, "Bericht," 35: "jeder Deputierte [sich] auf sein Ehrenwort reversiren sollte, seinen Committenten vor Beendigung des Convents Nichts von Dem, was darauf vorgeht, zu sagen."
59. See Wilhelm I. von Hessen, *Wir Wilhelm*, 183.
60. Ditfurth, "Bericht," 45: "über den Convent sehr aufgebracht [war], so daß er es gegen Profane nicht verbergen konnte."
61. See Hammermayer, *Wilhelmsbader Freimauerer-Konvent*, 71–72.
62. Ditfurth, "Bericht," 43: "Dann sagte ich Anderen: Ihr Leute, ich weiß mit Euch Nichts zu sprechen, ich weiß nicht, ob Ihr Alle Profane seid; aber es ist wenigstens eine ziemliche Menge Profaner im Convent, und wie kann man in Gegenwart solcher Leute deliberiren? Lasset uns lieber unter den Brunnen=Knechten, den Kutschers und dem Troß deliberiren!"
63. See Wilhelm I. von Hessen, *Wir Wilhelm*, 186, 188.

64. See Hammermayer, *Wilhelmsbader Freimauerer-Konvent*, 74–83.

65. See Trommsdorff, *Freimaurerei in Pyrmont*, 55.

66. See Hammermayer, *Wilhelmsbader Freimauerer-Konvent*, 74–83.

67. See Mühlphordt, "Europapolitik."

68. See Möller, "Bruderschaft der Gold- und Rosenkreuzer."

69. Gaber, "Nachwort," 543: "Gegeneinander von Spätaufklärung und Früh-konservativismus" – "Entstehung der politischen Strömungen in Deutsch-land." See Hardtwig, *Genossenschaft*, 330–359.

70. See Erker, Siebers, "'. . . von Pyrmont ab mit häßlichen Materialien beladen'"; Erker, "'Brunnenfreiheit',", 92–95; Kuhnert, *Urbanität*, 255–258; Rieck, "'Doctor Bahrdt mit der eisernen Stirn . . .'." My summary of the fallout from the publication of the Bahrdt pasquinade follows these works.

71. See in detail Mehrdorf, Stemler, *Chronik*, 272–277; Kuhnert, *Urbanität*, 63.

72. Quoted in Kuhnert, *Urbanität*, 257: "von allen Badegästen verschlungen, von Manchem mit Wohlgefallen belächelt."

73. See [Kotzebue], *Doctor Bahrdt.*

74. Bahrdt and Knigge were members of the German Union. See Erker, "'Brun-nenfreiheit'," 94.

75. See Strahlmann, "Heinrich Matthias Marcard"; Mehrdorf, Stemler, *Chronik*, 277–281; Kuhnert, *Urbanität*, 63.

76. Quoted in Kuhnert, *Urbanität*, 257: "verschiedene Nachrichten, Bemerkun-gen und ganz bekannte Anekdoten" – "Bekanntheit" – "im Vertrauen und auf Diskrezion."

77. On the definition of "spa freedom," see Chapter 5.

78. *Das Pyrmonter Brunnenarchiv*, 1782, 42: "Nicht leicht giebt es einen Ort in der Welt, wo sich mehr Stof zu Bemerkungen über die galante Welt darbietet, und über die mancherley Eitelkeiten der Menschenkinder, als vor dem Cof-feehause in der Pyrmonter grossen Brunnen-Allee. . . . Man denke sich eine gemischte Gesellschaft von Leuten aus den entfernten Provinzen, oft selbst aus mehrern Nationen; unter diesen manche von gutem Kopf, gründlicher Kenntniß und vieler Erfahrung, von denen jeder, vermöge der hergebrachten Brunnen-Freyheit, sich ohne Zurückhaltung mittheilt."

79. See *Das Pyrmonter Brunnenarchiv*, 1782, 42–46; *Allgemeine Deutsche Biographie*, vol. 34, article "Senckenberg, Renatus," 5–6; Aretin, *Das Alte Reich*, 186, 571–572, footnote 26; Aretin, contrary to the *Allgemeine Deutsche Biographie*, refers to Senckenberg as a "former Austrian archivist" ("früheren österreichischen Archivar"). This also contradicts the coffeehouse conversation in Pyrmont, which emphasizes that Senckenberg had "no spe-cial duties" ("keine besondre Pflichten") in relation to the Habsburg court and refers to him as councillor ("Regierungs-Rath"), a position Senckenberg held in the Hessian government in Gießen. *Das Pyrmonter Brunnenarchiv*, 1782, 44, 43. See also *Allgemeine Deutsche Biographie*, vol. 34, article "Senckenberg, Renatus," 5.

80. The dominant protagonist is of the opinion that Senckenberg acted correctly and honorably. Taking a decidedly anti-Habsburg stance, he describes Sen-ckenberg as a "benefactor of the human race, for whom the German empire should erect a monument" ("Wolthäter des menschlichen Geschlechts, dem das deutsche Reich Ehren-Säulen setzen sollte") because he prevented a full-blown war over the Bavarian succession and thus saved many lives. *Das Pyrmonter Brunnenarchiv*, 1782, 46.

81. See Zaunstöck, *Sozietätslandschaft*; Kuhnert, *Urbanität*, 80–81.

82. See Kuhnert, *Urbanität*, 16, 19.

83. See Hölscher, "Die Öffentlichkeit begegnet sich selbst."

84. Beermann, *Einige Historische Nachrichten*, 1706, 52: "Die Gelehrten sehen daselbst auf beyden Seiten den Buch-Laden/ und kan ein helluo librorum, oder wer sonsten an der Bücher-Krankheit danieder lieget/ in demselben seine Lust büssen."

85. Koromandel-Wedekind, *Der Brunnengast*, 1744, 15: "Wer ein Gelehrter ist, | An Büchern sich vergnügt und gern Journale liest, | Der findet Gelegenheit bey den Pyrmonter Linden, | Gar manchen klugen Kopf und guten Freund zu finden."

86. Pütter, *Selbstbiographie*, vol. 2, 552: "von der . . . Helwingischen Buchhandlung [aus Lemgo] mit einem zahlreichen Vorrathe von Büchern versehen . . . , und [lässt] selten eine Nachfrage unbeantwortet, oder doch in kurzem leicht Rath schaffen kann."

87. Deneken, "Bemerkungen bey dem Rehburger Gesundbrunnen," 1796, 205: "welcher zu Bällen – zum Lesen der Zeitungen und Monathsschriften und zu anderen gesellschaftlichen Unterhaltungen bestimmt seyn soll."

88. See Steudel, "Geschichte," 3–4; Palmer, "'In This Our Lightye and Learned Tyme'"; Park, "Natural Particulars."

89. See Probst, *Balneologie*, 14, 17; Fürbeth, "Bibliographie," 221–223, 232–236, 240–241; Steudel, "Geschichte," 6.

90. Fürbeth, "Bedeutung des Bäderwesens," 467: "Bädermonographien."

91. Fürbeth, "Bibliographie," 219: "Anleitung zur Selbstmedikation." See Fürbeth, "Bedeutung des Bäderwesens," 464–468; Lotz-Heumann, "Repräsentationen," 285–290; Martin, *Deutsches Badewesen*, 268, 272; Probst, *Balneologie*; Studt, "Badenfahrt," 33–34; Steudel, "Geschichte," 5–7.

92. See Gadebusch-Bondio, "Dietetics."

93. Planer, Planer, *Ausführlicher Bericht von dem Deinacher Sauer-Brunnen*, 1740, 47–61: "Von der Diaet in der Sauer-Brunnen-Cur."

94. Maskosky, *Im Namen JEsu! Das Göppingische Bethesda!*, 1688, ch. XIV: "Was in der Sauerbrunnen-Cur für eine Lebens-Ordnung zu führen."

95. Kestner, *Die wahre Brunnenfreiheit*, 9: "Ich soll Ihnen ein Journal liefern, ja ich soll *amusemens des eaux de Rehburg* schreiben. Eine harte Fodrung, da ich nicht der Baron von Pöllnitz bin und Rehburg kein Spa; noch mehr es sollen *amusemens* sein. Noch zur Zeit möchte ich nur *rêveries* zuschneiden."

96. Many spa publications used the genre of the epistolary novel as a model.

97. In his travelogue of 1754, Grundig also refers to the *Amusemens* genre in passing, thus implying that contemporaries were familiar with these publications. See [Grundig], *Beschreibung seiner, im Jahr 1751 in das Käyser Carls-Bad gethanen Reise*, 1754, 53.

98. See [Pöllnitz], *Amusemens des eaux de Spa*, 1734; [Pöllnitz], *Vermakelyke tydkortingen bij het gebruik der wateren te Spa*, 1735; [Pöllnitz], *Amusemens des eaux de Spa, oder Vergnügungen und Ergötzlichkeiten bey denen Wassern zu Spaa*, 1735; [Pöllnitz], *Amusemens des eaux de Spa: or the Gallantries of the Spaw*, 1737.

99. Several other *Amusemens* publications, both in French and English, and by different authors (among others J.P. de Limbourg) appeared over the course of the mid-to-late eighteenth century. These are not considered here because they did not deal with *teutsche* spas.

100. See [Pöllnitz], *Amusemens des eaux d'Aix la Chapelle, oder Zeit-Vertreib bey den Wassern zu Achen*, 1737.

101. See [Merveilleux], *Amusemens des eaux de Schwalbach, oder Zeitvertreibe bey den Wassern zu Schwalbach, denen Bädern zu Wisbaden, und dem Schlangenbade*, 1739 (French in 1738).

102. See [Merveilleux], *Angenehmer Zeitvertreib in den Bädern zu Baaden, in der Schweitz, zu Schintznach und Pfeffers*, 1739; Jasander, *Amusemens des eaux de Bade en Autriche*, 1747.

103. See [Schütte], *Amusemens des eaux de Cleve*, 1748. Schütte distinguishes his work clearly from other *Amusemens* publications: "Admittedly, I could have filled this work about Kleve with fictional and almost Romanesque descriptions of life, as other authors of *Amusemens* did; however, since authors are in the habit of using such descriptions when they do not have much that is realistic to write about a place, since such descriptions are to be found abundantly in novels, and since the work would be very extensive and annoying to read as a result, I have intentionally left them behind." ("Zwar hätte ich mit erdichteten und fast Romanischen Lebens-Beschreibungen, wie andere Verfasser der Amusemens gethan, auch diese Clevische anfüllen können; alleine da man sich dergleichen zu bedienen pfleget, wenn man nicht viel zu reelles von einem Orte zu schreiben hat, selbige in den Romanen überflüssig zu finden sind, auch das Werk dadurch sehr weitläufig und zu lesen verdrießlich seyn würde, so habe ich selbige mit Vorbehalt zurück gelassen.") Vorrede, 3v-4r. Schütte does indeed place greater emphasis on the description of the spa and its surrounding area, which, however, was also contained in other *Amusemens* works.
104. See Chapter 1.
105. See [Jormann], *Das Schwalbacher Sommer-wehrende Perpetuum Mobile*, 1690, 1701; *Aufgefangene Grillen bey der Brunnen-Cur zu Langen-Schwalbach*, 1737. "Aufgefangene Grillen" is a play on words. "Grillen" means both "crickets" and "antics" in early modern German, and "aufgefangen" means "caught," so the literal translation of the title is *Antics Caught at the Well-Cure in Langen-Schwalbach*.
106. Beermann, *Einige Historische Nachrichten*, 1706, title page: "Denen Brunnen-Gästen zu einiger Nachricht und Zeit-Verkürtzung."
107. See [Wasserbach], *Perpetuum mobile Pyrmontanum aestivum*, 1719.
108. See Koromandel-Wedekind, *Der Brunnengast*, 1744.
109. See [Möser], *Schreiben des Verfassers*, 1746.
110. See Donop, *Die Schönheiten Pyrmonts*, 1750.
111. See *Das alte teutsche ehrliche und liebliche Pyrmont*, 1752.
112. See *Neu-verbessert- und vermehrtes denckwürdiges Kayser Carls-Baad*, 1736, title page: "Allen Neubegierigen und respectivé hohen Baad-Gästen zu Belieben, und Zeit-Vertreib."
113. See [Lamprecht], *Moralische und Satyrische Nachrichten aus dem Carlsbade*, 1736.
114. See *Unschuldiger Zeitvertreib im Carlsbad*, 1751.
115. See [Grundig], *Beschreibung seiner, im Jahr 1751 in das Käyser Carls-Bad gethanen Reise*, 1754.
116. See Tralles, *Das Kaiser-Carls-Bad in Böhmen in einer Ode entworfen*, 1756.
117. See Tilling, *Nachricht vom Carlsbade*, 1756.
118. Frankenau, *Pyrmont*, 1799, 9–10: "'Wieder ein Scherflein von geringem Werth zu der grossen Summe von Reisebeschreibungen, welche in unserem schreibseligen Zeitalter so manchen Buchladen füllt' – höre ich einen oder den anderen Kritikaster murmeln – 'und dies Scherflein ist um desto unerwarteter, da der weit und breit berühmte Marcard bereits vor langer Zeit uns das berüchtigte Pyrmont als ein irdisches Paradies, als ein non plus ultra, geschildert hat.' – Ganz wahr gesprochen! Ich will daher dieses Mannes gar zu bezaubernde Beschreibung durchaus nicht wiederholen, sondern von diesem Bade eine Skizze entwerfen, wie es wirklich ist." (Italics by ULH.) See also Montag, *Das Schandauer Gesundheitsbad*, 1799.
119. See in general Müller, *Aufklärung*, 31–32.
120. See, e.g., Mosch, *Bäder und Heilbrunnen*, 1819; Reichard, *Passagier auf der Reise*, 1801.

121. See, e.g., Boclo, *Beschreibung einer Schülerwanderung im Jahre 1813*; Campe, *Reise von Braunschweig nach Karlsbad*, 1806.
122. See Chapter 6.
123. The didactic poem by Valerius Wilhelm Neubeck, *Gesundbrunnen*, 1798, is an exception to this rule, as is the novella *Dr. Katzenbergers Badereise* (first published 1809) by Jean Paul discussed later in this chapter.
124. See, e.g., Hohendahl, Lützeler, *Legitimationskrisen*.
125. See Frey, "'Offene Gesellschaft'."
126. Frey, "'Offene Gesellschaft'," 504: "Wegwerfliteratur, sondern um teure Statussymbole für eine zahlenmäßig kleine gesellschaftliche Elite handelte."
127. Frey, "'Offene Gesellschaft'," 505: "der bürgerliche Trivialroman ein bevorzugtes Kommunikationsmittel der gesellschaftlichen Eliten dieses Zeitraums gewesen ist" – "die Erwartungen der Leserschaft ungetrübt durch politische oder ästhetische Verbindlichkeiten zutage [treten], denn die Ansichten über die Neuordnung der sozialen Welt müssen . . . von den marktorientierten Autoren bruchlos an das Alltagsbewusstsein der Leserschaft angeschlossen werden."
128. Frey, "'Offene Gesellschaft'," 505: "den gültigen Normen verhaftet bleibt, . . . muß es sich bei den dort vertretenen Vorstellungen . . . um den Ausdruck des verbindlichen kulturellen Werthorizontes der Zeit handeln."
129. Du Mênil, *Rehburger Brunnen*, 1829, III: "Wer einen Badeort besuchen will, sieht sich gerne nach einer Schrift um, worin er Belehrung über das Nähere desselben findet; oder wer ihn besuchte, die ihm eine vollständige Rückerinnerung an alles, was er daselbst Interessantes fand, gewähren kann." See also Küttner, *Reise durch Deutschland*, 1801, part 1, 2–3.
130. See Ruppert, *Goethes Bibliothek*; online catalogues of the Herzogin Anna Amalia Bibliothek Weimar ("Sammlung Ausleihen Johann Wolfgang von Goethe") and of the Klassik Stiftung Weimar ("Sammlung Privatbibliothek Johann Wolfgang von Goethe"). Spa publications can be found in various categories, "balneology" ("Balneologie"), "geography" ("Geographie"), and "local and regional history" ("Lokal- und Regionalgeschichte"), thus reflecting modern distinctions rather than reading practices in the late eighteenth and early nineteenth centuries. Goethe also unsystematically collected lists of spa guest, especially from the Bohemian spas.
131. See Müller, *Aufklärung*, 32–33; Kiesel, Münch, *Gesellschaft*, 154–179.
132. See Fauser, *Einführung in die Kulturwissenschaft*, 52.
133. As explained in the Introduction, this purely balneological strand of spa publications is not a part of this study.
134. A typical example is Reichard, *Passagier auf der Reise*, 1801. This guidebook for "Germany and neighboring regions" ("Deutschland und einigen angränzenden Ländern") has a long section (351–393) on spas, covering Karlsbad, Franzensbad, Teplitz, Pyrmont, Doberan, Liebenstein, Lauchstädt, Alexandersbad, and Nenndorf.
135. For example, Springsfeld, *Abhandlung vom Carlsbade*, 1749, is an extensive balneological work about Karlsbad.
136. See, e.g., [Käppel], *Pyrmonts Merkwürdigkeiten*, 1800, 75–76. In this spa guide, a mere two pages at the end are dedicated to the "Rules for Spa Guests" ("Regeln für Brunnengäste").
137. See Stolberg, *Homo patiens*, 59–64; Sarasin, *Reizbare Maschinen*, 34–38. As late as 1831, Hufeland wrote about dietetics: "From ancient times, certain rules have been laid down for the use of mineral waters, with the intention of [controlling] time, measure, duration, diet, etc., which at first sight have the appearance of an old tradition or pedantry, and are therefore ridiculed

by some modern doctors, . . . that many of these ancient forms . . . are based on a very correct true reason will be revealed in the following examination." ("Es sind für den Gebrauch der Mineralwasser von alten Zeiten her gewisse Regeln in Absicht auf Zeit, Maaß, Dauer, Diät etc. festgesetzt worden, die auf den ersten Anblick den Schein eines alten Herkommens oder einer Pedanterie haben, und daher auch von manchem modernen Arzte verlacht werden, – . . . ob nicht viele dieser alten Formen . . . auf einem sehr richtigen Grunde beruhen, wird sich bei der folgenden Untersuchung zeigen.") Hufeland, *Praktische Uebersicht der vorzüglichsten Heilquellen Teutschlands*, 1831, 13–14.

138. Hufeland, *Praktische Uebersicht der vorzüglichsten Heilquellen Teutschlands*, 1831, 34: "Diätetik der Seele." The dietetic idea of the influence of emotions on health and illness also survived the change in discourse from the theory of humors and vapors to that of nerves. See also Marcard, *Beschreibung von Pyrmont*, vol. 2, 1785, 295–341; Duden, *Geschichte unter der Haut*, 163–172; Stolberg, *Homo patiens*, 229–233.

139. See Chapter 4.

140. [Käppel], *Pyrmonts Merkwürdigkeiten*, 1800, 76: "Während der Kur muss man alle Anstrengungen des Geistes und des Körpers, alle Sorgen und Bürden des Lebens, alle stürmischen Leidenschaften, alle Hazardspiele, alle Bachanalien, alle nächtlichen Ausschweifungen mit größter Sorgfalt vermeiden, und dagegen durch frohe Stimmungen der Seele, durch unschuldige, gesellige Freuden, durch den erquickenden Genuss der reizenden Natur, durch Musick, durch ein unterhaltendes Buch, und durch schickliche Wahl der Speisen und Getränke die heilsamen Kräfte des Gesundbrunnens so viel als möglich zu unterstützen suchen."

141. See Reichard, *Passagier auf der Reise*, 1801, 352–353.

142. See Hoser, *Beschreibung von Franzensbrunn*, 1799, which is an almost ideal-type example of a spa guide.

143. See Schreiber, *Handbuch für Reisende am Rhein*, 1822.

144. See Marcard, *Beschreibung von Pyrmont*, vol. 1, 1784; Marcard, *Beschreibung von Pyrmont*, vol. 2, 1785.

145. Frankenau, *Pyrmont*, 1799, 12–13: "Alle berufen sich auf des berühmten Marcards Zeugniss über die wundervollen Tugenden des Pyrmonter Gesundbrunnenwassers. Herrn Marcards Buche spreche ich durchaus seine Verdienste nicht ab; es verräth ganz vorzüglich, dass dieser Mann tief in das leichtgläubige menschliche Herz schauet: und das Buch hat ohne Zweifel manchen blanken Thaler in die Tasche des Herrn Leibarztes und der Einwohner Pyrmonts gezogen. Meine Feder wird, weder von Eigennuz geleitet, noch werde ich von irgend einem verschuldeten Fürsten besoldet."

146. "Review of Frankenau, *Pyrmont*, 1799," *Allgemeine Literatur-Zeitung*, 1800; "Review of Frankenau, *Pyrmont*, 1799," *Neue allgemeine deutsche Bibliothek*, 1803.

147. [Käppel], *Pyrmonts Merkwürdigkeiten*, 1800, VI: "Schmähschrift." The work was initially published anonymously, but a second edition appeared in 1810 with the author's name on the title page.

148. See Piepenbring, *Bemerkungen über die Schrift des Herrn Doctor Frankenau*, 1801.

149. "Review of Piepenbring, *Bemerkungen über die Schrift des Herrn Doctor Frankenau*," *Neue allgemeine deutsche Bibliothek*, 1802: "Mehr können wir von dieser kleinen Schrift, die natürlich jeder selbst lesen, und mit der von Frankenau vergleichen muß, nicht sagen."

150. See Marcard, *Kleines Pyrmonter Brunnenbuch*, 1805.

151. See Menke, *Pÿrmont und seine Umgebungen*, 1818.
152. See Sponagel, *Meine viertägigen Leiden im Bade Pyrmont* (first edition 1809, quotations from the reprint of the 3rd edition 1824).
153. See Sponagel, *Des Vetters Feldzug in die Seebäder von Doberan*, 1826.
154. See Sponagel, *Meine viertägigen Leiden im Bade Pyrmont*, 1824, 63–65.
155. Sponagel, *Des Vetters Feldzug in die Seebäder von Doberan*, 1826, 211: "'Es sind auch wohl nicht lauter Evangelia, die der Brunnenarzt schreibt,' brummte ich bei mir selbst, als ich mich schon ziemlich herumgetrieben hatte, und weder einen alten Freund noch Bekannten finden konnte. 'Hier sollen sich alte Freunde, Landsleute, Verwandte und Bekannte aus allen Gegenden zusammenfinden, und ich habe bei allem Suchen weder alte noch junge Freunde gefunden.'" Christiane von Goethe, in a letter to her husband from Lauchstädt in 1810, confirmed that spa guests did, in fact, meet old acquaintances and make new ones at the spa. She wrote, "Our stay in Lauchstädt is increasingly enjoyable because we daily make more acquaintances and have also found many old acquaintances again." ("Unser Aufenthalt in Lauchstädt wird immer lustiger, weil wir täglich mehr Bekanntschaft machen und theils auch viele alte Bekannte wieder gefunden haben.") Goethe, Vulpius, *Goethes Briefwechsel mit seiner Frau*, vol. 2, letter from Lauchstädt, 24 July 1810, 181.
156. See Stolberg, *Homo patiens.*
157. Sponagel, *Des Vetters Feldzug in die Seebäder von Doberan*, 1826, 7: "Badegäste" – "Geistes Erheiterung."
158. Sponagel, *Des Vetters Feldzug in die Seebäder von Doberan*, 1826, 7: "So möget Ihr denn nicht verschmähen I den Schwank, der zu erheitern strebt, I Mit Freundlichkeit den Geist erkennen, I Der bei der Dichtung mich belebt, I Der, unbekümmert um Kritiken, I Bei steifer Regel nicht verweilt, I Im Spiele zügelloser Laune I Mutwillig rastlos vorwärts eilt. I Gelingt es ihr, in trüben Stunden, I Wenn Unmut düster Euch umschleicht, I Ein Lächeln Euch abzugewinnen, I So ist der Posse Zweck erreicht."
159. See Paul, *Dr. Katzenbergers Badereise.*
160. Jean Paul was born Johann Paul Friedrich Richter.
161. See Paul, *Dr. Katzenbergers Badereise*, 8 (preface to the second edition, 1822); Miller, Taddey, *Handbuch der historischen Stätten: Baden-Württemberg*, article "Maulbronn," 517–518.
162. Jean Paul handles Dr. Katzenberger's alleged hometown in a similar way. He calls the university town "Pirma (in the principality of Zäckingen)" ("Pirma [im Fürstentume Zäckingen]"). Paul, *Dr. Katzenbergers Badereise*, 13.
163. Paul, *Dr. Katzenbergers Badereise*, 15–16: "nicht um sich – oder sie – zu baden, oder um da sich zu belustigen, . . . Katzenberger machte statt einer Lustreise eigentlich eine Geschäftreise ins Bad, um nämlich seinen Rezensenten beträchtlich auszuprügeln, und ihn dabei mit Schmähungen an der Ehren anzugreifen."
164. See Paul, *Dr. Katzenbergers Badereise*, 19.
165. Paul, *Dr. Katzenbergers Badereise*, 21: "einen täglichen Bericht ihrer Badereise."
166. The writer Theodobach, whom Theoda hopes to meet in Maulbronn, is actually the nobleman Theodobach von Nieß. Theoda initially does not recognize him because he travels to the spa as "Herr von Nieß." Also present in Maulbronn is Captain (*Hauptmann*) Theodobach, the man who ultimately wins Theoda's heart and marries her.
167. See Luhmann, *Liebe als Passion*; Maurer, *Biographie des Bürgers*, 548–549.
168. See, e.g., [Jormann], *Das Schwalbacher Sommer-wehrende Perpetuum Mobile*, 1690, 15–16.

169. By the late eighteenth and early nineteenth centuries, prostitution was either mentioned sarcastically (see, e.g., Sponagel, *Des Vetters Feldzug in die See-bäder von Doberan*, 1826, 169–177; Sponagel, *Meine viertägigen Leiden im Bade Pyrmont*, 1824, 24–33; Frankenau, *Pyrmont*, 1799, 29, 73–74) or authors of spa guides expressly denied the existence of prostitution at the spa, while at the same time hinting at opportunities for illicit sexual activity (see, e.g., *Reise nach den Badeörtern*, 1798, 135–137). This does not, of course, speak to the *actual* existence of prostitution at spas, but rather to the prevailing discourse and "regimes of sayability" in the context of spas and spa visits. The spa as a heterotopia was supposed to have neither beggars nor prostitutes.

170. See Bühren, *Vier Wochen in Pyrmont*, 1824.

171. See Schopenhauer, "Brunnengäste," 1828. The setting for this story is Wiesbaden, which at the beginning of the nineteenth century had risen to the top of the spa hierarchy. See also [Schulz], "Geheime Szenen aus Bädern," 1800; [La Roche], "Eine Baad-Bekanntschaft," 1781.

172. Paul, *Dr. Katzenbergers Badereise*, 77: "breite, beschattete, sich durch-kreuzende Kunststraßen."

173. Paul, *Dr. Katzenbergers Badereise*, 79: "in dem unmittelbaren Fürstentüm-chen Großpolei (jetzo längst mediatisiert) den letzten Berg hinab . . . ins Bad Maulbronn, das ein Städtchen aus Landhäusern schien."

174. See Chapters 3 and 4.

175. *Scènes à tiroir* or *pièces à tiroir* (literally "scenes in a drawer") are comedies "consisting of loosely affiliated scenes that are thematically linked, often with an actor playing multiple roles." Baldyga, *Hamburg Dramaturgy*, 397.

176. Paul, *Dr. Katzenbergers Badereise*, 126: "Tableau" – "der Landesherr des Badeortes" – "die Aussicht auf neue scènes à tiroir, auf neue Spektakelstücke und Szenenmaler für diese kleine Bühne; besonders die Aussicht auf die Erleuchtung der Höhle." (Italics by ULH.)

177. Paul, *Dr. Katzenbergers Badereise*, 162; "rings umher im Blätter-Dunkel ungesehen belauschen konnten."

178. See Paul, *Dr. Katzenbergers Badereise*, 69, 162–163.

179. See Chapter 4.

180. See Chapter 1.

181. Paul, *Dr. Katzenbergers Badereise*, 80: "Großpoleiische Zeitung."

182. See Paul, *Dr. Katzenbergers Badereise*, 87, 103, 117.

183. Paul, *Dr. Katzenbergers Badereise*, 27: "Ihr war nämlich ein unauslöschli-ches Bild von der Stunde geblieben, wo ihre Mutter sie als Kind in einer großen, mit Lampen erhellten Zauberhöhle des Orts – ähnlich der Höhle im Bade Liebenstein – umhergetragen hatte."

184. Paul, *Dr. Katzenbergers Badereise*, 64: "am Tage herab mit dem Bade-Ständchen angeblasen werden." See Campe, *Reise von Braunschweig nach Karlsbad*, 1806, 149–150; Sartori, *Taschenbuch für Carlsbads Curgäste*, 1817.

185. I.e., the relaxed customs and practices allowed at masquerades. On "spa freedom," see Chapter 5.

186. Paul, *Dr. Katzenbergers Badereise*, 22: "des vornehmen Morgen-Trinkgelags und der Maskenfreiheiten und des Kongresses des Reichtums und der Bildung."

187. Müller, *Welt des Baedeker*, 28: "Nur ein fertiges Format, das auf hinreichend bekannten Standardisierungen beruht, kann zum Gegenstand einer Satire werden."

Part II
Space and Time

Introduction to Part II

Research into landscape perception and its transformation during the eighteenth and early nineteenth centuries played an important role in the older cultural history at the beginning of the twentieth century.[1] In the 1970s and the 1980s, surveys and primary source collections on the introduction of the English landscape garden in Germany, the "discovery" of the Alps and of the seaside, and the development of Rhine Romanticism appeared.[2] In recent decades, literary scholars have researched the development of landscape perception in late eighteenth-century Germany, but the topic still receives only limited attention in cultural history.[3] In particular, we lack studies that explore how eighteenth-century changes in landscape perception that were initially driven by a few members of the learned elite became the dominant modes of perception in the early decades of the nineteenth century.

In the following two chapters, I will analyze the development of perceptions of space and time in the context of both spas and seaside resorts. In the published discourse, especially in spa guides and travelogues, we can see how spa visitors were gradually introduced to the new landscape perceptions. This process lagged behind the initial introduction of these new modes of perceiving the natural environment by elite authors, but through their wide distribution spa publications functioned as essential multipliers of the new perceptions during the late eighteenth and early nineteenth centuries. By closely examining this change in perception and practices, this study adopts a perspective on the late eighteenth and early nineteenth centuries that brings a fundamental cultural change into focus while also emphasizing its slow, meandering, and non-teleological nature. This gradual process resulted in a complete transformation of early modern perceptions of nature. The early modern ideal of an urban, "civilized" space, where nature was tightly controlled and mountains and the sea were regarded as "wild," was replaced by a positive, even rapturous, perception of mountains and the sea and by new practices of hiking and beach-going that to this day determine our modern notions of desirable views and an ideal vacation.

As Adrian von Buttlar and others have shown, the introduction of the English landscape garden in late eighteenth-century Germany marked a decisive shift. The adoption of the landscape garden meant a deliberate rejection of the geometric French garden and its attempt to control nature. Eighteenth-century contemporaries associated the new English landscape garden with the idea that a garden should look "natural" and, as a consequence, with Enlightenment concepts of freedom and rationality.[4] In his *Theory of Garden Art* (*Theorie der Gartenkunst*), published in five volumes between 1779 and 1785, Christian Cay Lorenz Hirschfeld, the leading German garden theorist of the time,[5] summarized these underlying ideas succinctly by arguing that the English landscape garden was "the taste of nature and reason, a taste directly opposed to the affectations and false wit of the old style [the French garden style]."[6]

In the empire, the princes introduced the landscape garden in their territories, residence towns, and summer residences and created the most outstanding examples thereof[7] – just as they built most of the spas. Numerous studies deal with individual gardens, in particular the Wörlitz Park, which was one of the first of its kind in Germany. Created by Prince Franz of Anhalt-Dessau, the Wörlitz Park was laid out between 1769 and 1773 and expanded in the 1780s and the 1790s.[8] Although studies about English landscape gardens in Germany rarely analyze spa gardens, they are nevertheless of value for placing the spa gardens in their contemporary context.[9]

Historians and literary scholars who research the perception of nature – especially mountains and the seaside – agree that a fundamental change took place during the eighteenth century. While mountains, first and foremost the Alps, and the sea had been perceived as wild and threatening during the early modern period, now they were viewed as sublime, picturesque, and romantic or, in contemporary terminology, "wild and romantic" (*wildromantisch*).[10] Traditionally, Albrecht von Haller's poem "The Alps" ("Die Alpen") of 1729 and Jean-Jacques Rousseau's novel *Julie, or the New Heloise* (*Julie, ou la nouvelle Héloise*) of 1761 and his battle cry "Back to Nature!" are regarded as pivotal moments in this development.[11] In contrast, Ruth and Dieter Groh have argued that the physico-theologians of the late seventeenth and early eighteenth centuries already paved the way for the modern, positive perception of mountains and "wild" nature via their definition of the "sublime."[12] More recent studies by literary scholars examine the perception of the landscape in travelogues and in the narrative prose of the late eighteenth and early nineteenth centuries.[13]

Concerning perceptions of the sea and the seaside, Alain Corbin's 1988 monograph *The Lure of the Sea: The Discovery of the Seaside in the Western World, 1750–1840* was groundbreaking and remains the leading work on this topic. On the basis of an in-depth study of early modern discourses and practices, Corbin succeeded in showing how attitudes toward the sea and the seaside gradually changed from negative to positive, with the Dutch and then especially the English spearheading this change in Europe.[14] The older perception of the sea as a terrible and ugly world populated by sea monsters[15] was gradually replaced by a more positive concept at the end of the seventeenth century.

Physicians began to propagate the healing effects of cold seawater, and a new "appreciation of dunes, sand, beaches, and views of the coast" developed.[16] This spatial perception took hold in the emerging English seaside resorts beginning in the middle of the eighteenth century and then gradually gained acceptance in other European countries.[17] By the 1820s, according to Corbin, "the lure of the sea" had led to new spatial ideals and new practices. Buildings at seaside resorts were oriented toward the sea, and visitors enjoyed walks on seafront promenades with a view of the beach and the ocean.[18] Finally, the Romantics no longer sought the view of the sea – the picturesque "frame" – but rather the immediate sensual experience of the beach and the ocean. Strolls along the seashore were accompanied by romantic meditations and regarded as deep emotional experiences. Islands in the sea were perceived as a refuge from society.[19] In the terminology employed here, a new spatial heterotopia had been born.

These changes in the perception of nature are closely related to the question of the development of modern tourism. It is striking that there is very little tourism research for the late eighteenth century. The concept and the phenomenon of tourism are generally assumed to have come to fruition in the nineteenth century, and only brief mentions point to earlier beginnings in the eighteenth century.[20] This assumption will be challenged in the following two chapters. Numerous elements of the tourist experience described by researchers for the nineteenth century can already be observed at the spas in the late eighteenth and early nineteenth centuries. Spas were, for all intents and purposes, tourist destinations. They were "particular places" outside of everyday life, where guests traveled "for regularised periods of time" to enjoy leisure activities, the consumption of culture and luxury goods, and "visual elements of [the] landscape."[21]

In particular, spas and the associated published discourse gave rise to a "tourist gaze," which entails looking at sights through the lens of "cultural styles, circulating images and texts . . . as well as personal experiences and memories."[22] As John Urry and Jonas Larsen have observed, "Gazing is not merely seeing, but involves cognitive work of interpreting, evaluating, drawing comparisons and making mental connections between signs and their referents."[23] The published spa discourse "guided the eye of the tourist" by standardizing viewing habits.[24] Just like the summer retreat (*Sommerfrische*) of the nineteenth century, it linked "notions of open spaces outside of urban everyday life, of idyllic country life and health."[25] And just like the seaside resort of the late twentieth century, a spa was a "liminal space, . . . which was characterized by fundamental otherness and enabled experiences that transcended everyday life."[26] As I will show in the next two chapters, the heterotopia of the spa represented the first stage of modern forms of tourism and vacationing not only in terms of spatial perception and leisure activities but also with regard to a specific experience of time.

Notes

1. See, e.g., Flemming, *Wandel des deutschen Naturgefühls*; Weiss, *Entdeckung der Alpen*. See also Maurer, "Reisen interdisziplinär," 311–312, footnote 78.
2. See Buttlar, *Landschaftsgarten*; Woźniakowski, *Wildnis*; Oppenheim, *Entdeckung der Alpen*; Faessler, *Bodensee und Alpen*; Seitz, *Wo Europa den Himmel berührt*; Corbin, *Lure of the Sea* (first published in French in 1988); Maurer, "Reisen interdisziplinär," 315–320.
3. See, e.g., Landwehr, Stockhorst, *Einführung in die europäische Kulturgeschichte*; Reinhard, *Lebensformen*; Münch, *Lebensformen*.
4. See Buttlar, *Landschaftsgarten*. See also Dülmen, *Das irdische Paradies*, 17–23; Lauterbach, "Der europäische Landschaftsgarten"; Gamper, *"Die Natur ist republikanisch"*; Schepers, *Hirschfelds Theorie der Gartenkunst*, 3–4; Bending, *Cultural History of Gardens*. See also Hirschfeld, *Theory of Garden Art*, 98: "To be honest, it was the report of garden improvements in England that animated this subject in Germany."
5. See Kehn, *Christian Cay Lorenz Hirschfeld*; Kehn, "Ästhetische Landschaftserfahrung"; Schepers, *Hirschfelds Theorie der Gartenkunst*.
6. Hirschfeld, *Theory of Garden Art*, 135. See also Hirschfeld, *Theorie der Gartenkunst*, vol. 1, 142.
7. See Martus, *Aufklärung*, 753–762.
8. The Wörlitz Park is part of the Dessau-Wörlitz Garden Realm (*Dessau-Wörlitzer Gartenreich*), today a World Heritage Site.
9. See Günther, *Gärten der Goethe-Zeit*; Kunst, "Delineatio"; Jöchner, "Geometrie"; Hirsch, "Hortus Oeconomicus"; Hirsch, "Utopia realisata"; Hirsch, "'Kron'zeugen"; Niedermeier, "Wörlitz"; Seng, "Wörlitzer Anlagen"; Trauzettel, "Gartenreich"; Mittelstädt, *Wörlitz*; Küster, "Gartenreich Dessau-Wörlitz."
10. See Raymond, *Von der Landschaft*, 120–165.
11. See Oppenheim, *Entdeckung der Alpen*, 41–42; Woźniakowski, *Wildnis*, 216; Stoffel, *Alpen*, esp. 90–171; Schaumann, "From Meadows to Mountaintops"; Ozturk, "Interlude: Geo-Poetics."
12. See Groh, Groh, *Weltbild*, 92–149. The distinctly teleological way in which Groh and Groh discuss this development is striking. They describe the "genesis of the modern experience of nature" ("Entstehungsgeschichte der modernen Naturerfahrung") as the "dismantling of barriers, which have long stood in the way of an aesthetic perception of nature" ("Abbau von Barrieren, die einer ästhetischen Wahrnehmung von Natur lange im Wege standen") and state that in 1823 Goethe "fell back into the old pattern of perception" ("in das alte Muster der Wahrnehnung"). Groh, Groh, *Weltbild*, 107.
13. See Jost, *Landschaftsblick*; Raymond, *Von der Landschaft*. Jost focuses on narrative prose, while also incorporating contemporary landscape painting. Raymond examines the new perception of the landscape in the travelogues of Sophie von La Roche, Fredericke Bruns, and Johanna Schopenhauer. See also Wunderlich, "Landschaft"; Stobbe, "Konkurrierende Wahrnehmungsmodelle."
14. See Corbin, *Lure of the Sea*. Corbin also comments on the influence of physico-theology on the emergence of a new conception of nature (see 22–32).

15. See Corbin, *Lure of the Sea*, 1–18.

16. Corbin, *Lure of the Sea*, 37.

17. See Corbin, *Lure of the Sea*, 57–73; Walton, "Coastal Resorts."

18. See Corbin, *Lure of the Sea*, 250–269.

19. See Corbin, *Lure of the Sea*, 163–183.

20. See Spode, "Die paneuropäische Touristenklasse"; Gyr, "Geschichte des Tourismus"; Urry, Larsen, *Tourist Gaze*, 6; Blackbourn, "Fashionable Spa Towns," 12.

21. Urry, Larsen, *Tourist Gaze*, 4. I concur with Karin Wurst who writes, "The spa culture with its many forms of entertainment represented an early form of the modern practice of vacationing, as it combined the spectacular entertainments of travel with unique forms of sociability, shopping, and dining experiences in addition to cultural practices such as dancing and walking." Wurst, *Fabricating Pleasure*, 258. Wurst does not, however, examine the role of landscape perception as a part of early tourist culture at the spas.

22. Urry, Larsen, *Tourist Gaze*, 17.

23. Urry, Larsen, *Tourist Gaze*, 17.

24. Kos, *Eroberung der Landschaft*, 23: "Blickleitung des Touristen."

25. Mai, "Touristische Räume," 13: "Vorstellungen von Freiräumen außerhalb des städtischen Alltags, vom idyllisierten Landleben und von Gesundheit."

26. Kolbe, "Strandurlaub," 189: "liminoiden Raum, . . . der sich durch grundsätzliche Andersartigkeit auszeichnete und alltagsüberschreitende Erfahrungen ermöglichte."

3 Reinventing the Eighteenth-Century Spa as a Leisure Space

The Early Modern Spa as an Urban Space

From the late Middle Ages to the middle of the eighteenth century, people expected the ideal spa to have the look and feel of an urban space surrounded by a landscape of gentle hills and fields as proof of human cultivation. This does not mean, however, that spas located outside of urban settlements or surrounded by mountains, such as Pfäfers in Switzerland, located in a deep gorge (Figure 3.1), or Karlsbad and Ems (Figure 3.6), both situated in valleys surrounded by rugged mountainous terrain, did not attract visitors. Rather, people went to these spas because the healing power of their waters had been proven by long experience. Nevertheless, contemporaries regarded the location of these spas as constraining and not conducive to positive emotions. In 1481, the two humanists Peter Schott and Johannes Geiler von Kaysersberg, while staying at Wildbad and Baden-Baden respectively, exchanged letters and "spa gifts" (*Badegeschenke*) between the two spas. Schott wrote to Geiler, expressing his hope that his spa gift would be "more civilized than the uninviting mountains full of rainfall where they had to take the exhausting bathing cure. After all, their minds should not be completely stifled by the wooded slopes of the surrounding mountains."[1]

By the late eighteenth century, a pleasing landscape surrounding the spa became a central demand in the published discourse. Hoser declared in 1799, "A spa, however great its medical reputation may be, if it does not possess some natural beauties, or, if lacking those, has not received some embellishments through artistry, remains a sad exile for anyone whose unfortunate health conditions force them to visit it."[2] But, as we will see in this chapter and the next, the definition of "natural beauties" changed dramatically between the late fifteenth and the late eighteenth centuries. What the humanists perceived as "uninviting" and "stifling" appeared as highly attractive to spa visitors of the early nineteenth century.

Before the middle of the eighteenth century, the representation of spas and their surroundings corresponded to generally accepted early

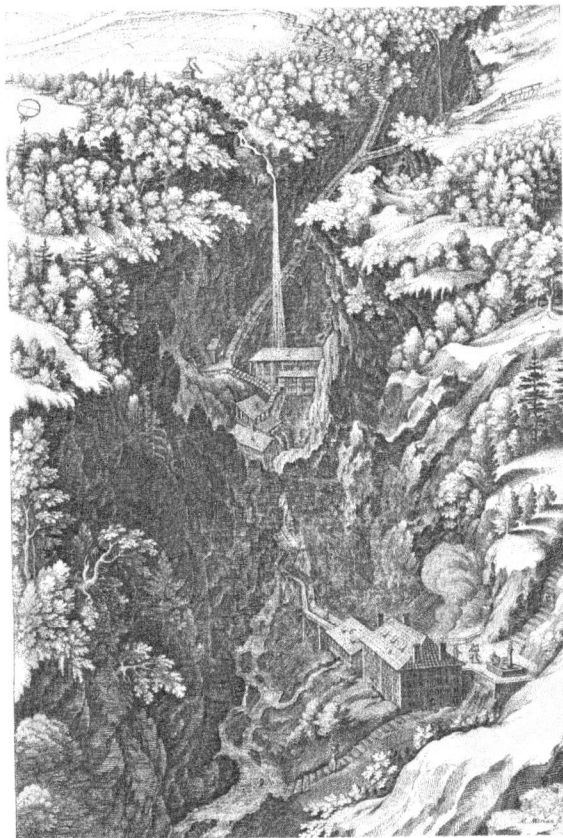

Figure 3.1 Pfäfers in Switzerland, engraving by Matthäus Merian the Elder, 1654. ("Wahre Contrafactur des Wunderlichen Bads zu Pfäffers in Ober Schweytz." In Merian, Matthäus, and Martin Zeiller. *Topographia Helvetiae, Rhatiae, et Valesiae*, after 42. Frankfurt a.M.: Meriansche Erben, 1654. Bayerische Staatsbibliothek, shelf mark Hbks/E 29–4#Beibd.3.)

modern ideals that were deeply rooted in both discourse and experience. Cities and towns were regarded as safe and "civilized" spaces, while a mountainous and rugged landscape was considered "wild" and dangerous. The ideal landscape was gentle, hilly, and, above all, recognizably cultivated by humans.[3] In the published discourse, especially in spa guides, authors did their utmost to persuade readers that a particular spa conformed to the ideal of an urban space surrounded by a cultivated landscape. Most spas located in the plains and rolling hills of northern and central Germany exhibited these attributes, and the authors only had to emphasize them. Spas situated in the higher elevations of the low mountain ranges (*Mittelgebirge*) of central and southern Germany did not meet these expectations, and authors accordingly took great pains to reinterpret these spas' surroundings, often employing rhetorical contortions.

Aachen, where the spa was embedded in the imperial city, fully met contemporary expectations. In Blondel's work on Aachen, published in 1688, a fold-out map of the city bound into the book opposite the title page immediately catches the eye of the reader (Figure 3.2). Moreover, Blondel describes the landscape surrounding Aachen in emphatic terms, dwelling on the fertile soil and agricultural activities. Notably, this was a landscape to be viewed from inside the city but not to be explored: "Although this city is situated in a valley, and surrounded by mountains

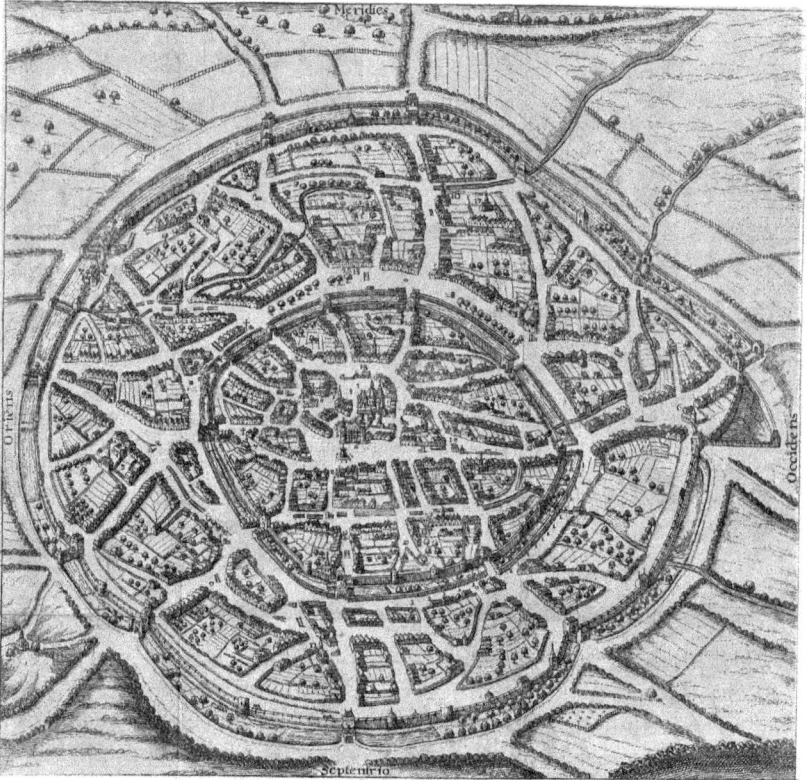

Figure 3.2 Fold-out map of Aachen, engraving, 1688. ("Urbis Aquensis urbs regalis, regni sedes principalis, prima regum curia." In Blondel, François. *Außfürliche Erklärung vnd Augenscheinliche Wunderwirckung Deren Heylsamen Badt- und Trinckwässern zu Aach*, before 1. Aachen: Clemens, 1688. SLUB Dresden/Deutsche Fotothek/DDZ.)

and woods, it is gifted with a very healthy air, and in particular fertility and gracefulness, so that wherever one turns one's eyes, one can see many and various wonders of nature at play, which are highly pleasing to the mind and eyes. Near the city one can see a valley far and wide in all directions, where cattle can graze comfortably. On the hills there are fertile fields that yield all kinds of fruits."[4] Pöllnitz's *Amusements at the Waters of Aix la Chapelle, or Pastimes at the Waters in Aachen* (*Amusemens des eaux d'Aix la Chapelle, oder Zeit-Vertreib bey den Wassern zu Achen*) of 1737 follows a very similar path, emphasizing urban characteristics. The first engraving at the end of the volume shows a map of the imperial city, enhanced by a detailed legend. Further engravings display the Aachen bathhouses and important buildings in the imperial city, among others the town hall and the Church of Our Lady, and the nearby spa of Burtscheid, underlining its small-town character.[5]

In his advertising pamphlet for Lauchstädt,[6] published in 1746, the Saxon mining director Johann Friedrich Henkel highlighted the urbanity of the spa and the advantages of its surroundings for potential spa guests: "The bathing spring itself is located inside the town, or at least in the garden next to it. This provides [Lauchstädt] with a not inconsiderable advantage over spas that are generally very isolated from towns and villages in fields, forests, even desolate places, and thus hardly profit from, or even have to do without, human services and other measures for enjoyment, which constitute half of the cure and the medicine."[7] Henkel's attempt to obscure the exact location of the healing spring in Lauchstädt reveals the considerable influence of the prevailing discourse. First he claims that the spa is situated in the town, and then he backtracks and admits that it is only nearby. Furthermore, Henkel stresses Lauchstädt's proximity to larger cities such as Merseburg, Halle, and Leipzig.[8] Lauchstädt's location is described as ideal: "The altitude is as beautiful as benevolent nature can make it, not mountainous, but also not swampy, not rough and sharp, but also not loamy and humid, but of a well-natured mixture."[9] Finally, Henkel praises the fertility of the fields surrounding the spa.[10]

In his *Amusements at the Waters of Kleve* (*Amusemens des eaux de Cleve*) of 1748, Schütte was even more emphatic: "What is more, there is probably no other place in Europe famous for its pleasant situation, where you can find so many avenues or walks, merry hills, immensely beautiful views, green mountains, shady valleys, fertile fields of grain and pastures, in such a wonderful order, all together, as at Kleve."[11] And in his poem *The Spa Guest* (*Der Brunnengast*) of 1744, Koromandel-Wedekind wrote in a similar vein, but at least he admitted that Pyrmont could not fulfill all contemporary expectations:

> Pyrmont is not big, and cannot even be described as a town,
> But one must grant it the fame of a Garden of Eden,

Which has much grace, enjoys the purest air,
Is endowed with animal husbandry, game and fish, and fruit.[12]

(See also Figure 3.9, an engraving of 1698 that shows Pyrmont embedded in softly undulating fields.)

Engravings of spas before 1750 also accentuate their urban character. The images published in Merian's *Topographia Hassiae* in the middle of the seventeenth century are typical examples. Wiesbaden embodies the contemporary ideal of the spa as an urban space: "An old, though not large, town, but famous for its wonderful and healing baths."[13] The entry for Wiesbaden includes an engraving that depicts the spa as a typical early modern town with surrounding walls, a church at the center, and embedded in a gentle, hilly landscape (Figure 3.3). The engraving for Schwalbach shows houses as densely built as in a small town as well as barriers and markers at the entrances to the village, lending the spa an urban character despite its lack of a wall.[14] The surrounding landscape looks gently undulating and largely cultivated (Figure 3.4).

When a spa and its surroundings did not conform to the early modern spatial ideal, authors and engravers tried to find ways to persuade readers and viewers of the spa's attractiveness. Count Wilhelm of Hanau, who in 1766 went to the spa of Ems with his wife to cure their infertility, uttered the hard judgment that it had been a "dull cure": "The location of the spa is hideous, squeezed between rocks and crevices of the [river] Lahn."[15]

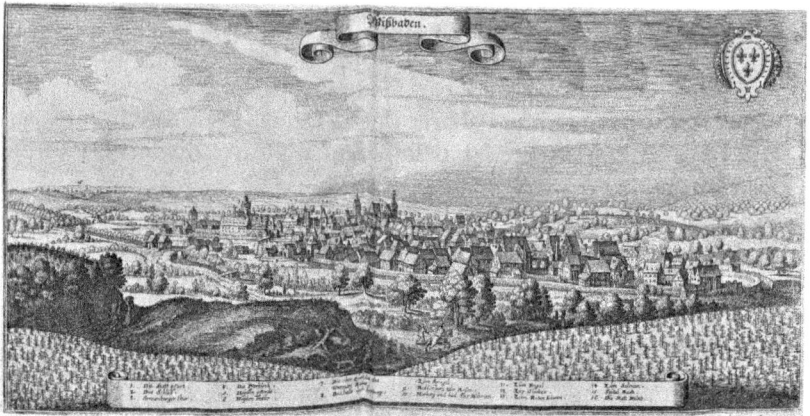

Figure 3.3 Wiesbaden, engraving by Matthäus Merian the Elder, 1655. ("Wißbaden." In Merian, Matthäus, and Martin Zeiller. *Topographia Hassiae, Et Regionum Vicinarum*, between 142 and 143. Frankfurt a.M.: Meriansche Erben, 1655. Bayerische Staatsbibliothek, shelf mark Hbks/E 30–8/9.)

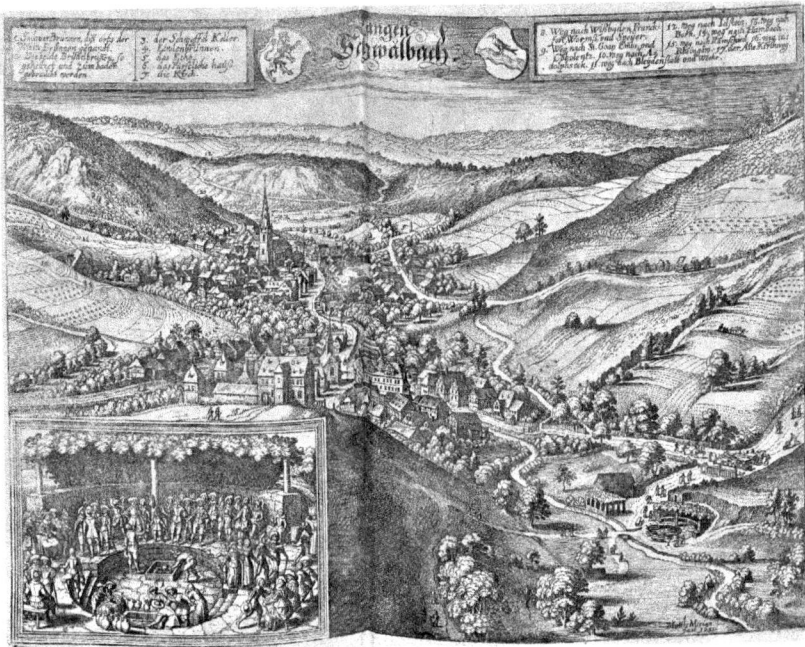

Figure 3.4 Schwalbach, engraving by Matthäus Merian the Elder, 1655. ("Langen Schwalbach." In Merian, Matthäus, and Martin Zeiller. *Topographia Hassiae, Et Regionum Vicinarum*, after 122. Frankfurt a.M.: Meriansche Erben, 1655. Bayerische Staatsbibliothek, shelf mark Hbks/E 30–8/9.)

In the Merian engraving of Ems (Figure 3.5), however, the spa looks far less "squeezed." Rather, the Lahn valley seems spacious and the spa buildings appear large compared to the mountains behind them. The "rocks and crevices" of the mountains appear more like gentle, rounded hills covered with vegetation. The location of the spa seems nonthreatening rather than "hideous." Clearly, the Merian depiction of Ems was beautified to conform to seventeenth-century expectations, as is obvious when we compare it to a view of Ems from the middle of the nineteenth century (Figure 3.6). Furthermore, in the Merian engraving the spa buildings of Ems resemble a castle, which can give the viewer a sense of the spa as a space that is at least safe, even if not urban.

It was particularly difficult for a spa like Schlangenbad to fit the prevailing discourse because it is literally squeezed in between mountains and had no urban features to recommend itself. In his advertising pamphlet of 1747, the Hesse-Kassel spa physician Johann Peter Welcker had to employ some rhetorical sugarcoating: "Schlangenbad is situated in a valley deeply

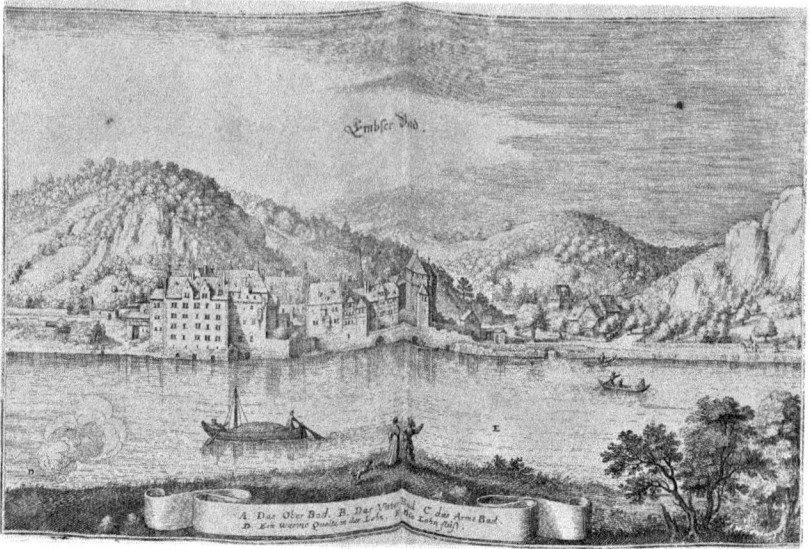

Figure 3.5 Ems, engraving by Matthäus Merian the Elder, 1655. ("Embser Bad." In Merian, Matthäus, and Martin Zeiller. *Topographia Hassiae, Et Regionum Vicinarum*, between 40 and 41. Frankfurt a.M.: Meriansche Erben, 1655. Bayerische Staatsbibliothek, shelf mark Hbks/E 30–8/9.)

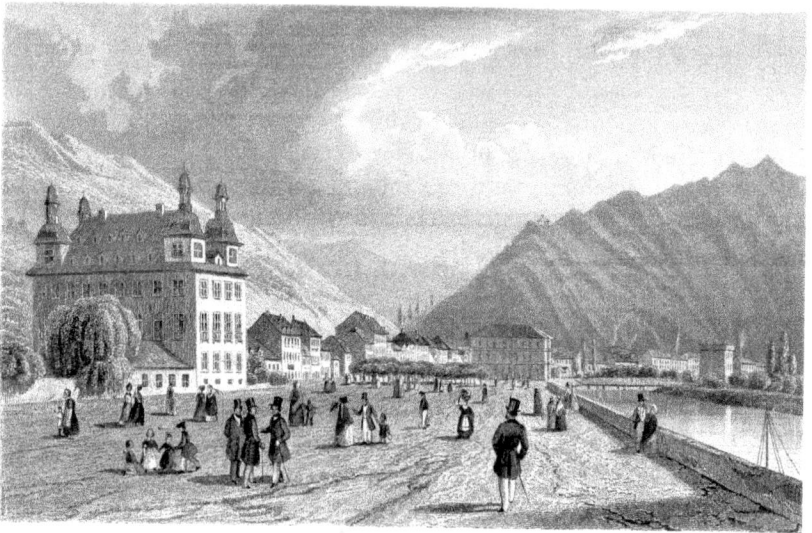

Figure 3.6 Ems, colored lithography, mid-nineteenth century. (Stadtarchiv Bad Ems.)

carved out by nature, which is surrounded by high mountains and forests full of trees. Hence the place is not particularly pleasant in itself, but through untiring diligence, through the beautiful buildings and the wide, delightful, and skillfully created avenue the natural situation has been improved, so that it can now rightly be counted among the most pleasant ones, and even though nothing but leaves and grass grow here, there is a great abundance of victuals."[16] In order to distract from the spa's surroundings, Welcker described the interior space of the small spa of Schlangenbad as well-ordered and "civilized" and, due to its proximity to the cities of Mainz and Frankfurt, as well-provided for. Johann Jacob Moser resorted to similar means in his 1758 description of Wildbad in the Black Forest. Moser admitted that "the surrounding mountains are high, and in many places rocks and large stones stick out."[17] He did not dwell on the spa's surroundings, however, and mainly devoted his attention to the *town* of Wildbad by inserting a map of the spa and describing in detail the lodging houses, avenues within the town, and the various bathhouses, as well as the surrounding towns.[18]

Karlsbad, one of the few spas in our sample with a long and unbroken history of success,[19] initially established itself in the published discourse by highlighting its urban space as a selling point. The landscape surrounding Karlsbad, however, had to be painstakingly redefined in order to conform to contemporary expectations. Since the town is located in a basin surrounded by mountains, authors emphasized its urban character, for instance by referring to urban development, trade, and the goods and services offered.[20] The author of *Newly Improved and Augmented Memorable Imperial Karlsbad* (*Neu-verbessert- und vermehrtes denckwürdiges Kayser Carls-Baad*), published in 1736, first described and praised the town and its urban features and then remarked, "Many people who have not experienced this town and the territory where it is located would hardly believe what I have described above, and that this town is so congenial, because of the surrounding hills and mountains."[21] An engraving shows Karlsbad situated in a spacious valley, similar to Ems in the Merian engraving of the mid-seventeenth century. "Despite" the mountains, the author argued, there were beautiful meadows, fields, gardens, and walks, providing the visitor with enjoyable views of the town. The author described the mountains surrounding Karlsbad as equivalent to urban bulwarks and ramparts.[22] Finally, the author – like Henkel in his description of Lauchstädt – pointed out the numerous towns in Karlsbad's vicinity.[23]

Christoph Gottlob Grundig's *Description of His . . . Journey to Imperial Karlsbad* (*Beschreibung seiner . . . in das Käyser Carls-Bad gethanen Reise*) of 1754 also references the expectations associated with a spa in the published discourse. The fold-out map opposite the title page does not hide the surrounding mountains, but its layout draws the viewer's

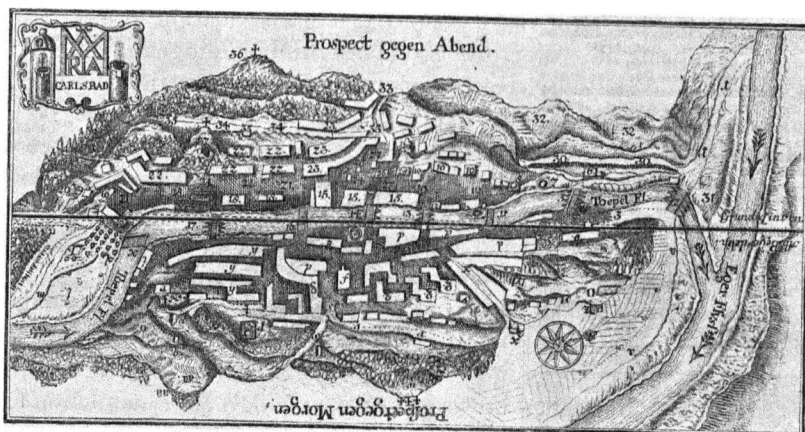

Figure 3.7 Fold-out map of Karlsbad (today Karlovy Vary), engraving, 1754. (In [Grundig, Christoph Gottlob]. *Mit nützlichen Nachrichten und Anmerkungen erläuterte Beschreibung seiner, im Jahr 1751 in das Käyser Carls-Bad gethanen Reise,* before A3r. Schneeberg: Fulde, 1754. SLUB Dresden/Digitale Sammlungen/Hist.urb.Germ.2169.)

attention to the town (Figure 3.7). All the buildings are detailed in a legend, presenting Karlsbad as an urban space. Accordingly, Grundig's description of the town is very comprehensive, and he gives many details about the buildings and the urban trades and crafts.[24] The landscape surrounding the spa was clearly not considered one of Karlsbad's attractions, "for so very narrow is the valley between the above-mentioned mountains, which I feel justified to call a gorge."[25] Moreover, Grundig described a walk on "steep tracks" (*Gemsensteigen*) in the vicinity of the town as a practice he himself enjoyed but that by no means appealed to most spa guests.[26]

From the sixteenth to the beginning of the eighteenth century, an avenue or a garden modeled on the Italian and French Renaissance gardens and the French Baroque gardens were the elements that brought nature into the interior space of a spa. Such small gardens and/or avenues, based on principles of symmetry, represented tamed nature in an urban space. They met the requirement of an appropriate space for walks and were regarded as a central feature of the spa, serving both health and recreational functions. In images of sixteenth- and seventeenth-century spas, for instance of Aachen (Figure 3.8, tree-lined walks) and Pyrmont (Figure 3.9, main avenue in the foreground, slightly right of center), these facilities are given a prominent place. The map of the spa of Boll ("Boller Landtafel"), included in the 1602 *New Spa Book* (*New Badbuch*) by Johannes Bauhin, depicts a large fenced-in spa garden in the formal

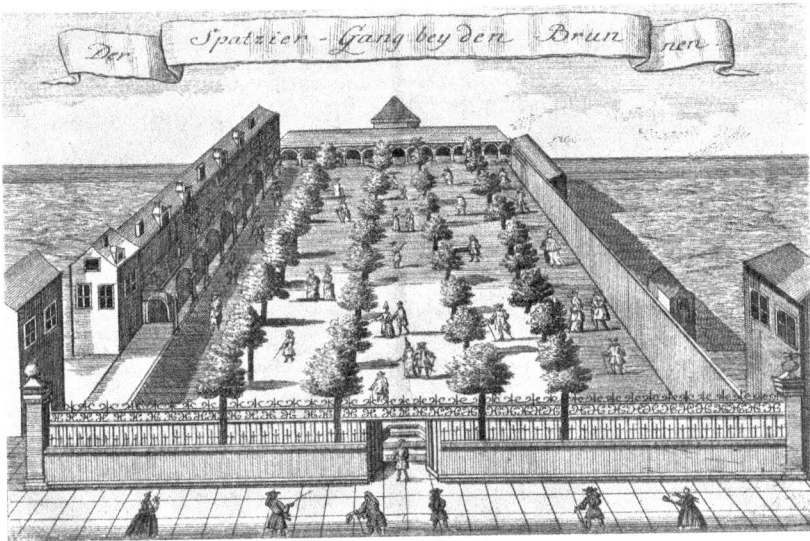

Figure 3.8 Aachen, tree-lined walks, engraving, 1737. ("Der Spatzier-Gang bey den Brunnen." In [Pöllnitz, Karl Ludwig Freiherr von]. *Amusemens des eaux d'Aix la Chapelle, oder Zeit-Vertreib bey den Wassern zu Achen*, figure VII. Berlin: Rüdiger, 1737. SLUB Dresden/Deutsche Fotothek/DDZ.)

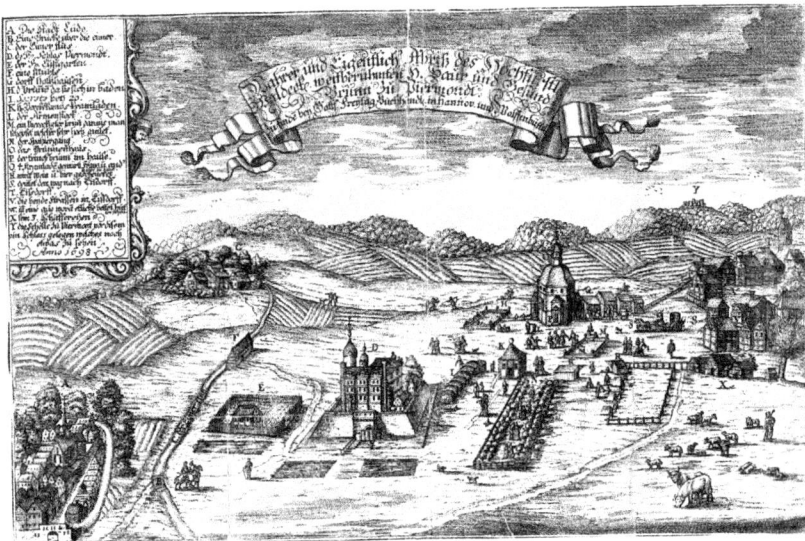

Figure 3.9 Pyrmont, engraving, 1698. ("Wahrer und Eigentlich[er] Abriß des Hochfürstl[ichen] Waldeck[ischen] weitberühmten H[eiligen] Saur[-] und Gesund-Brunn zu Piermondt." Hannover: Freytag, 1698. Museum im Schloss Bad Pyrmont.)

French style behind the complex of the lodging house and bathhouse (Figure 3.10). This ideal-type depiction also shows associated leisure activities: a form of bowling, two market stalls, dancing, an obstacle course, and hunting – an exclusively aristocratic activity.[27] An engraving of the Bavarian spa of Adelholzen[28] in Merian's *Topographia Bavariae* portrays both a fenced-in garden and a skittles (nine-pin bowling) alley at the center of the spa (Figure 3.11).

Until the middle of the eighteenth century, the spatial ideal of the spa prevalent in the published discourse was aligned with early modern perceptions of built and natural environments. A spa had to present itself as a space with urban features surrounded by a cultivated landscape of fertile fields and gently rolling hills. These ideals also influenced practices. Spa visitors were encouraged to take in the landscape, but from a vantage point inside the safe (urban) space of the spa. Nature was included in the interior spaces of the spa by means of formal French gardens or avenues; nature at the spa was tamed. Starting in the late 1770s, however, English landscape gardens were integrated into spas and thus the spatial construction of the ideal spa gradually changed.

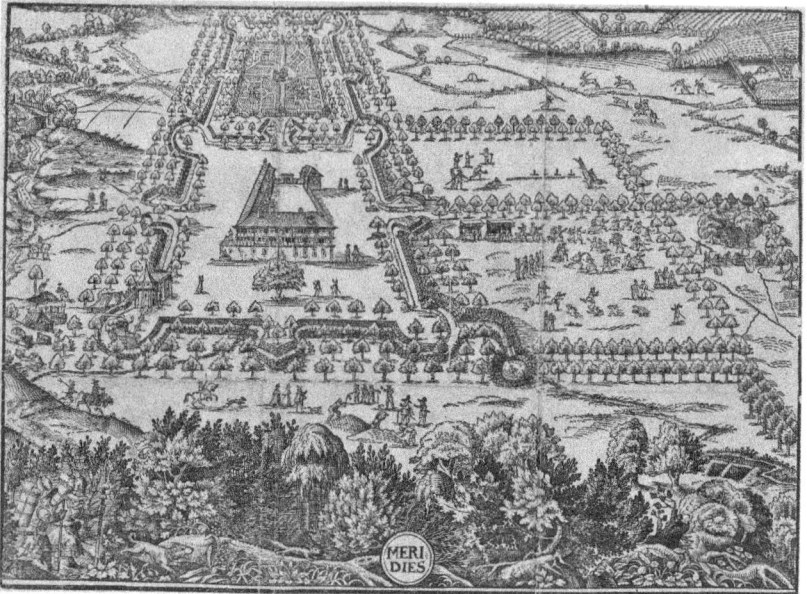

Figure 3.10 Boll, engraving, 1602. ("Boller Landtafel." In Bauhin, Johann. *Ein New Badbuch*, at end of volume. Stuttgart: Fürster, 1602. Württembergische Landesbibliothek, Stuttgart, shelf mark R 16 Bau 2.)

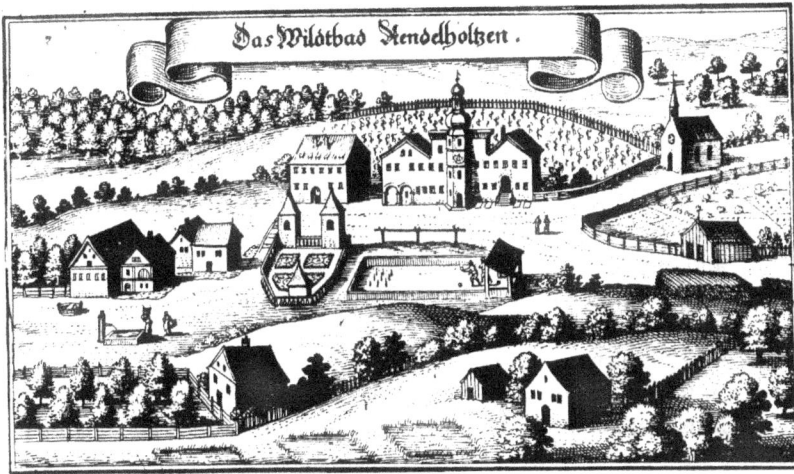

Figure 3.11 Adelholzen, engraving by Matthäus Merian the Elder, 1644. ("Das Wildtbad Aendelholtzen." In Merian, Matthäus, and Martin Zeiller. *Topographia Bavariae*, after 66. Frankfurt a.M.: Merian, 1644. Staats- und Stadtbibliothek Augsburg, shelf mark 4 K-K 116.)

The Spa as an Emerging Leisure Resort: Landscape Gardens, Vistas, and Recreational Spaces

Beginning in the late 1770s and the early 1780s, the early modern urban ideal of the spa was intensified and substantially modified at the same time. On the one hand, the spa was expected to provide services and leisure activities on par with larger towns. On the other hand, the spa was increasingly constructed as an idealized rural space, a retreat from urban life. The emphasis in the published discourse shifted from spas as actual towns to spas that provided urban amenities in spaces with a pastoral character. In this context, the new ideal of the English landscape garden replaced the old ideal of the formal French garden. As a result, many spa gardens were transformed to incorporate the new ideal, or new spas were designed with English landscape gardens as their central feature. While the adoption of the English landscape garden in spa design reflected general eighteenth-century trends, the expansion of the published spa discourse led to the dissemination of these new ideals to a growing audience of readers and spa visitors. Henceforth, the published discourse served as a multiplier of new ideas about the perception of nature and propagated the spa as a spatial heterotopia.

For a spa to be successful it had to be – or at least it had to present itself as – a multifunctional recreation space. The ideal spa had to offer not only an English landscape garden with convenient footpaths and various options for exercise and enjoyment but also an avenue, shops, a theater, and one or several spa buildings with halls for dancing, music performances, games of faro and billiards, smoking tobacco, and a reading library. It thus provided multiple opportunities for the consumption of culture and luxury goods.[29] Convenient lodging houses and a "spring temple" (*Brunnentempel*), where the visitors could drink their healing water in style, had to be in place. A pamphlet advertising Hofgeismar expressed all of this in a nutshell: "Here everything charming is lined up as if on a chain, and [the spa visitors'] senses and minds can find delight here."[30]

In the fifth volume of his *Theory of Garden Art* (*Theorie der Gartenkunst*), published in 1785, Christian Cay Lorenz Hirschfeld, in a detailed section on "Gardens at Spas" ("Gärten bey Gesundbrunnen"),[31] programmatically formulated the new demands that were at that time entering into the mainstream of the spa discourse.[32] In contrast to the small and strictly geometrical gardens of the older spa ideal, "gardens at spas" now had to meet different criteria: "They require numerous comfortable walks . . . as well as many spots for gatherings, social diversions, and for reposing in the shade."[33] In contrast to the strict limitations of the formal French garden, often embedded in an urban space, an important principle of the English landscape garden also became essential to the spa garden: "The garden area must not be closed off. One's gaze must move easily beyond borders that merge gradually into the surrounding countryside."[34] It is significant, however, that only the "gaze" of spa guests, but not their bodies, were to "move . . . beyond [the] borders" of the spa. Similar to the earlier period, the interior spaces of the spa remained more important than the surrounding landscape that usually only provided "open and cheerful views."[35] Spa guests were neither expected nor encouraged to physically move into this landscape.

Hirschfeld's remarks on the "gardens at spas" thus draw our attention to the direct linkage between spatial construction and social practices. Spaces are defined by practices of "spacing," by people's movements within spaces.[36] Hirschfeld systematically listed the elements of spa gardens intended to serve different social practices. First, a spa had to have "pathways, resting places, and arbors where one can retreat in raw and windy weather to be protected in the open air."[37] This was an essential requirement for a spa, where walking outdoors was one of the most important activities while drinking the healing water in the morning and at other times of the day. "Nature walks" in landscape gardens became an increasingly important spa practice at a time when walks emerged as a bourgeois practice in Germany.[38] Different types of shelter in spa gardens were pointed out in the published discourse.[39] Second, providing shade was also central to the spatial construction of the spa garden – another reminder that spa guests spent a lot of time outside.[40] Third, the spa should have "broad and level allées [avenues] . . . , especially close to the residential buildings, the pump room, or around the baths."[41] An avenue served the dual function of providing access to the spa and fostering social interaction: "[Avenues] are not only suitable as entrances, but are also convenient for sociable walks, for connecting the spa guests, and for entertainment."[42] Fourth, an English landscape garden with "serpentine paths"[43] was essential. While "the strollers disperse themselves among the advancing and retreating trunks"[44] of the trees, the garden also needed to be furnished with wooden benches and other seating for the convenience of the spa guests.[45]

In the published discourse, the garden was now constructed as the center of the spa, and it was increasingly described as a spatial heterotopia facilitating social interaction. Hirschfeld's fifth requirement for "gardens at spas," therefore, combined the idea of the spa garden with the concept of the spa as a social meeting place. He called for the creation of "large squares surrounded by plants, where groups [*Gesellschaften*] can gather in the open air, where they can drink their coffee in the morning, dine, play, dance, or socialize in the warm evenings."[46] At the same time, authors of spa guides emphasized that spa gardens were to offer guests the freedom to choose between being alone or being in company. For example, Waitz wrote in his spa guide for Hofgeismar in 1792, "Every spa guest will find sufficient opportunities to use the most beautiful walks, to choose them according to his [*sic*] preferences, depending on whether he is looking for company or prefers to be alone."[47]

Sixth, Hirschfeld demanded that buildings – "music halls, dance halls, dining rooms, drinking houses, gaming halls, or small assembly rooms" – offer further opportunities for social interaction and help embellish the interior space of the spa.[48] Seventh, he mentioned the buildings "that serve as apartments for guests and for drinking and bathing."[49] Eighth and finally, Hirschfeld pointed out that the surrounding area of the spa, usually only enjoyed as a view, can be useful to spa guests "who seek longer and stronger movements and diversion."[50] These guests are referred to the "many wild paths [*wilde Spaziergänge*] for walking, horseback riding, [and] carriage rides in the surrounding areas."[51] All in all, Hirschfeld described the spa as a spatial heterotopia with many different locations that offered spa guests a multitude of activities, with the spa garden at its center.

As this new ideal became deeply ingrained in the published discourse in the 1780s, established spas like Pyrmont had difficulties in meeting the new expectations. The gradual expansion of Pyrmont's gardens – from the middle of the eighteenth century onward – happened at such an early point in time that avenues and their geometric layout still dominated the spa, only supplemented by a small grove (*Boskett*). (In Figure 3.12, the grove is on the far left.) In 1784, Marcard argued that the main avenue (see Figure 2.1) was the spatial and social center of the spa: "This avenue is the general meeting place in good weather, and the center of everything in Pyrmont."[52] Only

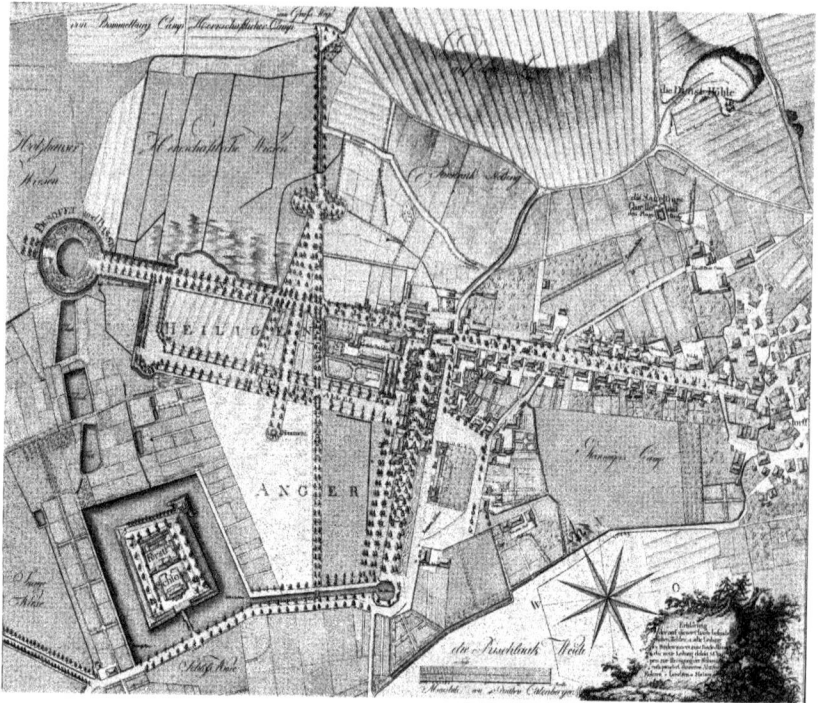

Figure 3.12 Map of Pyrmont, colored copperplate engraving by J.C. Dammert and F. Cöntgen, 1790. ("Plan von der Neustadt Pirmont mit ihrem Mineralbrunnen." Hannover, 1790. Museum im Schloss Bad Pyrmont.)

a year later, however, Hirschfeld made it clear that an avenue was not enough. He proposed to extend the grove (*Lustgebüsch*) in Pyrmont, to accentuate the view from the avenues into the grove, and even to enhance the accessibility and attractiveness of the walking trails around Pyrmont in order to facilitate the enjoyment of these views (*Aussichten*).[53]

Marcard was clearly aware of the change in the prevailing spatial ideal and of Pyrmont's shortcomings when measured against these new expectations. His *Description of Pyrmont* (*Beschreibung von Pyrmont*) contains some remarkably defensive passages:

> Comparisons have sometimes been made between other spas and Pyrmont, and people who are always filled up with the latest idea they have come across and who apply it with limited understanding to everything, have criticized about Pyrmont that it is not an English garden in its entirety and that one cannot leave the well and immediately lose oneself on a winding path and on narrow shady walking

trails near streams and groves. Such facilities are undoubtedly beautiful and pleasant, and can also be useful in such spas where a few dozen people gather, living like a family. But for Pyrmont, where everything is grand, such small-scale facilities would not be suitable, they would really be completely inappropriate and useless for a place where thousands gather during the summer.[54]

Marcard deliberately conceals the fact that the new spatial ideal of the spa included both an avenue and a landscape garden. He constructs the avenue and the landscape garden as opposites, only to downplay the landscape garden as the "latest idea," that is, a fashion that would pass, and to elevate the existing avenue in Pyrmont as the only possible way to design the interior space of a larger spa.

At the same time, Marcard's description of the landscape surrounding Pyrmont reveals that expectations about a spa's surroundings had not changed since the sixteenth and seventeenth centuries. With all its twists and contradictions, Marcard's depiction shows that gentle hills not encircling the spa too closely continued to be *de rigeur*: "The mountains that enclose the valley provide variety and beauty through their shapes and curves, through the considerable difference in their distance [from Pyrmont], and through their shades of green. But they do not enclose this valley in a basin, but it is completely open to the south and north, even if it does not seem so from some points of view. The free flow of the river proves it, and the high mountain that closes off the view, but not, in fact, the valley, in the south . . . is over two hours away from Pyrmont, far outside the valley."[55] The explanation of engraving no. VIII in Marcard's *Description of Pyrmont* (*Beschreibung von Pyrmont*), which shows a view of Pyrmont from afar, reinforces this traditional ideal of the landscape: "The area between the avenue [in Pyrmont] and that place [the nearby town of Lüdge] has the most beautiful meadows, and pastures dotted with cattle."[56]

Although Pyrmont lacked a landscape garden, it embodied the ideal late eighteenth-century spa in other ways, namely by offering a broad range of services and activities. As we have seen earlier, the ideal spa had to provide opportunities for entertainment, for the consumption of culture and goods, and for social interaction, thus combining a variety of spaces and practices in a small area. In Pyrmont, all activities were concentrated in a small space around the main avenue and the pump room (*Brunnenhaus*), which was located at one end of the avenue. Spa guests went for walks on the main avenue and in the adjacent avenues and grove; they drank the healing water and used the privies; they bought everything from medicine and books to fashion accessories in the sales boutiques along the avenue; they congregated in the coffeehouse, the theater, the ballroom, and the casino; and finally, they stayed in the lodging houses, many of them nearby. Unlike the sixteenth and seventeenth centuries, by the late eighteenth century spa guests no longer had to bring their own household goods and provide for their own needs because lodging houses were increasingly run like hotels.[57]

Marcard summarizes this in a few sentences: "On both sides [of the avenue] are the boutiques where all kinds of things are for sale. The pharmacy, the bookstore, the coffeehouse, the two large halls dedicated to entertainment and conversation, and where the faro bank is, the theater [*Komödienhaus*] and the well itself, everything is densely packed together here. The best apartments for the visitors are almost all very close to the avenue, and even certain conveniences [privies] that are very necessary for those who drink from the well are hidden from sight, but right next door."[58] Pyrmont's spatial construction, with an almost exclusive focus on its interior space, is underscored by the engravings included in Marcard's two-volume work. The spa guide contains seven engravings depicting Pyrmont itself – including a map of the spa – and only three engravings showing views of its surroundings.[59]

The development of Lauchstädt closely resembled that of Pyrmont. Lauchstädt was dominated by avenues and a pond in the geometric French garden style (Figure 3.13), but it also acquired a small English landscape garden.[60] Like Pyrmont, Lauchstädt provided a wide range of activities and amenities for spa guests in a very small space. Designed by the Merseburg architect Johann Wilhelm Chryselius from 1776 onward, Lauchstädt consisted of a series of pavilions built in the late Baroque style:

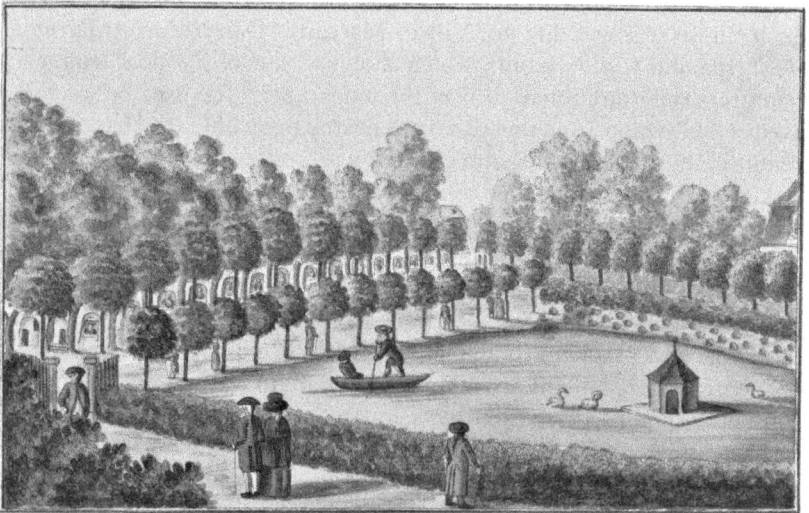

Figure 3.13 Lauchstädt, pond and avenue, colored etching by Friedrich August Scheureck, c. 1790. ("Die neue Allee am grossen Teich in Lauchstaed von der lincken Seite." Leipzig: Klein, c. 1790. Klassik Stiftung Weimar/Museums/shelf mark KGr/02570.)

the assembly hall (*Kursaal*) used as a ballroom and dining hall, flanked by a well pavilion doubling as a reading room and a bathing pavilion (Figure 3.14), and an older pavilion used as a games room (Figure 3.15). In addition, Lauchstädt offered colonnades with sales boutiques along the river Laucha (Figure 3.16).[61]

Karlsbad also faced similar challenges as Pyrmont and Lauchstädt. The descriptions of Karlsbad in the published discourse of the 1780s point toward the changing ideal of the spa. The spa offered ample entertainments and opportunities for consumption of culture and luxury goods,[62] but it only had an avenue and no landscape garden. In his 1780 travelogue, Johann Peter Willebrand provided a brief but revealing description of the entertainments (*Lustbarkeiten*) in Karlsbad. First, Willebrand mentioned the avenue, which, however, lacked benches and shelter from the rain. Strikingly, both were requirements mentioned by Hirschfeld. Next, Willebrand turned the reader's attention to the "spacious and glamorous coffee halls," the Saxon and Bohemian halls, "where one can play billiards and chess, get coffee, hot chocolate, lemonade, and raspberry juice."[63] Further entertainments were provided by the balls and the theater. Only at the end did Willebrand mention walks in the immediate surroundings of the spa, including to the garden of the spa physician Dr. David Becher, before returning to a description of goods like carved stones and artwork made from tin and iron that spa guests could purchase. Finally, the author

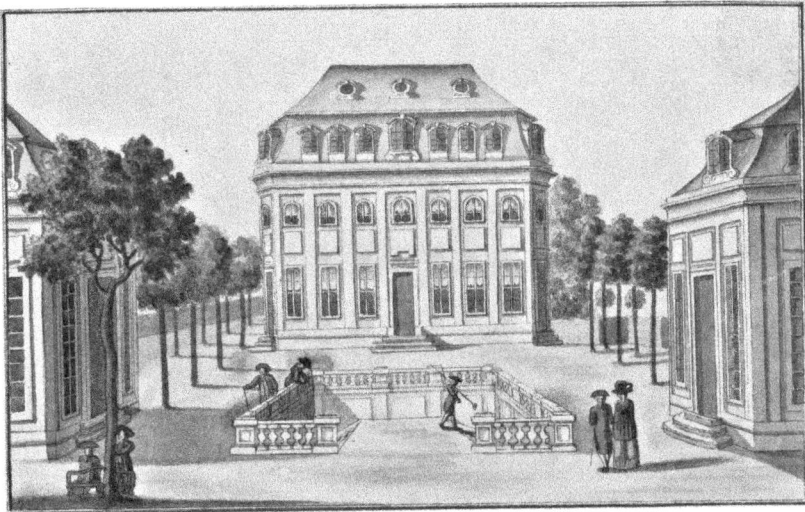

Figure 3.14 Lauchstädt, assembly hall (ballroom) and healing well, colored etching by Friedrich August Scheureck, c. 1790. ("Der neue Tanzsaal und der Brunnen in Lauchstaedt." Leipzig: Klein, c. 1790. Klassik Stiftung Weimar/Museums/shelf mark KGr/01916.)

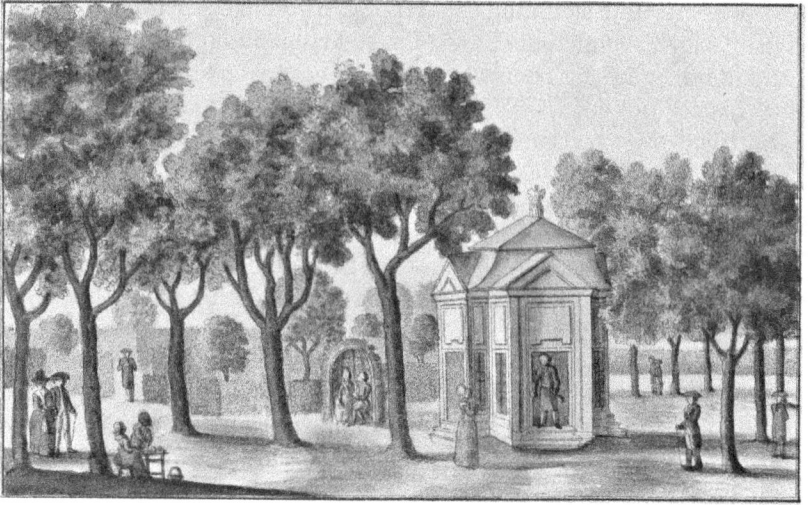

Figure 3.15 Lauchstädt, pavilion, colored etching by Friedrich August Scheureck, c. 1790. ("Der hinterste Pavillion in der großen Kastanien Allee." Leipzig: Klein, c. 1790. Klassik Stiftung Weimar/Museums/shelf mark KGr/02572.)

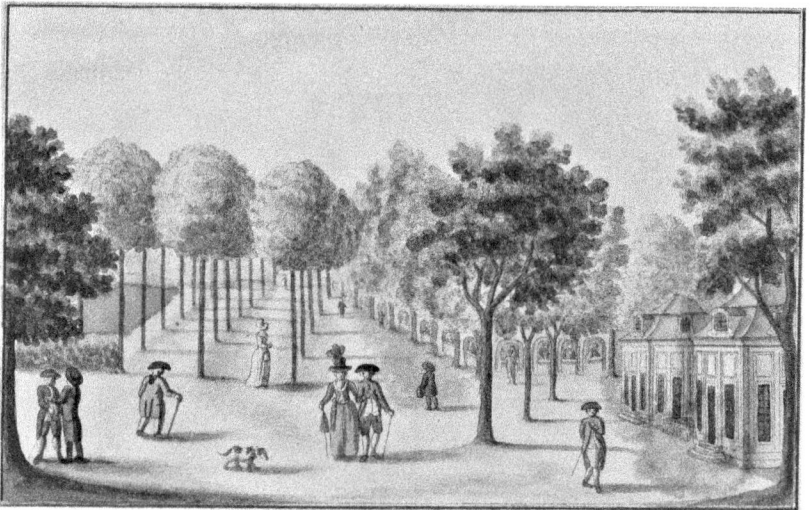

Figure 3.16 Lauchstädt, avenue with pond on left and sales boutiques on right, colored etching by Friedrich August Scheureck, c. 1790. ("Die neue Allee am großen Teich in Lauchstaedt von der rechten Seite." Leipzig: Klein, c. 1790. Klassik Stiftung Weimar/Museums/shelf mark KGr/00952.)

mentioned other (private) gardens that offered the opportunity for communal meals in the surrounding area.[64]

In the late eighteenth century, the new ideal of a spa's interior space that combined an English landscape garden with a wide range of facilities and buildings was put into practice at spas that were either completely redesigned or newly built. Wilhelm IX, count of Hanau and landgrave of Hesse, had the financial wherewithal to make Hofgeismar and Wilhelmsbad, and later also Nenndorf,[65] prime examples of this new ideal. Hofgeismar had originally been designed in the French garden style but was remodeled as an English landscape garden beginning in the late 1780s. The redesign included architectural changes according to plans by Wilhelm's court architect Simon Louis de Rys, in particular the construction of a new "spring temple" and a small palace named "Montcherie" as a summer residence.[66]

Wilhelmsbad was newly built in the 1780s and fulfilled all contemporary expectations. An extensive English landscape garden surrounded the spa on both sides of the avenue. Inspired by princely summer residences such as the Favorite in Mainz,[67] the spa buildings consisted of a series of pavilions along the avenue. Similar to Lauchstädt, Wilhelmsbad had a central spa building, the so-called colonnade building (*Arkadenbau*), that served as a dance and assembly hall and had two smaller assembly rooms for faro and billiards as well as guest accommodations. Other pavilions served as lodgings, shower and bath houses, and as the theater and stables. There was also a "spring temple" and boutiques.[68] (See Figures 3.17 and 3.18, the spring temple is in the center in Figure 3.18, between the trees, and the sales boutiques are on

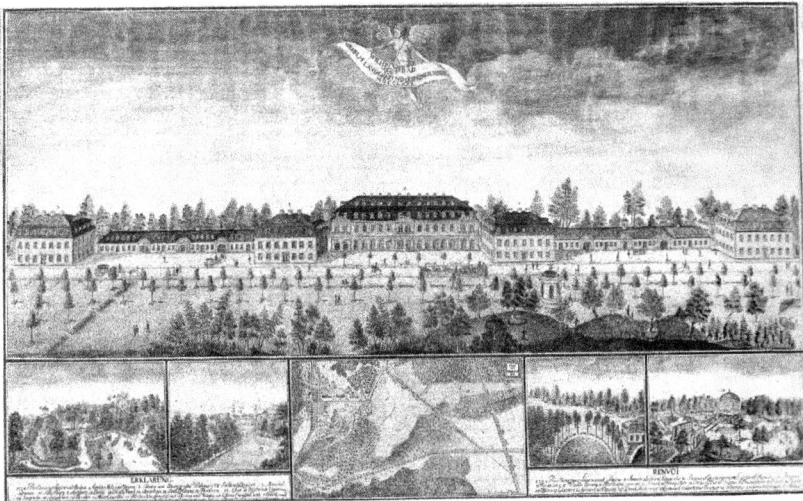

Figure 3.17 Wilhelmsbad, colored engraving, 1780. ("Wilhelmsbad. Gebaut von Wilhelm. Landgraf und Erbprinz zu Hessen. MDCCLXXX." Historisches Museum Hanau Schloss Philippsruhe.)

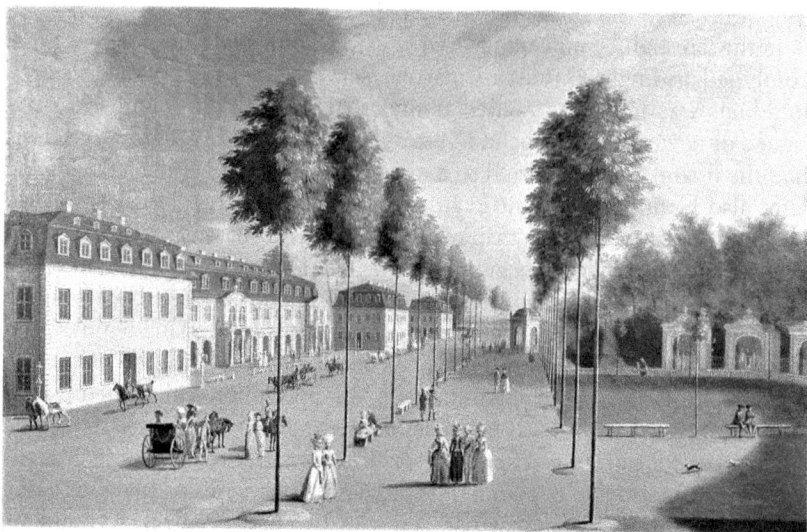

Figure 3.18 Wilhelmsbad, avenue, painting by Anton Wilhelm Tischbein, c. 1783. (Historisches Museum Hanau Schloss Philippsruhe.)

the far right.) The English landscape garden offered a wide range of choices for spa visitors: equipment for exercise and games, benches for resting, and a merry-go-round (Figure 3.19), a pond with boats (Figure 3.20), a grotto, a hedge theater (*Heckentheater*), an artificial hill that served as a lookout, a hermitage, and last but not least, a princely summer palace.[69] (All the amenities at Wilhelmsbad are shown in the small images at the bottom in Figure 3.17, an engraving commissioned to advertise the spa.)

Mid-sized and smaller spas that faced either spatial or financial constraints and were thus limited in their options for remodeling did what they could to conform to the new ideal. However, providing urban amenities *and* a full-fledged landscape garden proved difficult. Rehburg, Bertrich, Meinberg, Bocklet, Brückenau, and Godesberg are instructive examples of how this played out in individual spas during the late eighteenth century. In his spa guide of Rehburg, published in 1773, Christoph Weber claimed that Rehburg met general expectations regarding services and entertainments after improvements had been made: "In addition to the comfort of the already existing apartments, the spa guests at this place now find everything that is expected and required for the necessity and comfort of life at other spas. Food and drink are . . . available in abundance. One can find a billiard table, a bookstore, shops with millinery and other goods, and very good music. Games, dances, fireworks, and evening illuminations are frequent."[70] In the small spa of Bertrich, the elector of Trier built a coffee pavilion, various games, swings, as well as a

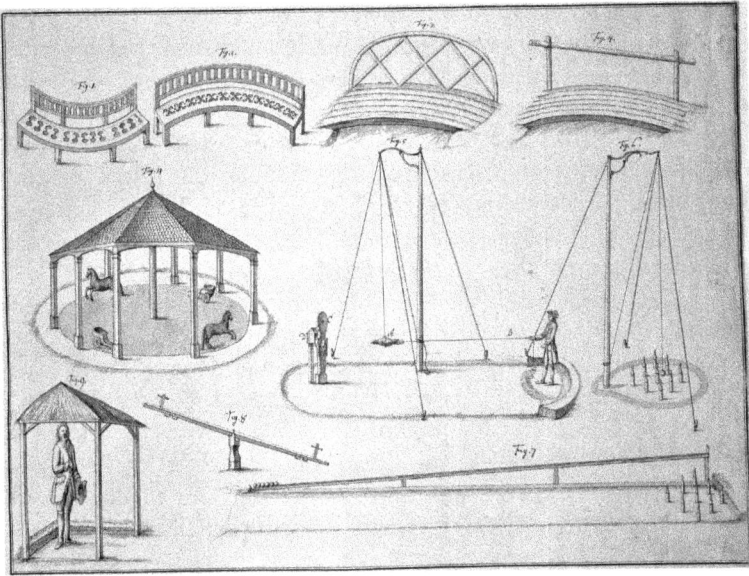

Figure 3.19 Wilhelmsbad, equipment for landscape garden including games and exercise, drawing, c. 1777. (Unbekannter Zeichner: Hanau, Wilhelmsbad, Entwurf für Spiele, GK II (1) 20847/Stiftung Preußische Schlösser und Gärten Berlin-Brandenburg/Fotograf: SPSG.)

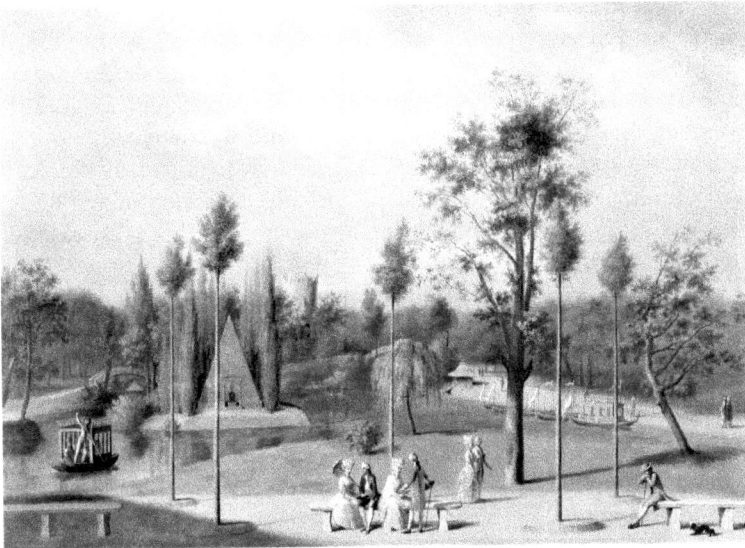

Figure 3.20 Wilhelmsbad, pond and island with pyramid, painting by Anton Wilhelm Tischbein, c. 1783. (© Kulturstiftung des Hauses Hessen, Museum Schloss Fasanerie, Eichenzell bei Fulda, FAS B 432.)

bowling alley and a billiard pavilion, among other facilities, in a narrow space along the Üßbach, a small stream running through the spa (Figure 3.21).[71]

Many spas aspired to integrate elements of the English landscape garden into their interior spaces. In Meinberg, groves reminiscent of landscape gardens were planted between the avenues connecting the spa buildings to reflect the new garden taste.[72] A similar solution was favored in Bocklet, where the spa complex consisted of two avenues that intersected in the center and thus created four equal-sized partitions. These squares were laid out as small English landscape gardens, each with its own specific feature like a pond and exercise equipment (Figure 3.22).[73]

In his 1782 article on Brückenau, Göckingk praised the avenues and the "pleasant walks" in the spa, including an "English path," which, however, was not circular, so one could only walk up and down.[74] As Brückenau lacked a full-fledged landscape garden, Göckingk suggested that the spa guests could dine from time to time in a small oak grove "barely 200 steps from the spa buildings." In spite of the short distance, he described this place as already "in the middle of the forest."[75] And finally, Göckingk recommended outings by carriage into the surrounding area, but the destinations were places perceived as "civilized": "the Hessian smalt or blue paint factory and mirror factory" or the "princely palace at Römershag."[76] Göckingk's suggestions again demonstrate that the spa discourse continued to place an emphasis on the interior spaces of the spa and that spa visitors were rarely encouraged to move beyond the boundaries of the spa district and into the open countryside.

A 1791 advertisement for the new spa of Godesberg also exemplifies the expectations, indeed requirements, for a spa to successfully inscribe itself in the published discourse, namely facilities for walking, shaded areas, an avenue as a social meeting place, "lovely views" (*reitzende Aussichten*) of the surrounding landscape, and proximity to the nearby town of Bonn. At the same time, the author used skillful rhetoric not only to downplay the fact that Godesberg did not have a landscape garden and that the walking trails led through existing, "wild" groves but also to reinterpret this as an advantage:

> The particularly lovely area around the well seems to have been created by nature especially for walking. Wild, isolated parts of this area have been connected by paths into a whole walking space, and thus the shade that is lacking in new gardens has been preserved. Also, the four avenues created close to the well do not deprive one of the invigorating view of surveying the well drinkers [*Brunnentrinker*]. The value of a stay at this spa is enhanced by the proximity of the river Rhine, the sweeping views of the same, and of the so-called Seven Hills [*Siebenberge*, today *Siebengebirge*], the picturesque location of the dilapidated Godesberg castle, a small stream flowing through the pleasant valley, [and] the short distance from the electoral residence town of Bonn.[77]

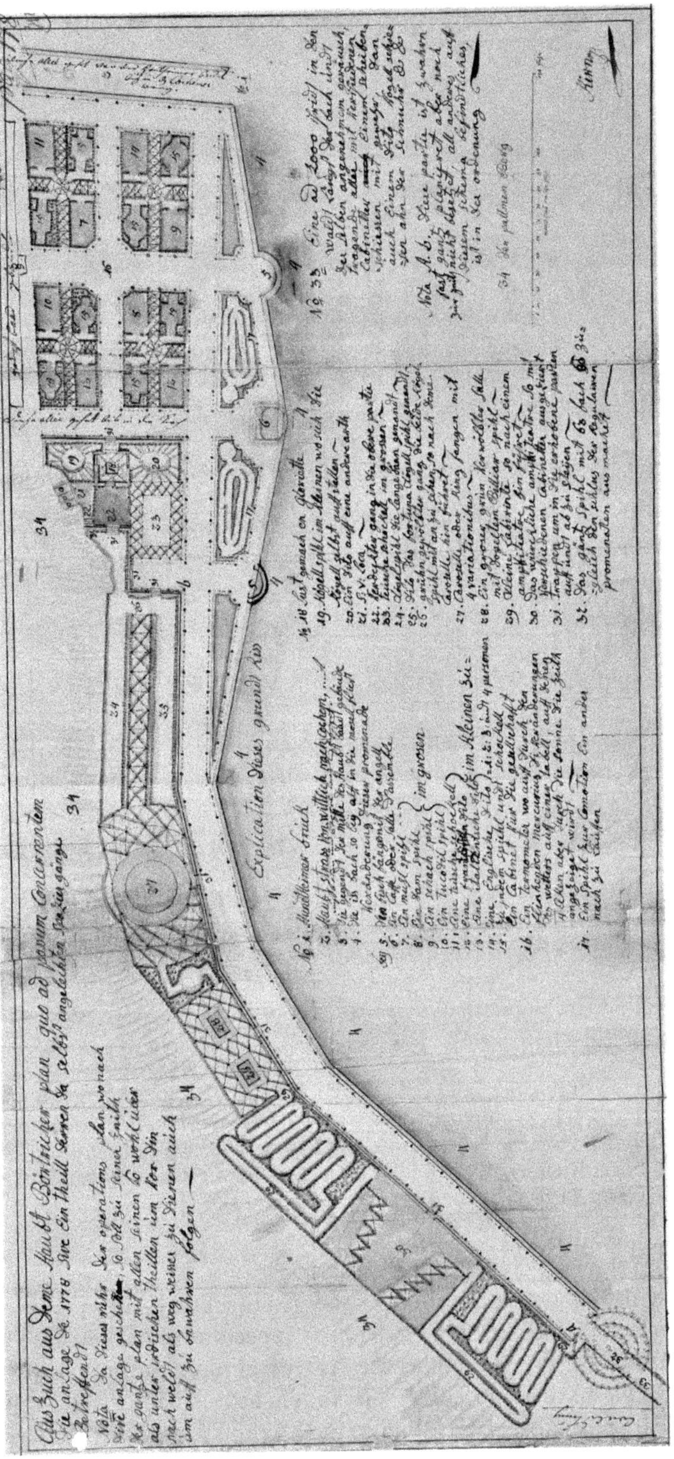

Figure 3.21 Bertrich, leisure facilities along the Üßbach, colored drawing by H. Kirn, 1778. (Landeshauptarchiv Koblenz, 1 C 2719 Bl. 318.)

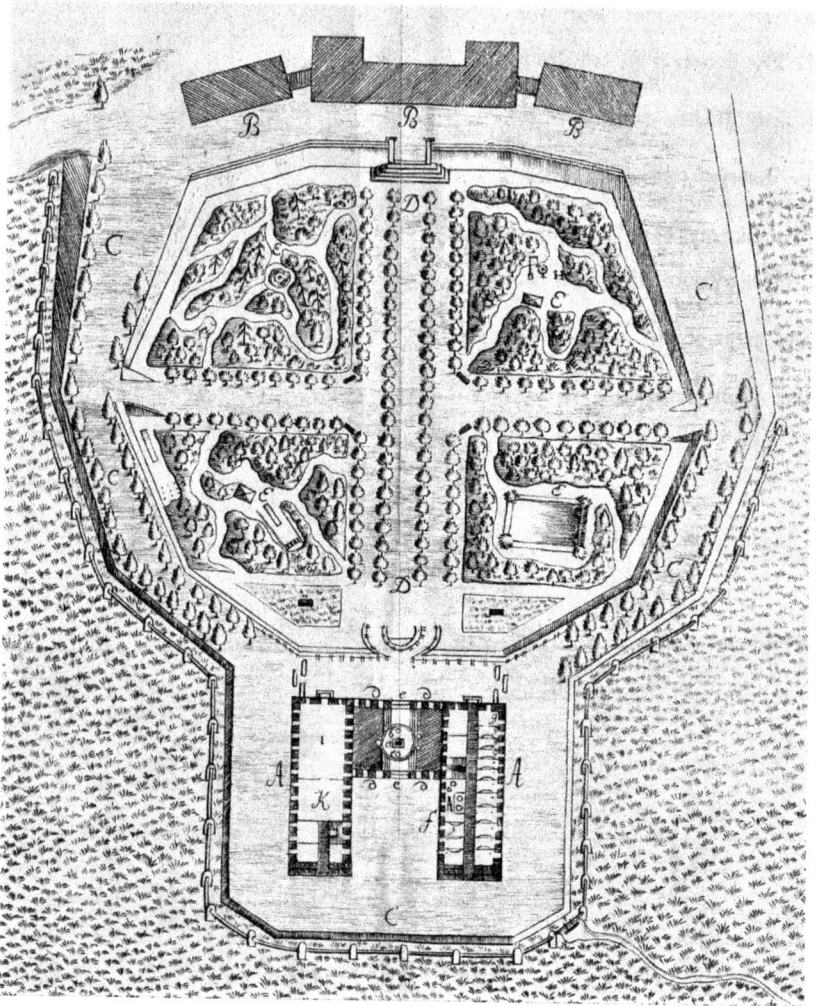

Figure 3.22 Map of Bocklet, engraving, 1793. ("Plan der neuen Anlage zu Bocklet 1793." In Goldwitz, Sebastian. *Die Mineralquellen zu Kissingen und Bocklet im Fränkischen Hochstifte Würzburg*, after 446. Würzburg: Rienner, 1795. SLUB Dresden/Digitale Sammlungen/Hist.urb. Germ.2190.)

In line with the article about Godesberg, Hirschfeld's descriptions of Wiesbaden and Ems confirm the prevailing expectations of the 1780s and the early 1790s. At the same time, they offer a glimpse of the changes yet to come. As we have seen earlier, Wiesbaden, as a (small) town, embodied the ideal spa before 1750 (Figure 3.3), while Ems was regarded as unattractive because of its location in a narrow valley of the river Lahn (Figure 3.6). By the 1780s, this had changed dramatically. Wiesbaden remained a densely built small town, but Hirschfeld described it as a "miserable little town with narrow streets." He continued, "Wiesbaden is situated on a low plain and in an area that does not have any particular charms. One has to look for them first in the neighborhood and at some distance toward the Rhine. It also lacks shady paths and notable facilities for decent public amusements."[78]

This does not mean, however, that Ems and its surrounding landscape were already regarded as attractive, as would be the case by the early nineteenth century. Rather, Hirschfeld's description of Ems demonstrates the slow and gradual change in the spa discourse during the 1780s: "The location of Ems deep between high rocky mountains is almost melancholy and desolate, yet the slopes are partly fertile and planted with grapevine; . . . But the location of Ems has some inconvenience, as the mountains enclose the valley too narrowly, . . . One sees here only one avenue, which furthermore is very narrow. The narrowness of the valley does not allow for the creation of more extensive walks. One has to look for these in the wilderness of the mountains and the neighboring area."[79] The location of Ems was far from desirable. Moreover, the interior spaces of the spa did not fulfill contemporary expectations. But – similar to the aforementioned article about Godesberg – Hirschfeld's reference to the surrounding landscape (a landscape one could not only look at but also walk through) indicates a gradual change in discourse and practice.[80]

In sum, the spa as a spatial heterotopia combined a variety of places and activities in a very small space. It was not the individual places and activities that constituted the spa as a spatial heterotopia but the diverse practices concentrated in one space that normally occupied several separate – urban and rural – spaces in late eighteenth-century society. The spa thus offered guests a unique combination of experiences in a space (and time) outside of everyday life. Foucault defines gardens, fairgrounds, and vacation villages as heterotopias of compensation.[81] By the end of the eighteenth century, the spa had also become such a heterotopia, its offerings anticipating what would become part of a typical tourist experience in the nineteenth and twentieth centuries. As we will see in Chapter 4, by the early nineteenth century the spa became a multiplier of even more aspects of modern tourist expectations and experiences.

Court, Town, and Countryside: Frictions and Contradictions

The combination of different spaces and practices that marked the spa as a spatial heterotopia also made for potential frictions and contradictions. Contemporaries focused on two aspects: the close proximity of courtly and bourgeois spaces and activities, and the spa's role in combining town and countryside, urban and rural life. Baggesen summarized Pyrmont's inherently contradictory character as a spatial heterotopia: "One is in a quiet shed far from the court and the city and large gatherings, but the court, the city, and the large gatherings are also in the shed. In the countryside one is surrounded by all the phenomena of the city."[82] Or, as Marcard put it in his *Description of Pyrmont* (*Beschreibung von Pyrmont*), the spa is "at the same time court, town, and countryside."[83]

As we have already seen, spas usually served as summer residences for their princely owners. Thus, the buildings designed for the entertainment and accommodation of spa guests were in close proximity to a princely palace, resulting in noble and bourgeois practices coexisting in a confined space. The importance of the spa as a space for princely representation found its expression in the way the palace always formed an essential part of the spa complex. In many cases, long vistas created a connection between the central areas of the spa and the palace. Examples of such spatial arrangements are legion. Pyrmont castle, a Baroque palace built on the base of a destroyed Renaissance castle (Figure 3.9),[84] has an elevated position and is connected to the spa by an avenue (Figure 3.12, the palace is in the bottom left corner). Following the Gothic fashion in eighteenth- and nineteenth-century architecture and based on the model of Shrubs Hill (today Fort Belvedere) in Windsor Great Park in England, the princely palace in Wilhelmsbad was built in the form of a decaying medieval castle. This spectacular building attracted immediate attention.[85] There was also a long vista from the avenue and main spa building (*Arkadenbau*) to the "castle,"[86] a constant visual reminder of the prince and his status in the central spa area. In Lauchstädt, the castle, which is located at some distance from the spa, was connected to the spa district through a walkway and a long vista. In Teplitz, the castle of the princes of Clary-Aldringen sits at the center of the spa town (Figure 3.23).

In some princely spas, the palace was, effectively, sending a mixed message about the ruler's role in the heterotopia of the spa. While the palace architecturally blended in with the other spa buildings, it was elevated and thus literally looked down on the spa. Bocklet (Figure 3.22, the steps up to the princely palace are visible at the top of the image) and especially Brückenau (Figure 3.24) are examples of this spatial construction. Göckingk wrote about Brückenau, "The princely dwelling-house [*Wohnhaus*] is characterized by nothing more than its exquisite location because one overlooks the entire spa from there."[87] The use of the term "dwelling-house" is telling here. Göckingk implied that the prince was a regular member of the spa society, who, almost like a member of the bourgeoisie, lived in a "dwelling-house." This reinforces the idea of the spa as a spatial heterotopia, with the prince and his palace blending into the larger space of the spa. At the same time, Göckingk subtly suggested that the location of the palace was an expression of the ruler's status; the palace's elevated position represented the prince's elevated position among the spa guests.[88]

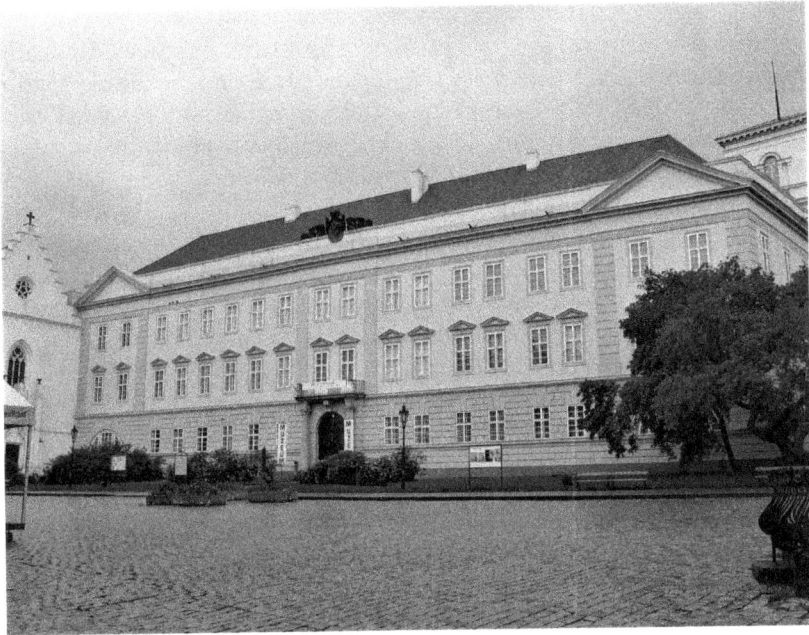

Figure 3.23 Teplitz (today Teplice), princely palace. (Photograph by author.)

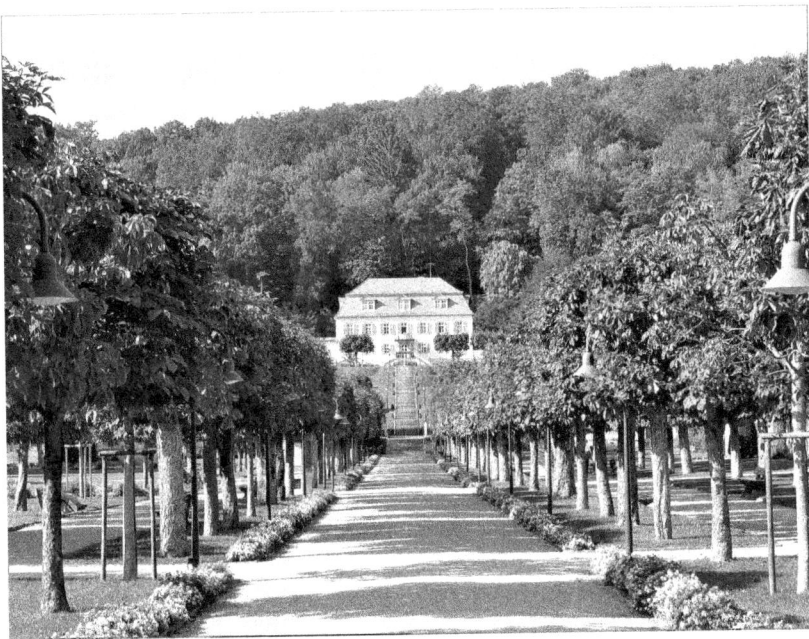

Figure 3.24 Brückenau, princely palace. (Photograph by author.)

This spatial constellation of princely spas was also reflected in the practices of spa visitors. Courtly practices and the activities of bourgeois spa guests coexisted at the spas and often occupied separate spaces, especially before the mid-eighteenth century.[89] At the same time, manifold spatial overlaps existed between these practices because they took place in a confined space. This gave rise to potential friction and conflict.[90] Hirschfeld's description of Hofgeismar alludes to these tensions:

> Several stalls selling fashion accessories extend from the gallery of the lower left wing [of the spa building]. People walk, play, and dance in between these stalls, and one almost always sees the landgrave, his court, or some other illustrious [noble] company. This place is therefore the liveliest part of the spa buildings. Although the greatest part of these buildings are occupied by the court when it is present [at the spa], guests can also take different rooms here, if they do not prefer to stay in the large nearby bathhouse. . . . The presence of the numerous and glamorous court may, of course, lead to some inconveniences for spa guests who wish to enjoy the peace and quiet here. But it is also certain that the court does not want to cause the slightest constraint, and that strangers can enjoy complete and agreeable freedom here under the court's eyes, if they so wish. The good prince provides for their comfort and pleasure at great expense. All spa guests can attend the French plays and public concerts, which the court constantly holds here, free of charge.[91]

Princes employed various practices to display their power and status at spas. The presence of the ruling prince at the spa was accompanied, for example, by illuminations, fireworks, and birthday celebrations for members of the princely family, and even military parades.[92] In these instances, the spa guests took on the role of spectators, like a prince's subjects did in his residence town. However, in the last third of the eighteenth century the spa reflected a broader process of change, when "the population, especially in and around the residence towns, came more into focus as an addressee of princely representation and as a consumer of courtly entertainment."[93] The princes' enlightened self-representation vis-à-vis their subjects in the residence towns manifested itself in allowing bourgeois access to the court theater and the palace gardens.[94]

By the late eighteenth century, the conceptualization of the spa as a spatial heterotopia led to bourgeois demands for access to spaces and activities that in the early modern period had been reserved for the exclusive use of the prince, the court, and the nobility. At the late eighteenth-century spa, gardens, balls, concerts, theater performances, billiards, gambling, and other spaces and practices – including the princely banquet table – were supposed to be open to the entire spa society of the upper middle class and the nobility. Because the spa was a place outside the limitations of everyday life, all spaces were to be accessible to the upper middle class without restriction. However, a fundamental tension that ultimately could not be resolved[95] remained between princely representation, even enlightened representation, and a bourgeois ideal of freedom projected onto the spas and the English landscape gardens.[96] As we will see in Chapter 6, the published discourse continued to grapple with these issues as it attempted to define the relationship between princes, the nobility, and the bourgeoisie in the late eighteenth and early nineteenth centuries.

The contrast between town and countryside constituted another sphere of tension that deeply impacted the perception of late eighteenth-century spas. As described previously, the urban ideal of the spa in the early modern discourse was modified during the late 1770s and 1780s. While a spa was still expected to provide urban amenities and services, the new English landscape gardens and pavilion-style architecture signified a shift toward a rural spatial ideal. Contemporaries were keenly aware of this tension and repeatedly addressed it in the published discourse. A travelogue about Pyrmont published in 1783 provides an example of a positive representation of this dual function of the spa: "The spa itself actually consists only of a long and wide tree-lined street; it has a rural character and resembles a Dutch village. The large double avenue, where the ball-comedy-coffee- and eating-house, the bookshop, and many boutiques are located, and which has the pump room [*Brunnenhaus*] and a basin with a fountain as its vantage point, is a wonderful piece."[97] Pyrmont, the author continued, offered "semi-urban, semi-rural promenades," "where country life and people of quality are so happily combined."[98]

In his 1790 advertising pamphlet for Lauchstädt, the spa physician Johann Ernst Andreas Koch also characterized this dual function as a positive feature. Koch defined Lauchstädt as a spa that offered both the sociability and amenities of a town and the solitude, simplicity, and tranquility of the countryside:

> For those who love noisy amusements and seek distraction and movement of the body in the bustle of society, the avenues of chestnut and linden trees, which have been extended and provided with new walkways, the band of musicians on the chestnut avenue, the daily and hourly opportunity to dance and play in the halls and pavilions designated for these purposes, the shops on the chestnut avenue with their covered walkway filled with all possible offerings, as well as the merry-go-round, which has been built in this area, the [communal] breakfasts, usually on Mondays and Thursdays, the five weekly plays, . . . the illuminations of the avenue, which often happen in the evening, and the fireworks in the meadow . . . provide ample opportunity. In contrast, the hill with a winding path [*Schneckenberg*] near the linden avenue, the beautiful path around the pond planted with flowers on the sides, the solidly built well and the castle garden, with

its shady walks, its graceful benches and niches, its kitchen garden, seemingly planted in careless order, and its fruit trees, provide quiet pleasure, peace, and cooling. Here it is lovely to watch the awakening of dawn, or to wander about in the evening air under the silver light of the moon, or to sit alone in sweet fantasies. . . . What art has done in consideration of the walkways around and at the well, nature has given in even greater measure outside of the circle of the avenue, and has ensured that even those who cannot or do not desire to participate in games and dances, and who like the simple things of the countryside more than the social noise, find their entertainment in walks near and far.[99]

In contrast, in 1788, an article entitled "Why not rural in the countryside?" ("Warum auf dem Lande nicht ländlich?") in the *Journal of Luxury and Fashions* (*Journal des Luxus und der Moden*) offered a negative assessment of the close connection between the urban and rural characteristics of spas. The anonymous author of this article criticized that the average spa guest "takes the city with him into the field": "So many . . . regularly travel . . . to the spa . . . , and even there they live as if within the town walls!"[100] The author unfavorably compared the urban lifestyle supposedly prevailing at the *teutsche* spas to a rural way of life ascribed to the spa of Baden in Switzerland.[101] This was, in fact, an entirely spurious argument. Baden was the most urban spa in Switzerland, a town where the Federal Diet of Switzerland (*eidgenössische Tagsatzung*) met repeatedly during the early modern period. The author, however, created an image of Baden for his readers that did not include the actual town. Rather, he focused on outings to the town's surrounding areas and views of the landscape, thus anticipating a change in the published spa discourse that began in the 1790s and came to fruition in the early nineteenth century.

These examples show that the urban and rural features of late eighteenth-century spas – often described in terms of "art" (*Kunst*) and "nature" (*Natur*) – could be construed in the published discourse as both complementary and opposing principles. However, positive interpretations of the combination of town and countryside, of art and nature, prevailed in the late eighteenth century. As research has shown, Enlightenment thinking of the late eighteenth century had not yet defined "art" and "nature" as opposites but as complementary principles. Only in the nineteenth century were they mainly defined in an antagonistic way.[102] This is reflected in the spa discourse: the spa as a spatial heterotopia was presented as a successful combination of the two principles of country and city life. At the same time, however, the idealization of the countryside in the article from the *Journal of Luxury and Fashions* (*Journal des Luxus und der Moden*) as well as the gradual change in the perception of the landscape surrounding the spa that we saw in

Hirschfeld's description of Ems point toward the radical reconfiguration of the spatial heterotopia of the spa in the 1790s and especially in the early nineteenth century.

Notes

1. Quoted in Studt, "Badenfahrt," 46: "zivilisierter als die wenig einladende, verregnete Bergwelt, in der sie die strapaziöse Badekur verbringen müßten. Denn schließlich sollten ihre Gemüter nicht ganz von den waldigen Abhängen der sie umgebenden Berge erdrückt werden."
2. Hoser, *Beschreibung von Franzensbrunn*, 1799, 114: "Ein Brunnenort so gross auch immer sein medizinischer Ruf seyn mag bleibt, wenn er nicht einige Naturschönheiten besitzt, oder in deren Abgang durch die Kunst einige Verschönerungen erhalten hat, ein trauriges Exil für Jeden, den seine misslichen Gesundheitsumstände ihn zu besuchen nöthigen."
3. See, e.g., Thomas, *Man and the Natural World*, 242–244; Dülmen, *Das irdische Paradies*, 156.
4. See Blondel, *Außfürliche Erklärung*, 1688, 8–9: "Ob nun zwar diese Statt in einem Thal gelegen/ und mit Bergen und Wäldern umbgeben ist/ so ist doch sie mit einer gar gesunde Lufft/ sonderlich fruchtbar- und anmüthigkeit begabet/ also daß wo man seine Augen hinwendet/ viele und unterschiedliche der spielenden Natur wunderwercken ersehen kan/ welche höchlich daß Gemüt und Augen erlustigen. Nechst bey der Statt seint hin und wieder weit und breite ebene zu sehen/ welchem die Vieh sehr bequemlich seint. Auff den Hügeln gitbs [*sic*] feiste zu allen Früchten dienliche äcker."
5. See [Pöllnitz], *Amusemens des eaux d'Aix la Chapelle*, 1737, engravings at the end of the volume.
6. Henkel, *Bethesda Portuosa*, 1746.
7. Henkel, *Bethesda Portuosa*, 1746, 6: "Der Bade-Brunnen selbst liegt im Städtgen drinnen, oder doch in dem nächsten Garten daran, wodurch denn nicht ein geringer Vorzug gegen diejenigen Bäder erhellet, welche insgemein von Städten und Dörfern in Feldern, Wäldern, ja wüsten Orten sehr abgeschnitten sind, und also wol der menschlichen Handreichung als andern Umgangs zur Ergetzlichkeit, welche die halbe Cur und Artzney ist, schwerlich geniessen können, ja wohl gar entbehren müssen."
8. Henkel, *Bethesda Portuosa*, 1746, 3.
9. Henkel, *Bethesda Portuosa*, 1746, 2: "Die Luft-Höhe ist so schön, als sie die gütige Natur nur verleihen kan, nicht bergigt, aber auch nicht sumpfig, nicht rauh und scharf, doch auch nicht letzschig und schwülig, sondern von einer wohlgenaturten Mischung."
10. Henkel, *Bethesda Portuosa*, 1746, 3.
11. [Schütte], *Amusemens des eaux de Cleve*, 1748, 58: "Wozu noch kommt, daß wohl kein Ort in Europa, der wegen seiner angenehmen Situation berühmt ist, zu finden; allwo man so viel Allees oder Spatzier-Gänge, lustige Hügel, ungemein ergötzende Aussichten, grüne Berge, schattige Thäler, fruchtbare Korn- und Weide-Länder, in einer so wunderbaren Ordnung, beysammen antrift, als zu Cleve."
12. Koromandel-Wedekind, *Der Brunnengast*, 1744, 8: "Pyrmont ist zwar nicht groß, auch keine Stadt zu nennen, | Doch muß man ihm den Ruhm vom Lustgefilde gönnen, | Das viele Anmuth hegt, die reinste Luft genießt, | Mit Viehzucht, Wild und Fisch, und Frucht versehen ist."
13. Merian, *Topographia Hassiae*, 142: "ein alte/ zwar nicht grosse/ aber ihrer herrlichen/ un[d] heylsamen Bäder halber eine berühmbte Statt."

14. See also the fold-out map in [Merveilleux], *Amusemens des eaux de Schwalbach*, 1739, that depicts Schwalbach in 1728. The map emphasizes the built environment and the two intersecting avenues, thus representing Schwalbach as an urban space. Compare this with the Merian drawings of Schwalbach in Diefenbacher, *Schwalbacher Reise*. The contrast between the published copperplate engravings in Merian and Merveilleux on the one hand and the decidedly rural character of the Merian drawings on the other is striking.

15. Wilhelm I. von Hessen, *Wir Wilhelm*, 75: "öde Kur" – "Das Bad liegt abscheulich, zwischen Felsen und Klüfte der Lahn eingezwängt."

16. Welcker, *Gründliche Beschreibung des Schlangen-Bads*, 1747, 9–10: "Es liegt das Schlangen-Bad in einem von Natur tieff eingesenckten Thal, welches um und um von hohen Bergen und Baum-reichen Wäldern umgeben ist; Dahero der Ort zwar an sich selbst eben nicht sonderlich angenehm ist; es hat aber der unverdrossene Fleiß, durch die schöne Gebäude und weitläufftige, und plaisirliche kunstreiche Allée die natürliche Situation also verbessert, daß man dieselbe nunmehr mit gutem Recht unter die angenehmste zählen kan, und ob auch gleich allhier nichts andres, als Laub und Gras wächset, so hat man doch an allerley Victualien einen grossen Uberfluß."

17. [Moser], *Brauchbare Nachrichten*, 1758, 8: "Das Gebürg herum ist hoch, und ragen an vielen Orten Felsen und grosse Steine heraus."

18. See [Moser], *Brauchbare Nachrichten*, 1758, 9–17.

19. See Chapter 1.

20. See, e.g., Schreber, *Reise nach Carlsbad*, 1771.

21. *Neu-verbessert- und vermehrtes denckwürdiges Kayser Carls-Baad*, 1736, 34: "Etlicher dieser Stadt und Landes Situation unerfahrne würden kaum glauben daß bereits beschriebene, und daß dieser Orth so Leuthseelig, um Willen der umliegenden Anhöhen und Bergen."

22. See *Neu-verbessert- und vermehrtes denckwürdiges Kayser Carls-Baad*, 1736, 34: "Ohnerachtet."

23. See *Neu-verbessert- und vermehrtes denckwürdiges Kayser Carls-Baad*, 1736, 36. See also Tilling, *Nachricht vom Carlsbade*, 1756.

24. See [Grundig], *Beschreibung seiner, im Jahr 1751 in das Käyser Carls-Bad gethanen Reise*, 1754, 88–95.

25. [Grundig], *Beschreibung seiner, im Jahr 1751 in das Käyser Carls-Bad gethanen Reise*, 1754, 80: "Denn so gar enge schließet sich zwischen besagten Bergen das Thal, welches ich mit allem Recht eine Schlufft nenne, zusammen."

26. [Grundig], *Beschreibung seiner, im Jahr 1751 in das Käyser Carls-Bad gethanen Reise*, 1754, 61, see 76.

27. See Bauhin, *Ein New Badbuch*, 1602. See also Rumpel, "Zwischen Kurvergnügen und Verkauf"; Mehring, *Badenfahrt*, 140–141.

28. Adelholzen is not on the map at the end of this book because it remained a spa with only local significance during the period covered in this study.

29. See the long list of luxury goods available in Nenndorf in [Springer], *Auch einige Worte eines Nieder-Deutschen*, 1795, 17–20.

30. Böttger, *Beschreibung der Gesundbrunnen und Bäder bey Hofgeismar*, 1772, 11: "Hier ist alles anmuthige in einer Kette gleichsam vereiniget, und Sinne und Geist können sich hier vergnügen."

31. See Hirschfeld, *Theorie der Gartenkunst*, vol. 5, 1785, 85–115. Hirschfeld, *Theory of Garden Art*, 414–417, provides a partial translation of the German original.

32. Kehn has shown that Hirschfeld's positive description of the spa of Wilhelmsbad in his section on "Gärten bey Gesundbrunnen" served as a kind of "letter of application" to Wilhelm, count of Hanau and

landgrave of Hesse-Kassel. See Kehn, *Christian Cay Lorenz Hirschfeld*, 99–100. This does not contradict the fact, however, that Hirschfeld's description of the "gardens at spas" reflects contemporary views and expectations. The order in which Hirschfeld discusses examples of spa gardens at the end of the section – Meinberg, Pyrmont, Hofgeismar, Wilhelmsbad, Ems, Schlangenbad, Schwalbach, Wisbaden, and Matlock – seems rather arbitrary (Hirschfeld mentions in a footnote that these are spas he has visited), and only Hofgeismar and Wilhelmsbad were owned by Count/Landgrave Wilhelm. In addition, Hirschfeld praises and criticizes these spas in accordance with the established discourse. Finally, during a visit to Meinberg in 1782, Hirschfeld had actually initiated the redesign of this spa with groves to suit contemporary taste. See Kehn, *Christian Cay Lorenz Hirschfeld*, 93.

33. Hirschfeld, *Theory of Garden Art*, 414. See also Hirschfeld, *Theorie der Gartenkunst*, vol. 5, 1785, 85.
34. Hirschfeld, *Theory of Garden Art*, 414. See also Hirschfeld, *Theorie der Gartenkunst*, vol. 5, 1785, 85.
35. Hirschfeld, *Theorie der Gartenkunst*, vol. 5, 1785, 85: "offene und heitere Aussichten." See also Hirschfeld, *Theorie der Gartenkunst*, vol. 5, 1785, 87.
36. See Löw, *Raumsoziologie*, 158–159.
37. Hirschfeld, *Theory of Garden Art*, 414. See also Hirschfeld, *Theorie der Gartenkunst*, vol. 5, 1785, 85.
38. See König, "Frei vom Gängelband?"; König, *Kulturgeschichte des Spazierganges*.
39. See, e.g., Böckmann, *Journal*, 11.
40. See, e.g., Hirschfeld, *Theorie der Gartenkunst*, vol. 5, 1785, 85, 86; Marcard, *Beschreibung von Pyrmont*, vol. 1, 1784, 13, 16.
41. Hirschfeld, *Theory of Garden Art*, 414–415. See also Hirschfeld, *Theorie der Gartenkunst*, vol. 5, 1785, 85–86.
42. Hirschfeld, *Theorie der Gartenkunst*, vol. 5, 1785, 86: "[Alleen] sind nicht allein als Zugänge schicklich, sondern auch bequem zum gesellschaftlichen Spaziergang, zur Verbindung der Brunnengäste und zur Unterhaltung."
43. Hirschfeld, *Theory of Garden Art*, 415. See also Hirschfeld, *Theorie der Gartenkunst*, vol. 5, 1785, 86.
44. Hirschfeld, *Theory of Garden Art*, 415. See also Hirschfeld, *Theorie der Gartenkunst*, vol. 5, 1785, 87.
45. See Hirschfeld, *Theorie der Gartenkunst*, vol. 5, 1785, 87–88.
46. Hirschfeld, *Theorie der Gartenkunst*, vol. 5, 1785, 87: "große umpflanzte Plätze, wo ganze Gesellschaften sich im Freyen versammeln können, wo sie am Morgen ihren Kaffee trinken, an warmen Abenden speisen, spielen, tanzen, oder sich gesellig unterreden."
47. Waitz, *Beschreibung der gegenwärtigen Verfassung des Curorts Hofgeismar*, 1792, 40: "Jeder Curgast findet also Gelegenheit genug, die schönsten Promenaden zu benutzen, sie nach Gefallen zu wählen, je nachdem, ob er Gesellschaft sucht, oder lieber für sich seyn will."
48. Hirschfeld, *Theorie der Gartenkunst*, vol. 5, 1785, 88: "Musikhäuser, Tanzhäuser, Speisehäuser, Trinkhäuser, Spielhäuser oder Kabinette."
49. Hirschfeld, *Theorie der Gartenkunst*, vol. 5, 1785, 90: "welche zur Wohnung der Gäste und zum Trinken und Baden dienen."
50. Hirschfeld, *Theorie der Gartenkunst*, vol. 5, 1785, 91: "die längere und stärkere Bewegungen und Zerstreuung suchen."
51. Hirschfeld, *Theorie der Gartenkunst*, vol. 5, 1785, 91: "in den umliegenden Gegenden umher" – "mancherley wilde Spaziergänge zum Gehen, zum Reiten, zum Fahren."

52. Marcard, *Beschreibung von Pyrmont*, vol. 1, 1784, 14: "Diese Allee nun ist der allgemeine Versammlungsort bey gutem Wetter, und der Mittelpunkt von Allem in Pyrmont."

53. See Hirschfeld, *Theorie der Gartenkunst*, vol. 5, 1785, 94–95.

54. Marcard, *Beschreibung von Pyrmont*, vol. 1, 1784, 25–26: "Man hat zuweilen Vergleichungen zwischen andern Bädern und Pyrmont angestellt, und Leute, die immer von der neuesten Idee, die sie erhielten, ganz angefüllt werden, und sie mit eingeschränktem Geiste auf alles anwenden, was vorkommt, haben an Pyrmont getadelt, daß nicht das Ganze ein englischer Garten sey, und daß man sich nicht gleich von der Quelle ab in einem gewundenen Gange auf schmalen schattigen Fußsteigen an Bächen und allenthalben Bosquetten verliere. Solche Anlagen haben unstreitig ihre Schönheiten und ihr Angenehmes, und können auch bey solchen Bädern allerdings statt finden, wo ein Paar Dutzend Menschen sich versammlen, die wie eine Familie leben; aber für Pyrmont, wo alles ins Große geht, würden sich solche kleinliche Einrichtungen nicht schicken, sie wären für einen Ort, wo im Sommer Tausende zusammenkommen, würklich ganz zweckwidrig und unbrauchbar."

55. Marcard, *Beschreibung von Pyrmont*, vol. 1, 1784, 7: "Die Berge, welche das Thal einschließen, geben durch ihre Formen und Biegungen, durch beträchtliche Verschiedenheit ihrer Entfernung und durch die Schattirungen des Grüns, Mannigfaltigkeit und Schönheit. Sie schließen aber dieses Thal nicht in einen Kessel ein, sondern es ist nach Süden und Norden völlig offen, wenn es auch in einigen Standpunkten nicht so scheint; der frey durch hinströmende Fluß beweist es, und der hohe Berg, welcher im Süden die Aussicht, aber nicht das Thal, schließt, ... liegt über zwey Stunden von Pyrmont, also weit außerhalb dem Thale."

56. Marcard, *Beschreibung von Pyrmont*, vol. 1, 1784, 322: "die Fläche, welche zwischen der Allee und jenem Orte liegt, sind die schönsten Wiesen, und mit Vieh bedeckten Weiden."

57. See [Hassencamp], *Briefe eines Reisenden von Pyrmont*, 1783, 20–21; Kuhnert, *Urbanität*, 115–117.

58. Marcard, *Beschreibung von Pyrmont*, vol. 1, 1784, 15: "Zu beyden Seiten liegen die Boutiquen daran herunter, in denen allerley erdenkbare Dinge feil sind. Die Apotheke, der Buchladen, das Kaffeehaus, die beyden großen Säle, die den Lustbarkeiten und den Conversationscirkeln bestimmt sind, und worin die Pharobank ist, das Comödienhaus und der Brunnen selbst, alles ist hier dichte bey; auch die besten Wohnungen der Fremden sind fast alle ganz nahe um die Allee her, und sogar gewisse für Brunnentrinker sehr nothwendige Bequemlichkeiten sind, zwar ungesehn, aber gleich dabey."

59. Marcard, *Beschreibung von Pyrmont*, vol. 1, 1784, map, title page engraving, and engravings I-VIII at the end of the volume. See also the explanation of the engravings, 308–323, where it says about engraving no. VII on p. 318: "Even if one sees little or nothing of the spa and the facilities of Pyrmont on this sheet, I have included it here with pleasure, partly because it is beautiful and true to nature." ("Ob man gleich auf diesem Blatte wenig bis gar nichts von dem Orte und den Anlagen von Pyrmont selbst wahrnimmt, so habe ich es doch gern hier aufgenommen, theils weil es mahlerisch schön und der Natur getreu ist.")

60. See Günzel, *Bäder-Residenzen*, 80–82.

61. See Heimühle, *Historische Kuranlagen*, 8–12; *Dehio – Handbuch der deutschen Kunstdenkmäler: Sachsen-Anhalt II*, article "Bad Lauchstädt," 39–43.

62. During the season, tradespeople came to Karlsbad from Prague and Vienna, so there was a wide range of goods for sale, rivaling the offerings in a city. For a summary of luxury goods available in Karlsbad, see [Schulz], *Reise eines Liefländers*, 1795, 63–69; *Karlsbad: Beschrieben zur Bequemlichkeit der hohen Gäste*, 1788, 33–34, 37–38; Bürger, *Lilien-Blätter*, 1826, 139.

63. Willebrand, *Carlsbader Brunnenreise*, 1780, 196: "geräumige und prächtige Caffeesäle, wo man Billard und Schach spielen, Caffee, Chocolate, Limonade und Himbeersaft . . . bekommen kann."

64. See Willebrand, *Carlsbader Brunnenreise*, 1780, 196–197.

65. See Weinland, "Geschichte des Bades Nenndorf," 390–392.

66. See Hirschfeld, *Theorie der Gartenkunst*, vol. 5, 1785, 93–101; Röhring, "1639–1989: 350 Jahre Gesundbrunnen bei Hofgeismar"; Bott, *Gesundbrunnen zu Hofgeismar*.

67. See Wegner, "Staatsbad Brückenau," 269–270.

68. See Clausmeyer-Ewers, Löw, *Staatspark Wilhelmsbad Hanau*, 18–19; Bott, *Heilübung und Amüsement*, 90–123.

69. See in detail Clausmeyer-Ewers, Löw, *Staatspark Wilhelmsbad Hanau*, 34–66; Bott, *Heilübung und Amüsement*, 124–201.

70. Weber, *Nachrichten von der Lage*, 1773, 19–20: "Außer der Bequemlichkeit der bereits vorhandenen Wohnungen finden die Brunnengäste an dem Orte nunmehro alles dasjenige, was bey andern Gesundbrunnen zur Nothwendigkeit und Bequemlichkeit des Lebens gerechnet und erfordert wird. Speisen und Getränke sind . . . im Ueberfluß vorhanden. Man findet hier ein Billard, einen Buchladen, Krambuden mit Mode- und anderen Waaren und eine sehr gute Music. Spiele, Tänze, Feuerwerke und Abenderleuchtungen fallen häufig vor."

71. See Wackenroder, *Kunstdenkmäler*, article "Bad Bertrich," 83–85.

72. Compare the description of the avenues in Trampel, *Beschreibung des Bades zu Meinberg*, 1770, 77–78 with the depiction of the avenues and the "pleasure grove" (*Lustgebüsch*) in Hirschfeld, *Theorie der Gartenkunst*, vol. 5, 1785, 93. Hirschfeld was responsible for the redesign of Meinberg.

73. See Wegner, "Staatsbad Bocklet," 259.

74. Göckingk, "Von dem Kurbrunnen bei Brückenau," 1782, 334: "angenehmen Spaziergänge" – "englischen Spaziergang." See also 330–331, 334–335.

75. Göckingk, "Von dem Kurbrunnen bei Brückenau," 1782, 343: "kaum 200 Schritte von den Kurgebäuden" – "mitten im Wald."

76. Göckingk, "Von dem Kurbrunnen bei Brückenau," 1782, 335: "die hessische Schmalten- oder blaue Farbfabrik und Spiegelfabrik" – "fürstlichen Schlosse zu Römershag."

77. "Anzeige [Godesberg]," 1791, 9: "Die besonders reitzende Gegend um die Quelle scheint von der Natur eigens zum Spazieren angelegt; wilde einzeln gelegene Theile derselben sind durch Verbindungswege zum Ganzen des Spazier-Raums gezogen; und auf diese Art ist der bei neuen Holzanlagen mangelnde Schatten erhalten worden. Auch ist nahe am Brunnen durch vierfach gesetzte Alleen dem belebenden Anblick von Ueberschauung der Brunnentrinker nichts dadurch entzogen. Den Werth des Aufenthalts an diesem Orte erhöhet die Nähe des Rheinstromes, die reitzenden Aussichten auf selbem, und gegen die sogenannten Siebenberge; die mahlerische Lage des altverfallenen Schlosses Godesberg; ein kleiner durch das angenehme Thal fliessender Bach; eine kurze Entfernung von der kurf[ürstlichen] Residenzstadt Bonn."

78. Hirschfeld, *Theorie der Gartenkunst*, vol. 5, 1785, 111–112: "elendes Städtchen mit engen Gassen" – "Wiesbaden liegt in einer niedrigen Ebene,

und in einer Gegend, die keine besondern Annehmlichkeiten in sich faßt, sondern sie erst in der Nachbarschaft und in einiger Entfernung gegen den Rhein hin suchen muß. Auch fehlt es an schattigen Spaziergängen und an merkwürdigen Anstalten zu anständigen öffentlichen Vergnügungen."

79. Hirschfeld, *Theorie der Gartenkunst*, vol. 5, 1785, 107: "Ems hat in Tiefe zwischen hohen felsigen Gebirgen eine fast melancholische und einsame Lage; doch sind die Abhänge zum Theil fruchtbar und mit Wein bepflanzt; . . . Doch hat die Lage von Ems einige Unbequemlichkeit, indem die Berge das Thal zu enge verschließen, . . . Man sieht hier nur eine Allee, die noch dazu sehr schmal ist. Die Enge des Thals verstattet keine Anlagen ausgebreiteterer Spaziergänge. Man muß sie in der Wildniß der Berge und der benachbarten Gegend suchen."

80. See also [Grävemeyer], "Fortgesezte Auszüge aus dem Tagebuche eines Frauenzimmers," 1781, 197–198.

81. See Foucault, "Of Other Spaces," 25–26.

82. Baggesen, *Labyrinth*, 168: "Man ist so weit entfernt von Hof und Stadt und den großen Gesellschaften in einem ruhigen Verschlag – doch der Hof, die Stadt und die großen Gesellschaften sind auch mit darin. Man ist auf dem Lande umgeben von allen Phänomenen der Stadt."

83. Marcard, *Beschreibung von Pyrmont*, vol. 1, 1784, 61: "zugleich Hof, Stadt und Land."

84. See *Dehio – Handbuch der deutschen Kunstdenkmäler: Bremen, Niedersachsen*, article "Pyrmont," 170–172.

85. See Bott, *Heilübung und Amüsement*, 181.

86. See Clausmeyer-Ewers, Löw, *Staatspark Wilhelmsbad Hanau*, 145.

87. Göckingk, "Von dem Kurbrunnen bei Brückenau," 1782, 332: "Das fürstliche Wohnhaus zeichnet sich durch weiter nichts, als seine vortreffliche Lage aus, denn man übersieht von da den ganzen Kurbrunnen."

88. See also Chapter 6.

89. See Chapter 5.

90. See Chapter 6.

91. Hirschfeld, *Theorie der Gartenkunst*, vol. 5, 1785, 96–97: "in dem untern linken Flügel laufen aus der Gallerie dieser Seite mancherley Galanteriebuden fort, zwischen welchen spaziert, gespielt und getanzt wird, und man fast immer den Landgrafen, seinen Hofstaat, oder eine andere glänzende Gesellschaft erblickt. Dieser Platz ist daher der lebhafteste Theil der Brunnengebäude. Obgleich bey der Gegenwart des Hofes ihr größter Theil von ihm eingenommen wird, so können doch auch Brunnengäste hier verschiedene Zimmer haben, wenn sie nicht lieber in dem großen nahen Badehause wohnen wollen. . . . Die Gegenwart des zahlreichen und glänzenden Hofes mag freylich für Brunnengäste, sie sich hier ganz in dem Genuß der Ruhe zu erfreuen wünschen, einige Unbequemlichkeit haben. Allein es ist doch auch gewiß, daß der Hof nicht den geringsten Zwang machen will, und daß Fremde hier unter seinen Augen eine vollkommene anständige Freyheit genießen können, wenn sie wollen. Der gute Fürst sorgt mit vielen Kosten für ihre Bequemlichkeit und für ihr Vergnügen. Alle Brunnengäste können ohnentgeltlich den französischen Schauspielen und den öffentlichen Concerten beywohnen, die der Hof hier beständig erhält."

92. See "Badechronik," *JLM* (October 1800), 515; Wilhelm I. von Hessen, *Wir Wilhelm*, 163; Goethe, Vulpius, *Goethes Briefwechsel mit seiner Frau*, vol. 1, letter from Lauchstädt, 4–10 July 1803, 408.

93. Daniel, *Hoftheater*, 28: "auch die Bevölkerung vor allem in und um die Residenzen als Adressat fürstlicher Außendarstellung und als Konsument höfischer Vergnügungsangebote stärker in den Blick [kam]."

94. See, e.g., Daniel, *Hoftheater*, 28, 127–130; Blanning, *Culture of Power*, 431; Hirsch, *Dessau-Wörlitzer Reformbewegung*, 419; Niedermeier, "'Die ganze Erde wird zu einem Garten'," 122.

95. See Lotz-Heumann, "Daheim und auf Reisen"; Mittelstädt, *Wörlitz*, 32–39.

96. See Seng, "Wörlitzer Anlagen"; Hirsch, "Utopia realisata"; Niedermeier, "Wörlitz"; Hirsch, *Dessau-Wörlitzer Reformbewegung*; Niedermeier, "'Die ganze Erde wird zu einem Garten'"; Umbach, "Visual Culture."

97. [Hassencamp], *Briefe eines Reisenden von Pyrmont*, 1783, 8: "Der Kurort selbst besteht eigentlich nur aus einer langen und breiten auf beyden Seiten mit Bäumen besetzten Strasse, hat etwas ländliches und mit einem Holländischen Dorfe einige Aehnlichkeit. Die große doppelte Allee worinnen das Ball-Comödien-Caffe- und Tracteurhaus, der Buchladen und viele Boutiquen sich befinden, die oben das Brunnenhaus und ein Basin mit einer Fontaine zum Point de Vue hat, ist eine herrliche Piece."

98. [Hassencamp], *Briefe eines Reisenden von Pyrmont*, 1783, 9: "halbstädtische, halbländliche Promenaden" – "wo Landleben und große Welt so glücklich verbunden sind."

99. Koch, *Der Gesundbrunnen und das Bad zu Lauchstädt*, 1790, 35–36: "Denen, welche lärmende Vergnügungen lieben, und Zerstreuung und Bewegung des Körpers im Geräusch der Gesellschaft suchen, giebt die erweiterte, und mit neuen Gängen versehene Castanien- und Linden-Allee, das auf der erstern befindliche Chor Musikanten, die tägliche und stündliche Gelegenheit zum Tanz und Spiel in den dazu bestimmten Saal und Pavillons, die auf der Castanien-Allee mit allen ersinnlichen Bedürfnissen angefüllten Crambuden mit ihrem verdeckten Gange, wie auch das in dieser Gegend angelegte Carousell, die Montags und Donnerstags gewöhnlichen Dejeunès [sic], die wöchentlich fünfmaligen Schauspiele, . . .; die öfters des Abends angestellten Erleuchtungen der Allee, und die Feuerwerke auf der Wiese, . . . hinlängliche Gelegenheit. Hingegen gewährt der an der Linden-Allee befindliche Schneckenberg, der schöne an den Seiten mit Blumen bepflanzte Weg um den Teich, der gut angelegte Brunnen und Schloßgarten, mit seinen schattigen Gängen, mit seinen anmuthigen Bänken und Nichen, mit seinen in nachlässig scheinender Ordnung hingepflanzten Küchengewächsen, und Fruchtbäumen, stilles Vergnügen, Ruhe und Kühlung. Hier ist es lieblich, die Morgenröthe erwachen zu sehen, oder in der Abendluft unter dem silbernen Lichte des Monds zu wandeln, oder in süßen Phantasien einsam zu sitzen, . . . Was die Kunst in Rücksicht der Spatziergänge um und bey der Quelle gethan, hat die Natur ausser dem Zirkel der Allee in noch reicherem Maaße gegeben, und dafür gesorgt, daß auch diejenigen, welche an Spiel und Tanz nicht Theil nehmen wollen oder können, und denen das Einfachländliche mehr, als das gesellschaftliche Geräusch, gefällt, in nahen und entfernten Spatziergängen ihre Unterhaltung finden."

100. "Warum auf dem Lande nicht ländlich?," 1788, 473: "führe die Stadt mit sich aufs Feld" – "Wie viele . . . ziehen nicht regelmäßig . . . nach dem Bade . . ., und auch da leben sie wie innerhalb der Stadt-Mauern!" On this contradiction in English spas, see Benedict, "Consumptive Communities," 206.

101. See "Warum auf dem Lande nicht ländlich?," 1788, 473–480.

102. See Kehn, "Gartenkunst," 209, 213; Umbach, "Visual Culture," 138.

4 Spas and Seaside Resorts on the Cusp of Modern Tourism
New Perceptions of Nature and a Daily Routine

The Spa and the Landscape: A New Perception of Mountains

Starting in the late 1780s and especially the 1790s, the inclusion of the surrounding landscape became an integral part of the spatial ideal of the spa. This development was closely associated with a positive perception of mountains and thus with the Alpine euphoria initially propagated by elite authors.[1] At the same time, the spas also reflected a contemporary development in towns, especially in princely residence towns. As Edith Ennen has noted, "The residence town . . . [was] the center of a residence area that consciously incorporate[d] the landscape."[2] At the end of the eighteenth and the beginning of the nineteenth centuries, towns opened up to their surrounding landscape by razing town walls and creating large parks.

These developments also resulted in new practices of experiencing the landscape at spas. Outings into the open countryside, the so-called *Partien*,[3] vastly expanded the space for spa visitors' activities. The associated practices – walking and also increasingly "hiking,"[4] horseback riding, and carriage rides – created a completely new spatial heterotopia of the spa that was now constructed as a rural space embedded in a mountainous natural environment. These fundamental changes were inscribed into the spa discourse at the same time as spa publications diversified and reached a wider reading public.[5] Consequently, the published spa discourse became a multiplier of the new landscape perception and new practices of leisure.

In the published spa discourse of the last decade of the eighteenth century, we can observe the emergence of new statements and the gradual transformation of discursive formations. The limits of what was "sayable" shifted slowly, and authors were engaged in training the eyes and minds of spa visitors. Many spa publications read like instruction manuals on how to see and feel differently, on how to develop a new, positive view, both literally and figuratively, of mountainous landscapes.[6] The "Letters about Karlsbad" ("Briefe über Carlsbad") – published anonymously

by Ludwig Giseke, a Braunschweig privy councillor, in the 1793 issue
of the *German Magazine* (*Deutsches Magazin*) – provide an example of
discursive change in action. Giseke starts with a description of his arduous journey to Karlsbad, a journey through "many mountainous valleys
between terrible stones and depths."[7] While this statement obviously
aligns with the older discourse about spas – and thus with the expectations of Giseke's readers – his rationale shifts when he begins to describe
Karlsbad and its immediate surroundings. He states, "By the way, the
area here is extremely pleasant and romantic." And offering a description
of "mossy cliffs" and "dark fir trees" – elements of the natural environment that were not counted among the advantages of Karlsbad just a few
decades earlier – he informs his readers that "benevolent nature even in
its beautiful wildness" compensates them for many things, "if only we
have a feeling for it and know how to deal with it in a familiar way!"[8]
Reinforcing this new idea, he again assures his readers: "The whole shape
of the local area is very charming. One is entranced at first sight, and is
happy to find nature, despite all the wildness it has here, so friendly."[9]

Giseke's landscape description clearly marks a period of transition in
the published spa discourse. He employs the term "wildness" in the older,
negatively charged sense and at the same time he links "wildness" to
highly positive terminology like "beautiful," "charming," and "friendly,"
offering the reader a positive reinterpretation of Karlsbad's surrounding
landscape. Similarly, the discourse that brought about Alpine euphoria
had introduced the new terminology "wild and romantic" (*wildromantisch*).[10] "Untouched nature" was thus gradually reinterpreted from being
threatening to being perceived as beautiful and admirable.[11] Repeatedly,
Giseke not only guides his readers in this process but also accommodates
the older perception: "A small peaceful meadow, enclosed on all sides,
but not in a frightening way, grants precisely that restriction which is so
benevolent to us because it does not cut off, but invites us to the actual
enjoyment of what reality is offering. On one side, fir trees cover the
peaks, while on the other, fields, meadows, and strangely shaped rocks
shimmer between green bushes. Single scattered small houses distract
from the wildness of the area."[12] Again, Giseke's text exemplifies discursive change in action. The small meadow is enclosed on all sides, but the
author immediately assures his readers that this is not threatening and
that fields, meadows, and houses stand next to "wild" fir trees and rocks
as signs of tamed nature and human civilization.

Giseke also introduces his readers to two other typical aspects of the
new perception of the landscape, namely the recurring references to
Switzerland or analogies with the Swiss Alpine landscape, and the new
practice of hiking. He writes, "Whoever has not yet had the luck to see
Helvetia can get a taste of it here."[13] And he continues, "Here rises a
high, isolated rock, which surprises the lonely walker with its picturesque
shape."[14] At the same time, however, Giseke also employs the spatial

construction of earlier depictions of Karlsbad by beginning his "Letters" with an extensive description of the spa town.[15] He justifies this by referring to the "ordinary order," that is, the rules of the older spa discourse: "Although the town of Karlsbad, its houses, streets, and squares cannot be regarded as especially remarkable, it seems to me that I would be well advised to stick to the ordinary order and to introduce you, my friend, to it first."[16]

In the published spa discourse of the 1790s, the old and the new landscape perception coexisted. In the same year, publications that focused on the interior spaces of a spa, on urban features and landscape gardens, appeared alongside texts that propagated the new spatial ideal, praising mountains and the new practice of hiking, and referencing the Alps. Two journal articles, published in 1796 in the *Journal of Luxury and Fashions* (*Journal des Luxus und der Moden*) and the *German Monthly* (*Deutsche Monatsschrift*) respectively, exemplify this synchronicity of the nonsynchronous. An article about Nenndorf and Rehburg in the "German Spa Chronicle" ("Teutsche Badechronik") of the *Journal of Luxury and Fashions* adheres to the traditional spatial ideal of the spa and its surrounding landscape: "Nenndorf. In 1788, the landgrave of Hesse-Kassel had a wilderness turned into a charming spa close to this little village. . . . The surrounding mountains are at such a distance that the place, far from being frightening and enclosed, rather offers the most open, cheerful views."[17] The article goes on to describe in detail the interior space of the spa of Nenndorf and the amusements offered, including an amateur play "by a group of nobles from Celle."[18] The surroundings and the interior space of the neighboring spa of Rehburg, in contrast, are described in negative terms: "The spa facilities are located half an hour from the small town of Rehburg, which is situated in a valley enclosed by mountains and forests like a cauldron. The place where the bathhouses etc. are located is not beautiful."[19]

A completely different – and utterly positive – picture of Rehburg, however, is presented in an article published in the same year in the *German Monthly* (*Deutsche Monatsschrift*). According to this article, Rehburg is situated "in an extremely romantic area."[20] The author praises the "unfolding, picturesque landscape" that evokes in him "the images of the views of Switzerland, which had already been half obscured by time."[21] He continues, "I thought I saw a miniature painting of some Swiss region in the lovely variety of woodlands . . . , but especially in the view of Lake Steinhude . . . and in the mountains, which in the twilight distance enclose this charming landscape."[22] These statements comparing Rehburg's surrounding landscape to the Swiss Alps show how spa publications functioned as "visual aids." These visual aids "form perceptual dispositions and become the foundation of a visual and spatial order that is superimposed on reality," similar to the discursive practice of later guidebooks like the *Baedeker*.[23]

The contradictory depictions of Rehburg that appeared in the same year in the *Journal of Luxury and Fashions* and in the *German Monthly* illustrate the degree of change in the spatial ideal of the spa in the 1790s. Considering the differences in the descriptions – "a valley enclosed by mountains . . . like a cauldron" on the one hand and mountains that form a "picturesque landscape" on the other – it is hard to believe that these authors are talking about one and the same spa. By 1811, however, at the time when the spa physician Wilhelm Anton Ficker published the *Driburg Pocketbook* (*Driburger Taschenbuch*), the transformation in landscape perception and associated practices was complete. "Hiking" in the surrounding mountains was given preference over "walking" or "strolling" in the interior space of the spa: "The venerable chain of mountains surrounding Driburg . . . gives the area the romantic beauty that the inhabitants of the plains so admire, the nature lover likes to climb them, . . . But even the walks near the spa of Driburg are sufficiently extensive to provide the weaker spa guest with . . . a substitute for the high level of pleasure that the faster mountain climber can have every day."[24]

In the spa discourse of the early modern period, readers and spa visitors were "guided" through towns and urban spaces, and in the spa discourse of the late 1770s and 1780s they were guided through English landscape gardens and entertainment spaces. The new spatial heterotopia of the spa, however, shifted the focus away from the spa itself. Spa guides figuratively accompanied readers and spa visitors on walking or even hiking tours through the (mountainous) countryside, and the spatial heterotopia of the spa was no longer primarily defined by its interior spaces, but by the surrounding landscape. The extensive descriptions of the practices of walking, hiking, and mountain climbing in the spa publications served as models for the realization of these practices by spa guests.[25] Goethe, in a letter written at Wiesbaden to his wife Christiane in 1814, described in detail how outings, both on foot and by carriage, had become standard practices among the spa visitors there: "Four chaussées that lead from hills and mountains into the depths where the place [Wiesbaden] is situated are full of people coming and going, of people who go on pleasure outings. They go to Mainz, Biebrich, Elfeld, Schlangenbad, Schwalbach, and wherever else. There are ruins of castles for walkers to explore, with refreshment places, in the nearby mountain range. There, and so on! [Carl Friedrich] Zelter, a formidable hiker, has already roamed through all of that."[26]

During the long, unbroken success story of the spa of Karlsbad between the seventeenth and the early nineteenth century, several different "Karlsbads" were created in the published discourse. Over the centuries, the spa was thus inscribed in the discourse in radically different ways: the "formulas of success" ranged from Karlsbad as a town to Karlsbad as a rugged, mountainous landscape. While Giseke's article discussed earlier still exemplified the shifting discourse of the late 1780s and 1790s, an article about Karlsbad in the *Journal of Luxury and Fashions* (*Journal des Luxus und der Moden*) in 1796 already focused entirely on the new spatial construction of the spa.[27] In contrast to Giseke, the author no longer provides a description of Karlsbad as an urban space but instead discusses the "walking trails" (*Promenaden*) surrounding the spa, thus drawing the reader's attention to the location and the landscape. The anonymous author addresses a fictitious friend: "You will not, dear friend, find the detailed description of Karlsbad's walking trails too long, if you know that they are one of the main amenities of this beautiful spa, and no other spa can boast of them. Karlsbad does not have any artificial facilities, but nature has created a large park of beautiful mountain forests, magnificent views, and valleys around the spa, where it [nature] shows itself in such a charming, free, and genuine grace."[28] This statement is supplemented by references to the "beautiful, narrow Töpel [Teplá river] valley,"[29] to Switzerland,[30] and the practice of "mountaineering."[31]

By the early nineteenth century, this spatial construction of Karlsbad prevailed in the published discourse and in personal narratives. In his 1801 spa guide *Karlsbad and the Surrounding Area* (*Karlsbad und die umliegende Gegend*), Hubert von Harrer gave the following description: "The natural location of the town is made for a spa. A narrow, romantic valley, with the Töpl [Teplá] river cutting through it, surrounded by mountains."[32] Johanna Schopenhauer's article on "Spa Life in Karlsbad" ("Badeleben in Karlsbad"), published in 1815, also paints the spa's surroundings in a completely positive light. Karlsbad, she writes, "may dispute the rank of any spa with regard to its location" because, "almost as if wedged into the lovely valley that the Töpel [Teplá] river flows through, surrounded by magnificent forest-crowned rocks, it offers an endless variety of the friendliest and most sublime scenes."[33]

By 1821, Schopenhauer saw this new ideal of Karlsbad threatened by the building activity in the town: "In the town itself, every place even remotely suitable is built on, almost every green garden spot, and namely with houses two or three stories high, so that one loses much of the view of the magnificent rocks that surround Karlsbad so beautifully, which, if this continues, will soon only stand out with their peaks above the mass of houses."[34] Schopenhauer's comment shows how the spatial ideal of the spa had been completely transformed since the early modern period. By the early nineteenth century, this led to the rejection of any further urban development of the spa – a discursive statement about the "perfect" vacation spot that continues to be used to this day.

In contrast to the abundance of statements about the spa as a spatial heterotopia in the published discourse, authors of personal narratives rarely commented on their perception of nature and the landscape during spa visits. Pütter's autobiography, for example, provides us with many details about social interactions at the spa, but lacks reflections on his perception of the landscape. In light of the slow pace of this kind of cultural change, this is not surprising. Letters, diaries, or autobiographies are much more likely to reflect on events, both personal and historical, and on social and economic developments that had an immediate impact on people's lives. In contrast, gradual changes in cultural practices, for instance the way people perceive nature or how their bodies move in different spaces, are difficult to notice, and even more difficult to reflect upon while they are happening. Beyond the elite authors who actively pushed the discourse in a certain direction – the "trendsetters" or "gatekeepers" – most people were gradually, and largely unconsciously, acculturated to a new cultural trend.

Accordingly, few authors of personal narratives mention landscape perception. The Danish-German writer Jens Baggesen and the writer and frequent spa guest Elisa von der Recke are exceptions. They were members of the social and cultural elite who had adopted the new spatial ideal and its associated practices early on, but their descriptions also illustrate that this process largely happened on an unconscious level. Baggesen published a travelogue about Pyrmont in 1789. He calls Pyrmont's interior spaces "boring"[35] and prefers exploring the surrounding area on foot.[36] When Elisa von der Recke visited Pyrmont in 1791, she too had already internalized the new landscape ideal. She commented on how she perceived the landscape during an outing from Pyrmont to Meinberg: "The forms of these mountains are very uniform and have no romantic beauty. To an eye accustomed to the plains, this region will . . . offer a pleasant change, but anyone who has recently seen the Bohemian mountains, who is coming from Dresden, will find this area insignificant."[37] In 1795, during her visit to Karlsbad, she recorded almost daily walks in the spa's surroundings. Her diary is filled with detailed descriptions of the landscape, using terms like "beautiful rock masses,"[38] "romantic valleys,"[39] and "innocent joys of nature."[40] Recke describes two experiences in her diary that illuminate how contemporaries became aware of their own changed perceptions of nature and how changes in the prevailing discourse reached different social groups at different times.

On 2 May 1795, Recke's social circle went on an outing from Karlsbad to Ellenbogen (today Loket in the Czech Republic). Dr. Bernhard Mitterbacher (1767–1839), spa physician in Karlsbad, had hired a guide to show them Ellenbogen's surroundings, but the guide's performance caused deep disappointment in Recke's circle: "Young Mitterbacher had procured a guide for us, who he believed would show us the most beautiful areas around Ellenbogen. But this man had absolutely no sense for beautiful landscapes and rocky areas. He led us . . . up a steep, shadowless mountain, from which one could overlook the town, and there he said with self-possessed simplicity: 'You see here, there one can see our town gate . . . ' Mitterbacher, the good man, was quite ashamed that instead of picturesque rocky areas, we were shown only this miserable gate after such an arduous walk."[41]

There is clearly more to this incident than a "simple man" who had no sense of beauty. Rather, it highlights social differences in perception: the tourist guide (most likely a member of the urban middle or lower middle class) had not yet internalized the new landscape perception that his elite visitors already took for granted. The man's eagerness to show the spa guests a town gate – the ultimate symbol of an urban space – is strikingly reminiscent of the early modern spatial ideal discussed in Chapter 3. Without realizing it, Recke provides us with a glimpse into a perceptual gap between two social groups. In fact, we have evidence in another personal narrative, the spa diary of Imperial Count Heinrich XXVI of Reuß Younger Line, that a generation earlier, Recke's circle would have wanted to see the town gate: Count Heinrich reports that during his visit to Karlsbad in 1766, he took a walk to the garden of Dr. David Becher, the spa physician, and "looked at the beautiful view down into the town."[42]

On 7 May 1795, Recke recorded another observation about landscape perception in her diary. She describes a walk with several gentlemen in Karlsbad's surroundings: "Then we walked up a steep, high hill, which was densely covered with dark fir trees and where jumbled masses of rocks were piled up in an eerie way. [Count] Nieuport told me that he feels more attracted to such wild, eerie areas than to gentle, cheerful landscapes. For me, too, the roughest rocky patches have the greatest appeal – why rugged rocks fill my soul with greater ideas than beautiful, cheerful areas, *I cannot account for that*."[43] And in 1816, Adele Schopenhauer made the following observation about Schlangenbad in her diary that 40 years earlier would not have been conceivable, either in the published spa discourse or in a personal narrative: "I feel very good here, *I don't know* what I like so much about this quiet green forest area."[44] Both Recke and Schopenhauer had clearly internalized the new landscape ideal. Recke's spa practices – going for walks in "wild areas" – and Schopenhauer's perception of Schlangenbad as an attractive location reflect this change. At the same time, however, they explicitly stated their inability to explain their own sentiments. Considering that Recke and Schopenhauer were very well-educated women, it is hard to imagine that other contemporaries were able to reflect on this discursive change on a more conscious level. This again demonstrates the largely subconscious nature of a cultural change of this kind.

The change in landscape perception had far-reaching consequences for both the number and the location of *teutsche* spas that garnered attention in the published discourse. The map of fashionable German spas thus changed considerably in the early nineteenth century. Existing spas unable to provide the facilities and services that had become *de rigeur* since the late 1770s advertised their mountainous surroundings in order to establish themselves in the published discourse. In the same vein, new spas were able to inscribe themselves in the discourse. As a result, several spas and spa clusters appeared in the published discourse for the first time.

This development fit into the larger context of Alpine euphoria during the late eighteenth and early nineteenth centuries, when central European mountain ranges like the Elbe Sandstone Mountains came to be associated with the Swiss Alps and were called "Saxon Switzerland" (*Sächsische Schweiz*) and "Bohemian Switzerland" (*Böhmische Schweiz*).[45] Spas located in the higher elevations of the low mountain ranges (*Mittelgebirge*) of central and southern Germany successfully imprinted themselves on the perception of spa visitors through references to Switzerland and the Alpine regions. Examples thereof are Schandau and other spas in Saxon Switzerland,[46] Imnau in the Swabian Alps, Alexandersbad in the Fichtel Mountains, Alexisbad in the Harz Mountains, and Baden-Baden, Wildbad, Teinach, Rippoldsau, Langensteinbach, Liebenzell, Huber Bad, and the Renchtal spas in the Black Forest.[47] Often spas in existing clusters were able to attract more attention, such as Schlangenbad as part of the Taunus spa cluster and Marienbad (today Mariánské Lázně in the Czech Republic), founded in 1818, as part of the Bohemian spa cluster that also included Karlsbad, Franzensbad, and Teplitz. Spas like Baden-Baden and Ems took advantage of the new landscape ideal, and thus their rise to international fame began. Last but not least, the map of German spas represented in the published discourse expanded[48] as spas in the Giant Mountains (*Riesengebirge*) in Silesia were now perceived supra-regionally.[49]

The shift in spatial perception that focused spa visitors' attention on the surrounding landscape rather than the interior spaces of the spa became an essential advertising argument for spas at the end of the eighteenth and the beginning of the nineteenth centuries. For instance, in an advertising pamphlet for the spa of Teinach in the Black Forest, published in 1789, we find a completely new line of argument: "For Teinach itself, nature has done very much, but art has done only as much as is necessary to enable [spa guests] to stay here comfortably. . . . It is true, in comparison with Pyrmont, Spa, and if one takes these places as a standard, that Teinach is of course lacking in amusements. . . . But whoever finds pleasure in contemplating nature, which can never be seen in its purity near towns and where it is at best artificially recreated in English gardens, . . . whoever wants to withdraw his mind from the noise [of towns], . . . should come here and enjoy nature."[50]

In these passages, the new spatial heterotopia of the spa is presented in an almost pure form. In contrast to the earlier discourse, the new landscape ideal is based on the construction of an opposition between art and nature.[51] The author propagates a positive perception of "pure nature" and contrasts it with the urban character of spas like Pyrmont and with English landscape gardens – thus he rejects both spatial ideals that preceded the new landscape ideal. The author argues that Teinach is worth a visit not because of its interior spaces, but because of the surrounding landscape. This became the standard argument for smaller spas that sought to inscribe themselves in the published discourse.

The pamphlet advertising the spa of Imnau, published in 1795 by the privy councillor and spa physician Franz Xaver Mezler, is an example of the new discursive strategy that smaller spas employed at the end of the eighteenth century. Strikingly, Mezler reverses the established textual order of spa guides. He begins with a description of the area surrounding the spa and only mentions the facilities and services at Imnau, which did not meet contemporary expectations, much later in the text. Throughout his pamphlet, Mezler emphasizes the new spatial ideal: "It [Imnau] is situated in a valley with meadows, which is very lovely due to its natural beauty and very charming because of its apparent seclusion. . . . The mountains surrounding it are at rather close distance . . . and combine their black fir-tree green in different bosoms and curves with the beautiful light green of the meadows in the valley."[52]

The author then guides his readers through this landscape and recommends outings that include the mountainous countryside as well as castles and small towns in the surrounding area. He emphasizes that "the spa guests . . . have the advantage that through small excursions they can become acquainted with excellent people, with beautiful nature sceneries, and various curiosities."[53] Mezler no longer recommends that spa guests view the countryside from inside spa towns, but rather encourages his readers to explore the countryside.[54] And the author argues, "In the afternoon, when the hours are really dull at other spas, one party takes an outing walking, riding, or driving to one place, and a different party takes an outing to another place."[55] The practice of the afternoon outing that Mezler describes as unique to Imnau in fact became a standard practice at all spas.[56]

Beginning in the early nineteenth century, suggestions for outings became a central element in spa guides. The spa practice of taking outings extended the spa's reach far into its surrounding area and offered new experiences of nature to spa visitors. In 1812, Wilhelm Lebrecht Götzinger published *Schandau and its Surroundings or Description of So-Called Saxon Switzerland* (*Schandau und seine Umgebungen oder Beschreibung der sogenannten Sächsischen Schweiz*). As the title suggests, this work was primarily a guidebook to Saxon Switzerland and only secondarily a spa guide for Schandau. Götzinger systematically lists "suggestions for Schandau's spa guests for small outings into Saxon Switzerland during their spa visit."[57] He also provides information about the length of the outings.

Similarly, in Johann Friedrich Krieger's 1812 spa guide *Alexisbad in the Lower Harz with its Surroundings* (*Das Alexisbad im Unter-Harz mit seinen Umgebungen*), a chapter entitled "Recreational Outings in the Neighborhood of Alexisbad" ("Erholungsparthien in der Nachbarschaft des Alexisbades") takes up more than half of the book.[58] Krieger even plays with the old urban ideal of the spa by stylizing Alexisbad's surrounding landscape as the spa's "house-neighbor" (*Haus-Nachbarn*). He also mentions the creation of "vacation" memories and of relaying these memories to friends and acquaintances at home and thus references another practice that became typical of the modern tourist experience:

> A good neighborhood, whether it be dead or living nature, who does not count it among the greatest comforts of life, the creator of pure pleasures? . . . Alexisbad enjoys having such a neighbor in all directions, accessible at any time of day, appealing to every inclination, often without house and roof, yet still making the most beautiful house. If you want to get to know only those who are closer and more attractive, and limit yourself to one acquaintance each day, you can easily fill your entire spa visit with such one-day excursions, so that you have happy memories and lots of material to talk about at home.[59]

In his 1799 advertising pamphlet for Franzensbad, Joseph Karl Eduard Hoser follows a similar line of argument. The pamphlet was published when the spa was still under construction. Therefore, Hoser refers potential spa guests to hikes in the surrounding countryside in order to distract from the fact that the spa's interior spaces including its garden did not (yet) meet their expectations: "Notwithstanding that the area closest to Franzensbrunn [Franzensbad] does not yet deserve to be called picturesque, and will only have a claim to this label in a few years' time, the location of more distant villages and the entire circle of mountains surrounding this fertile little country are full of picturesque beauty in every respect, and every person whose feeling for nature has not yet vanished will certainly derive genuine pleasure and pure enjoyment from his hikes through them in more than one way."[60]

The new spatial heterotopia of the *teutsche* spa downplayed the role of interior spaces and defined a spa as attractive if it had mountainous surroundings and offered spa guests opportunities for outings into the countryside. Thus, it served as a multiplier of the ideals of Alpine euphoria among spa guests and readers of spa guides. These changes were reflected both in the titles and in the engravings of the spa guides that appeared in the early nineteenth century. Many spa guides already announced the new spatial ideal in their titles. To name just a few examples: *Schandau and its Surroundings or Description of So-Called Saxon Switzerland (Schandau und seine Umgebungen oder Beschreibung der sogenannten Sächsischen Schweiz)*;[61] *Alexisbad in the Lower Harz with its Surroundings (Das Alexis-Bad im Unter-Harz mit seinen Umgebungen)*;[62] *Description of Augustusbad near Radeberg: Especially for Spa Guests and also as a Guidebook to its Surroundings (Beschreibung des Augustusbades bey Radeberg: insbesondere für Kurgäste und zugleich als Wegweiser in den Umgebungen)*;[63] *Description of Teplitz and its Picturesque Surroundings*

(*Beschreibung von Teplitz und seinen pitoreskischen Umgebungen*);[64]
Karlsbad and the Surrounding Area (*Karlsbad und die umliegende Gegend*);[65] *Description of Baden near Rastatt and its Surrounding Area* (*Beschreibung von Baden bei Rastatt und seiner Umgebung*).[66]

In addition, the images and maps in spa guides focused on the surrounding area of a spa rather than its interior spaces. Especially the publications about spas that had not entered the published discourse before the beginning of the nineteenth century often included images showing only a view of the spa from a distance and images of the destinations of outings. The two fold-out engravings in Krieger's *Alexisbad in the Lower Harz with its Surroundings* (*Das Alexis-Bad im Unter-Harz mit seinen Umgebungen*) focus on the spa as a rural idyll and fulfill the visual expectations of Romanticism: the image of Alexisbad depicts the spa as a small village of half-timbered houses deeply embedded in the landscape and the second fold-out image shows the ruins of the monastery Hagenrode, one of the recommended destinations for outings (Figure 4.1).

Carl Friedrich Mosch's spa compendium *The Spas and Healing Springs of Germany and Switzerland: A Pocketbook for Spa and Bathing Guests* (*Die Bäder und Heilbrunnen Deutschlands und der Schweiz: Ein Taschenbuch für Brunnen- und Bade-Reisende*), published in 1819 and reprinted

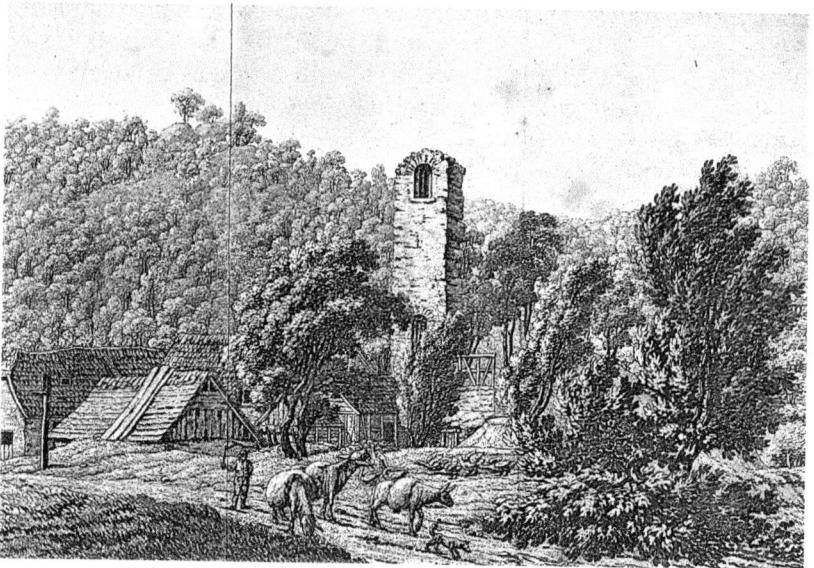

Figure 4.1 Monastery Hagenrode near Alexisbad, engraving by Johann Friedrich Klusemann, 1812. ("Kloster-Ruine beim Alexis-Bade im Unter-Harz." In Krieger, Johann Friedrich. *Das Alexisbad im Unter-Harz mit seinen Umgebungen*, after 154. Magdeburg: Creutz, 1812. Collection of the author.)

several times in the early nineteenth century,[67] also exemplifies this trend. In Mosch's work, three images accompany the entry for "Baden in Swabia" (Baden-Baden), all in the style of Romanticism: a view of the spa from a distance with a hiker as a staffage figure in the foreground, an image of the ruins of the old castle (Hohenbaden) among overgrown foliage and trees, and a view of the waterfall near Geroldsau. Franzensbad is represented by three images, all showing destinations for outings in the surrounding area: Hochberg, Seeberg, and Maria-Culm. Griesbach, as an emerging spa in the Renchtal, is depicted as a small village with five houses and a chapel, dwarfed by the surrounding mountains (Figure 4.2). And, strikingly, an established spa like Teplitz is represented by images of the ruins of Castle Daubersberg (today Doubravská hora) on an isolated mountain near the spa (Figure 4.3) and the ruins of Castle Rosenburg (today Hrad Krupka) in the nearby small town of Graupen (today Krupka in the Czech Republic) (Figure 4.4) – both quintessential Romantic ruins – rather than by the magnificent princely palace situated at the center of Teplitz (Figure 3.23).

Johann Isaak von Gerning's didactic poem *The Spas at the Taunus Mountains* (*Die Heilquellen am Taunus*) of 1814 includes engravings of

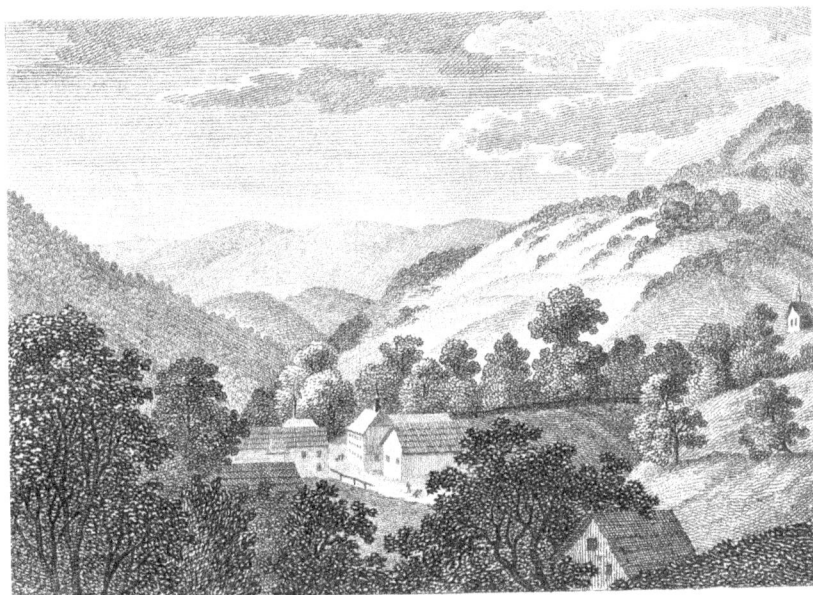

Figure 4.2 Griesbach, engraving by F. Rosmäsler junior, 1819. ("Griesbach." In Mosch, Carl Friedrich. *Die Bäder und Heilbrunnen Deutschlands und der Schweiz: Ein Taschenbuch für Brunnen- und Badereisende.* Vol. 1, unpaginated, in article "Griesbach." Leipzig: Brockhaus, 1819. Collection of the author.)

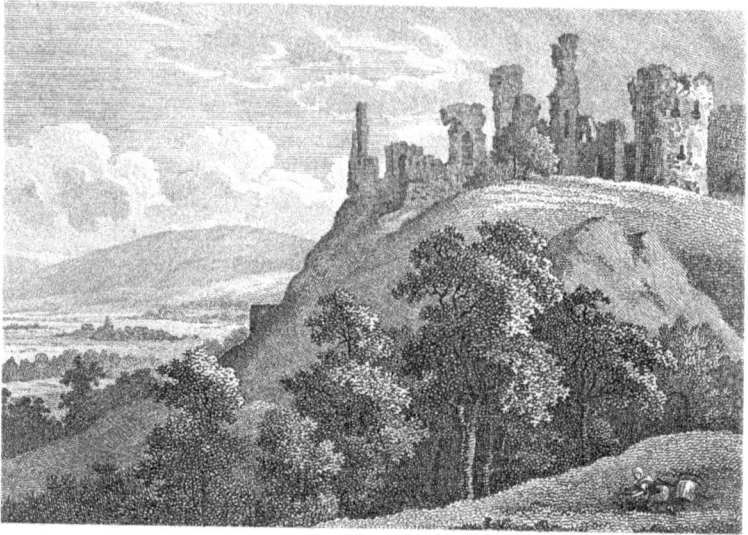

Figure 4.3 Castle Daubersberg (today Doubravská hora) near Teplitz (today Tep-
lice), engraving by F. Rosmäsler junior, 1819. ("Ruine des Töplitzer
Schlosses." In Mosch, Carl Friedrich. *Die Bäder und Heilbrunnen
Deutschlands und der Schweiz: Ein Taschenbuch für Brunnen- und
Badereisende*. Vol. 2, unpaginated, in article "Teplitz." Leipzig: Brock-
haus, 1819. Collection of the author.)

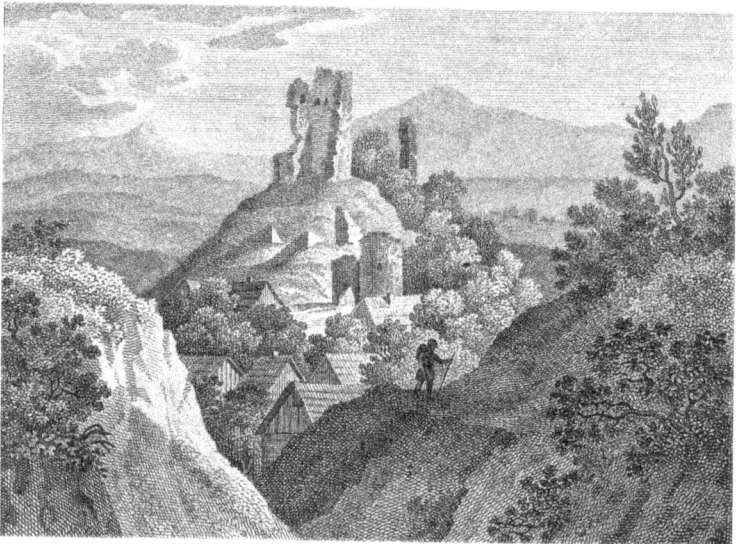

Figure 4.4 Castle Rosenburg (today Hrad Krupka) in Graupen (today Krupka)
near Teplitz (today Teplice), engraving by F. Rosmäsler junior, 1819.
("Graupen." In Mosch, Carl Friedrich. *Die Bäder und Heilbrunnen
Deutschlands und der Schweiz: Ein Taschenbuch für Brunnen- und
Badereisende*. Vol. 2, unpaginated, in article "Teplitz." Leipzig: Brock-
haus, 1819. Collection of the author.)

the emerging spa of Soden,[68] and of Ems, Schlangenbad, Schwalbach, and Wiesbaden. While the difference between the landscape surrounding Ems, situated deep in a Lahn valley, and the other four spas is recognizable, the images of Schlangenbad, Schwalbach, Soden, and Wiesbaden look similar enough to make it hard to discern, at a cursory glance, the individual features of these spas and their natural environments. Thus, these engravings almost give the impression of stock images conforming to the new spatial ideal of a spa embedded in a mountainous environment. The volume is completed by an image of the striking rock formation of the "Brunehildis-Stein" (today *Brunhildisfelsen*) on the Great Field Mountain (*Großer Feldberg*), the highest mountain in the Taunus range.[69]

Fold-out maps showing spas and spa clusters embedded in the surrounding area became a standard feature of spa compendia in the early nineteenth century. Gerning's *The Spas at the Taunus Mountains* contains a fold-out map of the larger area where the spas are situated.[70] Similarly, Mosch's *The Spas and Healing Springs of Germany and Switzerland: A Pocketbook for Spa and Bathing Guests* (*Die Bäder und Heilbrunnen Deutschlands und der Schweiz: Ein Taschenbuch für Brunnen- und Bade-Reisende*) offers its readers a "Map of the Healing Springs at the Taunus Mountains" ("Carte zu den Heilquellen am Taunusgebirge").[71] Another example is Johann Ludwig Klüber's 1810 *Description of Baden near Rastatt and its Surrounding Area* (*Beschreibung von Baden bei Rastatt und seiner Umgebung*).[72] These maps are striking representations of the new spatial ideal of the spa. It is actually difficult to locate the spas mentioned in the titles of these volumes on the accompanying maps because they are dwarfed by other features, especially mountains. In Klüber's volume, the fold-out map represents the Murg river valley (Figure 4.5) and at first glance it is difficult to locate Baden-Baden (it is in the top right-hand corner).

In 1805, an article in the *Journal of Luxury and Fashions* (*Journal des Luxus und der Moden*) commented on the transformation of the spatial heterotopia of the spa and the resulting changes of the German spa map. With an ironic undertone, the anonymous author observes that the new spas in Saxon Switzerland came into being because enterprising Saxons wanted to attract spa guests from Dresden who otherwise visited the Bohemian spas: "Where only nature revealed some mineral content in the springs that burst forth here and there, where one could hope that the charming region, even more than the [healing] powers of the spring, . . . would attract spa guests, a new spa was created, and it is this [the charming region] we have to thank for the creation of Tharand and Schandau, which have flourished so quickly."[73] As the nineteenth century progressed, this new perception of mountainous landscapes as sublime, picturesque, and romantic, or "wild and romantic," and the accompanying Romantic ideal of the lonely hiker in "untouched" nature, gradually solidified and became a cliché.[74] By 1831, Christoph Wilhelm Hufeland, in his *Practical*

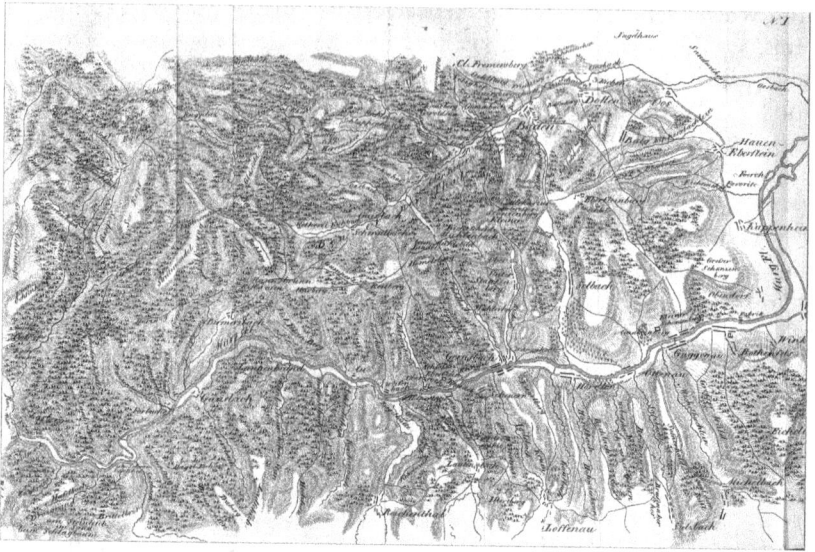

Figure 4.5 Map of the surroundings of Baden-Baden and the Murg river valley, engraving by Carl Ausfeld (one half of a two-part map), 1810. ("Karte der Umgebungen von Baden und des Murg Thales." In Klüber, Johann Ludwig. *Beschreibung von Baden bei Rastatt und seiner Umgebung.* Vol. 2, *Umgebung, nähere und entferntere*, after 282. Tübingen: Cotta, 1810. Collection of the author.)

Overview of the Most Prominent Healing Springs in Germany (*Praktische Uebersicht der vorzüglichsten Heilquellen Teutschlands*), claims, without distinction, that spas are situated in "romantic" surroundings.[75]

Seaside Resorts in Their Infancy

The rise of seaside resorts on the Baltic and North Sea coasts in the early nineteenth century led to another fundamental change in the map of summer resorts in Germany. Over time, sea bathing, enjoying the view of the sea, and strolling along the beach became standard practices associated with seaside resorts that to this day continue to be part of a typical tourist experience. However, people were acculturated to these ideas during the first decades of the nineteenth century through a slow and meandering process. The establishment of seaside resorts in Germany was thus a development with many twists and turns, similar to, but in some significant ways also different from, the changes in landscape perception that affected the inland spas between the early modern period and the early nineteenth century. The creation of seaside resorts was part of a long-term change in the perception of the sea and the seaside, not unlike the changes in spatial perceptions impacting inland spas in the late eighteenth and early nineteenth centuries that had been based on "the discovery of the Alps." And, similar to the published discourse about inland spas, a significant part of the discourse about seaside resorts engaged in training the eyes and minds of visitors. At the same time, however, the published discourse about seaside resorts had to contend with the powerful existing discursive regime about spas and confront the ideals of spatial arrangements, services, and practices that prevailed at the inland spas. And, finally, in contrast to the spa discourse, the discourse about seaside resorts had an important proponent who acted as a "gatekeeper" by pushing western European ideas into the German discourse: the Göttingen professor Georg Christoph Lichtenberg.

In 1793, Lichtenberg published a programmatic article in the *Göttingen Pocket Calendar* (*Göttinger Taschenkalender*) titled "Why Does Germany Not Yet Have a Large Public Seaside Resort?" ("Warum hat Deutschland noch kein großes öffentliches Seebad?").[76] Informed by his travels to the English seaside resorts of Margate and Deal in 1774–1775,[77] he made the case for the establishment of a seaside resort on the German North Sea coast. With his article, Lichtenberg abruptly shifted the direction of the discourse on the sea and seaside resorts in Germany by opening new possibilities for what was "sayable." On the one hand, he offered his readers positive descriptions of the sea that had so far been unfamiliar statements in the published discourse. He even went so far as to declare his preference for the North Sea over the Baltic Sea.[78] (The North Sea has tidal flows and a stronger surf, and contemporaries thus perceived it as "wilder" than the Baltic.) On the other hand, Lichtenberg offered comparisons with the inland spas that cast them in an unfavorable light, again changing what could be said in the spa discourse.

Lichtenberg's article was in stark contrast with the depiction of the sea that Christian Cay Lorenz Hirschfeld offered in his *Theory of Garden Art* (*Theorie der Gartenkunst*) in 1779. Even though, according to Corbin, attitudes toward the sea had already changed fundamentally in western Europe at the time, Hirschfeld's ambivalent perception of the sea focused on containing "nature" through "art." He clearly still perceived the sea as a threat: "Man cannot tame the sea; he can force no part of it into his designs. He can, however, join a view of it to his scenes and make use of this prospect. Meanwhile, through shaping and planting the shore, the perspectives can be changed in various ways, and thus art can achieve a kind of dominion over the prodigious element."[79]

In his 1793 article, Lichtenberg propagates a completely different view of the sea and the coast. First, with a good dose of irony, Lichtenberg expresses his astonishment that in Germany, where "almost every decade"[80] a new spa was established, no seaside resort had yet been founded: "Why is it that, with this willingness of our countrymen and -women to not only recommend new spas, but also to actually let themselves be cured at them, no enterprising mind can be found that thinks of establishing a seaside resort?"[81] Second, Lichtenberg lists a veritable catalogue of the advantages and the "indescribable attraction that a stay on the shores of the world's oceans in the summer months has, especially for people from landlocked regions."[82] Third, he combines a positive perception of the sea that is free from any threat with proposals for numerous new practices at seaside resorts. The sight of the waves, their shimmer, and their thunderous rolling are described as utterly positive – the Rhine Falls of Schaffhausen are a "tumult in a washbasin" by comparison.[83] And fourth, Lichtenberg prefers the North Sea to the Baltic Sea because of the "indescribably great spectacle of the tides."[84] All this, according to Lichtenberg, has an effect on the "sensitive person with a power that does not find its equal in nature."[85]

Lichtenberg dramatically shifted the discourse about the sea and seaside resorts not only by describing the sea in positive terms, without fear, and full of fascination, but also by proposing new practices. "A walk along the shore of the sea" is to be preferred to the "dull avenues of the inland spas."[86] In fact, avenues were still regarded as essential elements of spas at that time, even if they were becoming less fashionable in the published discourse. In light of this, it becomes clear how much Lichtenberg shifted the boundaries of the existing discourse. He calls swimming in the sea a "pleasure,"[87] and argues that a trip to Heligoland as a new practice at seaside resorts is preferable to the typical practices at spas, "balls and faro."[88] In his conclusion, Lichtenberg addresses – again with ironic exaggeration – the fear his contemporaries still had of the sea and sea creatures: "The fish that could eat a prophet are there [in the sea] as rare as the prophets. One could rather warn the fish there of the sea bathers. Since time immemorial, the fish there have been eaten with great predilection, especially by visitors, but I am not aware that any of them ever returned the compliment."[89]

One author alone, however, was not able to create a new discursive formation. This becomes clear by looking at the development of the published discourse about seaside resorts after 1793. Although Lichtenberg shifted the boundaries of what was "sayable," the inscription of seaside resorts in the published discourse took decades, and authors advertising seaside resorts had to defer to the assumptions and rules of the older spa discourse. Apart from that, more than Lichtenberg himself, it was Lichtenberg's social network that was instrumental in the foundation of seaside resorts in Germany. Samuel Gottlieb Vogel, a former student of Lichtenberg's in Göttingen and later spa physician of the first German seaside resort in Doberan-Heiligendamm on the Baltic Sea, personally sought advice from Lichtenberg in 1793.[90] Friedrich Wilhelm von Halem, who in 1797 founded the first North Sea resort on the island of Norderney, was also Lichtenberg's student.[91] And last, but certainly not least, the idea of establishing seaside resorts was already "in the air" in the 1780s, especially on the North Sea islands close to the Netherlands. In 1783, the Protestant pastor on the East Frisian island of Juist, Gerhard Otto Janus, had written a letter to King Frederick II of Prussia in which he shared his experiences of sea bathing and proposed the foundation of a seaside resort in Juist.[92] However, the project did not come to fruition before the mid-nineteenth century.

When Duke Friedrich Franz of Mecklenburg-Schwerin arrived at his summer residence in Doberan on 8 September 1793, he received a memorandum by the Rostock professor of medicine Samuel Gottlieb Vogel, in which the latter explained to the duke the advantages of a seaside resort on the Baltic coast.[93] Vogel praised the benefits of bathing in the sea, while at the same time he pointed out that women in particular found the sea air too rough and the water too cold. Vogel argued that a bathhouse for warm baths in sea water would solve this problem, and he proposed to build such a bathhouse in Doberan – an hour's carriage ride from the sea! Vogel also emphasized the advantages of the duke's summer residence as a spa *cum* seaside resort. He pointed out that Doberan already had a reputation as a small spa among guests from Rostock, Schwerin, and Hamburg. And he described Doberan as situated in a charming landscape, with a number of facilities in place. In order to convince the duke, Vogel also employed mercantilistic arguments.[94] He emphasized that the prince as the owner of a successful spa could not only keep the money otherwise spent at spas in other territories in his own lands, but that he could also expect additional income.[95]

Duke Friedrich Franz found Vogel's arguments convincing; he responded immediately and accepted Vogel's proposal to draw up a plan, explicitly referring to Vogel's mercantilistic reasoning.[96] Vogel's next step is telling. He embarked on a journey to the spas of Lower Saxony, especially to Pyrmont,[97] in the company of the duke's architect Johann Christoph Heinrich von Seydewitz. Vogel met Lichtenberg in Göttingen on this trip, but Doberan-Heiligendamm did not become the kind of seaside resort that Lichtenberg had envisioned. On the contrary, the differences between Lichtenberg's vision of a North Sea resort and the first Baltic seaside resort founded in Doberan-Heiligendamm could hardly be more pronounced. Although Doberan-Heiligendamm quickly became a success, and in its first season in 1794 it already attracted 300 guests,[98] it remained, for all intents and purposes, a spa.

In its early years, Doberan-Heiligendamm was far from the prototype for the modern seaside resort focused on the sea and the beach. Rather, it was a spa that provided visitors with the opportunity for sea bathing. Doberan was almost entirely modeled on the spatial ideals prevailing at the inland spas. Surrounded by gentle hills, Doberan corresponded to the earlier landscape ideal, an ideal that had begun to change but had not yet been fully replaced in the discourse. Subsequently, Doberan was equipped with all the necessary buildings for a typical spa. The lodging house (*Logierhaus*), erected in 1796, was designed by Seydewitz. Numerous buildings designed by Carl Theodor Severin in the style of early Classicism followed: a salon building with a dining hall (1801/1802), two pavilions in the so-called Chinese taste (1808/1809), a princely palace (1806–1810), and numerous residential buildings. Doberan acquired a casino in 1802 and a theater in 1805/1806.[99] Balls, concerts, and fireworks were organized. There were colonnades with shops and a reading library. The so-called Kamp, created on public pasture lands, combined the main avenue with an English landscape garden.[100] All the buildings and facilities in Doberan corresponded to what contemporaries expected to find at spas like Pyrmont or Wilhelmsbad.[101]

Spa practices in Doberan also mirrored the activities at the inland spas. Visitors stayed in Doberan and spent most of their days engaging in the customary leisure pursuits of playing games and attending communal meals, balls, and the theater.[102] One did not take walks on the beach or even on a seafront promenade, but wandered through an English landscape garden under trees at a safe distance from the sea. Early nineteenth-century spa publications about Doberan that included recommendations for outings into the spa's surroundings did not recommend the seaside. Rather, proposals for "pleasure outings over land" were limited to walks in the countryside, to overlooks in the surrounding area, and to the nearby towns of Rostock and Warnemünde.[103] In sum, Doberan, usually considered the first German seaside resort, in its early years was anything but.

A comparison between Lichtenberg's article of 1793 and Vogel's 1798 advertising pamphlet for Doberan is a study in contrast. Vogel's description of Doberan adheres to traditional expectations for inland spas.[104] In fact, there is not the slightest hint at a consideration of the seaside in his text; Vogel does not mention the sea or the seacoast at all. He describes Doberan as "this beautiful healing spring" and points out that at the spa "art rushes in from all sides to help nature," thus harking back to the earlier discourse.[105] The seaside is not part of the landscape that Vogel's readers are encouraged to explore; it is not even part of the described views. Vogel advertises bathing in seawater, and thus replaces spring water with seawater, but he does *not* propagate a seaside resort, a new form of summer retreat by the sea, or a new perception of the sea. In contrast to Lichtenberg, Vogel is not interested in inscribing Doberan as a new type of seaside resort into the established discourse. While Lichtenberg condemned the "dull avenues of the inland spas,"[106] Vogel praises "the quantity and variety of shaded promenades"[107] in Doberan.

If Vogel's original plan to transport seawater to a bathhouse in Doberan had been feasible,[108] the spa might never have become the first German seaside resort. But Vogel's plan had to be abandoned, and, as a result, in 1795/1796 a bathhouse designed by Seydewitz was built on the "Heiligen Damm."[109] A painting from the early nineteenth century shows that the new bathhouse, which was extended in 1820, did not face the sea

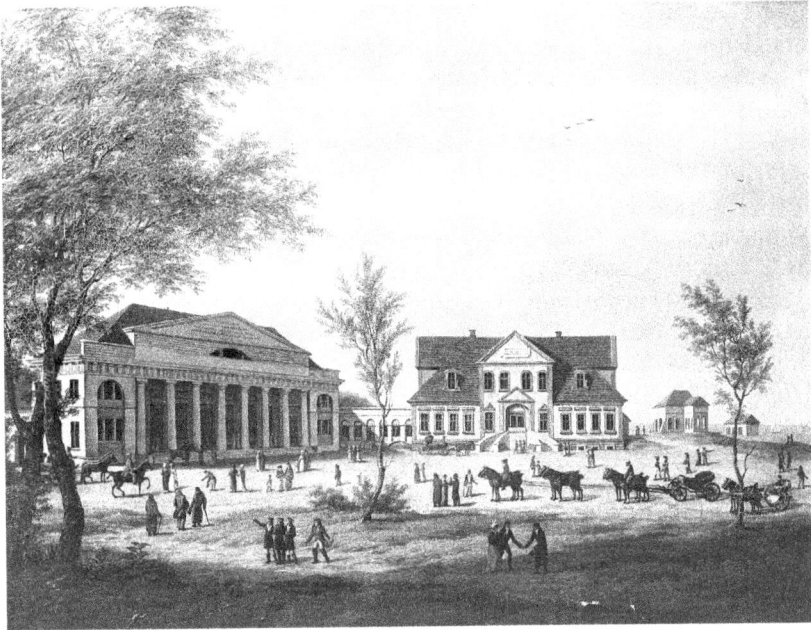

Figure 4.6 Heiligendamm, painting, first quarter of nineteenth century. (SLUB Dresden/Deutsche Fotothek/Beckmann, ?, um 1900.)

(Figure 4.6, the bathhouse is the building on the right, the building on the left was constructed later.) The concept of a bathhouse on the beach was clearly still new and unusual, and the orientation of the bathhouse did not encourage spa guests to take in the view of the sea. If spa guests spent time at the seaside at all, they did so as part of an outing to Heiligendamm in the morning for the sole purpose of bathing in seawater. In addition to the bathhouse, Heiligendamm offered guests "bathing sloops" (*Badeschaluppen*), which resembled the bathing ships on rivers that had been common in Germany since the 1760s. However, these obviously did not inspire much confidence among guests. In his "General Bathing Rules" ("Allgemeines Bade-Reglement") of 1798 Vogel thus tried to reassure bathers: "Also, there is no need to fear any misfortune in the bathing sloops."[110] From 1803 onward, Heiligendamm offered its guests so-called bathing machines, which were common in England. Bathing machines were carts with a cloth cover and stairs at the back, from which a bather could climb into the sea.[111]

Doberan-Heiligendamm attracted 480 guests in 1797, but only about 100 of them took hot or cold seawater baths.[112] As in most spas of this period, the leisure function held sway over the health function in Doberan. In other spas, however, most of the guests – even the healthy ones – drank the healing water as part of a social ritual. In contrast, the mistrust of bathing in seawater was so pervasive in late eighteenth-century Germany that this practice was not part of a daily routine shared by all spa guests. In his advertising pamphlet, Vogel's detailed "General Bathing Rules" speak to this uneasiness. He endeavors to dispel the fear of the cold seawater by arguing that the "worry" people felt should be countered by positive thinking: "The more cheerful and fearless one climbs into the bath, the better."[113]

Starting in the 1810s, the changes in perception and practices identified by Corbin in his work *The Lure of the Sea* began to take hold in Germany. After tentative beginnings, Heiligendamm developed into a seaside resort. A central spa building (*Kurhaus*) designed by Carl Theodor Severin was built in 1814–1816. Its main facade with a triangular gable faces the sea (Figure 4.6, building on the left). As new seaside resorts were founded on the North and Baltic Sea coasts – the island of Norderney, Travemünde, Cuxhaven/Ritzebüttel, Putbus on the island of Rügen,[114] and the island of Föhr – a new discourse about the sea and the seaside emerged. In the same way that the discourse about inland spas was first influenced by the adoption of Alpine euphoria and then served as a multiplier for the new appreciation of mountains, the discourse about seaside resorts originated with elite authors, but soon functioned as a multiplier for the ideas and practices associated with the "discovery of the seaside."

These new ideals, however, were conveyed to the reading public through a slow and meandering process. Authors of guidebooks for seaside resorts succeeded only gradually in extending the boundaries of the established discourse about inland spas. Carl Friedrich Mosch's spa compendium of 1819 shows that the published discourse about seaside resorts was in a transitional phase. In the description of Doberan, the images do not show the Baltic Sea or even the buildings in Heiligendamm, but rather a view of Doberan from a distance (Figure 4.7) and the church of its former Cistercian monastery. The choice of illustrations takes up both the earlier ideal of the spa as well as the Gothic Revival aesthetics: Doberan, with substantial buildings but open to the surrounding countryside and without walls, looks like a village with urban amenities, and the impressive Gothic church is depicted in its park-like surroundings. At the same time, however, the text recommends outings on foot and by carriage into the surrounding countryside as well as by ship on the Baltic Sea.[115] The author points out that these "water outings" were made possible by the grand duke of Mecklenburg-Schwerin who invited spa guests from the educated elite to accompany him on his frigate.[116]

The sea now became an integral part of the view that visitors could enjoy. At the very beginning of the description of Doberan in Mosch's compendium, the reader is informed that one has "a beautiful view of the mirrored surface of the sea."[117] The sea is "covered with ships," which one can observe while enjoying "the pure sea air in the morning."[118] A

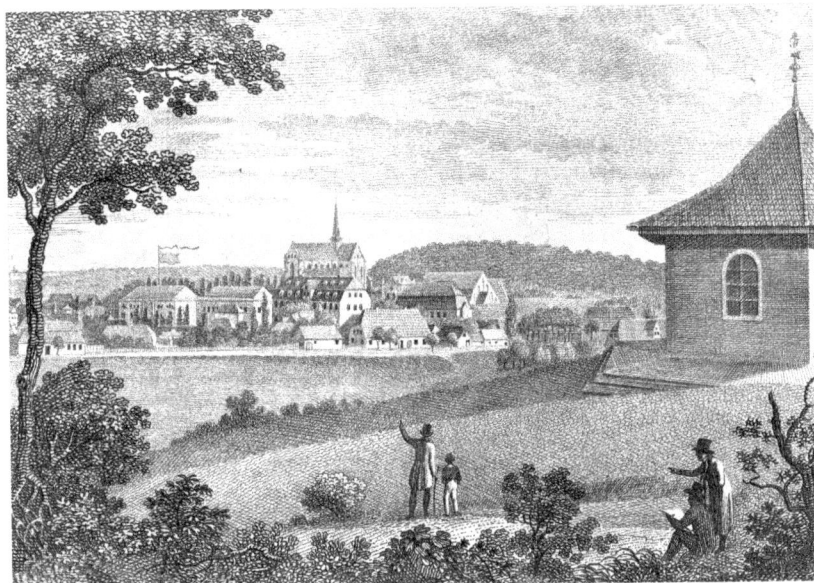

Figure 4.7 Doberan, engraving by F. Rosmäsler junior, 1819. ("Doberan." In Mosch, Carl Friedrich. *Die Bäder und Heilbrunnen Deutschlands und der Schweiz: Ein Taschenbuch für Brunnen- und Badereisende.* Vol. 1, unpaginated, in article "Doberan." Leipzig: Brockhaus, 1819. Collection of the author.)

"Dollond" to watch the ships, a telescope named after the eighteenth-century British optician John Dollond, had been installed "at the beach" in Heiligendamm, and a chart of flags was displayed in the bathhouse, so that guests could "find out the people [*Volk*] to whom the ship belongs."[119] The description of Travemünde, also on the Baltic Sea, tells the reader that guests at this new seaside resort can see the "billowing" cornfields on one side and the "billowing" sea on the other side.[120] The author also highlights how "interesting" it is for the "inhabitants of landlocked areas" to view the sea and the spectacle of arriving and departing ships, visible from the patio in front of the dining hall.[121]

The repeated use of the term "interesting,"[122] however, expresses the mental distance still present in the perception of the sea, even the Baltic Sea, that shaped the emerging discourse about seaside resorts. In Mosch's compendium, the area around Doberan is described in a rather ambivalent way, with only the English landscape garden and the surrounding landscape receiving unmitigated approval, while the sea is described in negative terms: "One of the closest and shadiest [promenades] is the one on the Kamp connected to an English garden. The nearby park with its water basin is very pleasant, as is the Jungfernberg [literally: Maiden

Mountain] with its splendid grove and beautiful walkways. Doberan is picturesquely situated at the foot of the latter and embellishes by its location the coastal area that otherwise has little charm. . . . seawards the eye loses itself in the vast desert of the sea covered with ships."[123] In a similar vein, the article about Cuxhaven/Ritzebüttel praises the small bathhouse at this seaside resort, especially for its location, "placed on a dam between two small lakes connected to the port of Hamburg." Thus, the author argues, guests could "enjoy the effect of bathing in the open sea without exposing oneself to it."[124]

Contemporaries' persistent mental distance from the sea is most noticeable in the descriptions of North Sea islands. In many ways, these islands embodied the new spatial ideal of the seaside advocated by Lichtenberg. North Sea islands, surrounded by sea water, waves, and tides, and made up of nothing but sand dunes, could not differ more from the "avenues of the inland spas."[125] Authors advertising North Sea islands like Norderney and Föhr constantly had to accommodate the expectations of their readers that were clearly defined by the published discourse about inland spas. At the same time, they tried to push the limits of that discourse.

The article about Norderney in Mosch's compendium is an example thereof. It addresses the danger of traveling through the Wadden Sea by ship or carriage at low tide, and the tides are described as a "strange spectacle" that is "particularly interesting."[126] Norderney is judged by the standards of inland spas and therefore falls short of expectations: "There is not much variation in walks. One generally hikes along the seashore, or in the grove, the only one on the island. Climbing up the dunes is generally hampered by the difficulty of wading in the sand, although the panorama of the sea and the view into the inner overgrown gorges of the dunes is worth the effort."[127] The gradual change in the discourse is tangible here. On the one hand, the author still criticizes the lack of footpaths and gardens, but at the same time he discovers the specific appeal of walking in the dunes. The description of dunes as having "overgrown gorges" can be interpreted as an attempt to reference mental images of the Alpine euphoria.

In his 1822 guidebook, Friedrich Wilhelm von Halem, the founder of Norderney, also tried to respond to the spatial ideal of the inland spas. Halem repeatedly references the dominant discourse about inland spas. He proudly reports that the "conversation house" (*Conversations-Haus*) in Norderney, built around 1800, had "large bright dining and dancing halls, billiards and games rooms, [and] a room where newspapers and journals are available."[128] He diligently explains Norderney's perceived shortcomings compared to inland spas. For instance, Halem observes that it would be perfectly possible to plant a grove next to the conversation house, "if it is done with patience and adapted to the individuality of the island."[129] With regard to accommodations, Halem resorts to a similar

line of argument: "Large lodging houses admittedly have a more impos-
ing appearance than the small one-story houses on our island. But those
who have once experienced the flurry and inconvenience of such large
establishments will, in light of the good-natured and friendly service of
the inhabitants [of the island], soon wean themselves from the purported
advantages of such modern facilities."[130] He sums up in a slightly defensive tone: "Our little island is not such a desolate heap of sand, as the
ignorant would like to think, and even if it lacks the shady avenues of
many inland spas, these spas lack the invigorating sea air."[131] At the same
time, Halem – in contrast to Vogel some twenty years earlier – applies
discursive statements about "sublime nature" (*erhabene Natur*) to the sea
in an attempt to acculturate his readers to a new spatial perception: "It
is the pleasure that the simple sublime nature here on the beach offers its
admirers in the highest perfection."[132]

The 1824 guidebook *The Island of Föhr and the Wilhelmine Seaside
Resort* (*Die Insel Föhr und das Wilhelminen See-Bad*) by Friedrich von
Warnstedt is another example of the discursive twists, sometimes even
contortions, that authors propagating seaside resorts had to make in order
to cater to their readership. Warnstedt argues that Föhr does not need the
"exhilarating amusements" of other "glamorous bathing facilities," that
is, the inland spas.[133] At the same time, however, he describes in great
detail the efforts made to adapt the interior spaces of the village of Wyck
to the expectations associated with these "glamorous" spas. Examples
of these efforts are the extension of the assembly rooms (*Gesellschafts-
haus*)[134] and the planting of an avenue of poplars that is described as "a
nearly always dry sand path." It is striking that Warnstedt still mentions
an avenue in the 1820s. This is another reminder of the enduring influence
of the inland spas on the published discourse: invoking an avenue of trees
that drains well can only be read as a reference to the main avenue in
Pyrmont and its drainage capabilities, praised by Marcard in his famous
spa guide.[135]

Similar to Halem, Warnstedt guides his readers' perception of the seaside. He uses emotive language and encourages guests to emulate these
emotions. Warnstedt also propagates a transfer of the practice of hiking
to the seaside. His description of a "hike"[136] along the avenue with a view
of the sea is both utterly positive and full of Romantic tropes. These were
soon to become clichés, as we have already seen in the case of inland spas
and the perception of mountains: "Nature in its infinite greatness seizes
the lonely hiker, the steady roaring and rolling of the waves from the
deep dark distance beneath him [*sic*] enchants him wonderfully, immerses
him in the infinity of serious thought, and in unspeakable bliss he feels
wrested from the petty tangle of life, freer, and closer to the great infinite
universe!"[137] The author even invites guests to try out the new practices
of "walking, [horseback] riding, [and] carriage rides on the beach itself,"
describing them as "among the most inviting and beneficial pleasures."[138]

And yet, Warnstedt felt it necessary to evoke the established discourse about Alpine landscapes in his attempt to attract visitors to the island of Föhr. He constructs a striking parallel between the Swiss mountains and the dunes of the neighboring North Sea islands of Sylt and Amrum: "These two . . . islands protect Föhr in particular with their high sand dunes, which in their shapes and their crests overgrown with pale green sand-sedge and . . . rugged white sand slopes present the most striking resemblance to Swiss mountainous regions in miniature."[139]

In sum, beginning in 1793/1794, the new perception of the sea and the seaside that first developed in western Europe was gradually established in Germany over a period of more than two decades. Like the transformation of the published spa discourse and its function as a multiplier of "Alpine euphoria," the change in the discourse about seaside resorts did not progress in a straightforward manner. Rather, the discursive change took shape through a circuitous and slow process. Advertising pamphlets and travel guides reflect the patterns of perception among the majority of readers interested in the new seaside resorts, who were most likely also visitors of inland spas. These sources show that Georg Christoph Lichtenberg's article of 1793 did not represent a broadly shared perception, but was, in effect, a discursive anomaly in Germany at the time.

Initially, authors advertising seaside resorts struggled to make their argument. Clearly catering to the expectations of their readers, they consistently emphasized that seaside resorts offered similar, if not the same amenities as inland spas. This included spa buildings and services as well as avenues and English landscape gardens. The enduring power of this ideal is demonstrated by the fact that seaside resorts in the 1790s and beyond aspired to emulate inland spas that were themselves undergoing fundamental changes at the time. Authors propagating seaside resorts engaged in direct comparisons with the statements of the published discourse about spas and did not attempt to construct a new spatial ideal. Samuel Gottlieb Vogel's 1798 description of Doberan was an example of this. Even in the early nineteenth century, seaside resorts were still listed alphabetically alongside inland spas in spa compendia.[140] This also indicates that seaside resorts were not yet regarded as an independent type of summer resort.

Ultimately, however, German authors promoting seaside resorts succeeded in establishing a new discursive regime about "the lure of the sea" and the seaside in their readers' minds, thereby multiplying a spatial ideal that continues to deeply affect tourist experiences until this day. During the 1820s, seaside resorts emerged as a new type of spatial heterotopia in the published discourse. The sea had become a "picturesque view," and the beach, the dunes, and the seascape were now considered worthy of admiration. As the discourse about seaside resorts caught up with the parallel discourse about spas, the Romantic "lonely hiker" in nature was encouraged to explore both the mountains in the vicinity of an inland spa and the dunes of a North Sea island. Nevertheless, a residue of mental distance from the sea and seaside practices among the reading public can still be observed in the way authors guide their readers' perceptions. So it comes as no surprise that Wilhelm von Humboldt remarked about Norderney as late as 1833: "The sea and having a constant view of the sea, however barren the beach and the island may be, is a nice bonus."[141]

Time at the Spa: An Annual Ritual and a Daily Routine

The temporal aspect of the spa as a heterotopia – Foucault calls this "heterochrony" – refers to two different characteristics of a spa visit: spa trips as annual occurrences and the daily routine at the spa. *First*, spa trips occurred during a clearly defined time of the year. For the upper middle class and the nobility, the spa trip meant a change of location lasting several weeks, carefully planned, and usually repeated annually during the summer months.[142] This makes spa visits precursors of modern summer vacations. Spa visits differed from the so-called summer retreat (*Sommerfrische*) that also emerged in the late eighteenth century. During summer retreats, families spent the time from May to October in a place in the countryside outside (but close to) the city, while the housefather usually continued to move back and forth to do his work. In contrast, spa visits were limited to a few weeks and required absence from work due to the greater distance traveled.[143] *Second*, the spa as a heterotopia, as life outside of everyday life, also made for a particular experience of time. As we shall see later, spa days were defined by a rather rigid daily routine. In theory, a spa visitor could be overwhelmed by the many activities offered by the heterotopia of the spa, but the daily routine that characterized life at the spa limited the number of options at any given time of the day. The goal was to still leave guests with choices, but prevent them from being overwhelmed. Thus, while staying at a spa was in many ways an exceptional situation, the ritualization of daily life through a social routine served to stabilize this open and potentially unstable heterotopia.

First, in the sixteenth and seventeenth centuries, spring and autumn were also considered appropriate times for spa visits, but by the eighteenth century the custom of summer trips prevailed. The main season at the spas generally lasted from June to August. The highest number of guests came in June and July,[144] and the month of July was generally regarded as the peak of the season.[145] In 1785, Joachim Christoph Friedrich Schulz observed the ebb and flow of the season in Karlsbad and the change in the social composition of the spa society over the course of each season:

> This bustle lasts from the first days of June until about the last of July, when it ends all at once, almost always within three days, because the members of the society that made it [the bustle] seemed to have promised each other to come and go at the same time. Now the remaining

spa guests draw breath again, and their number is increased by those businessmen, who now – during the dog days of summer – can take care of their health; . . . This period lasts until the beginning of September, when yeomen, priests from the neighborhood, shopkeepers with their wives and children, and peasants come to Karlsbad.[146]

The length of a spa visit usually fluctuated between three and six weeks; a four-week stay was the most common.[147] University professors, for example, were granted leaves of absence for the purpose of spa-going. Pütter, who had visited Pyrmont for three weeks almost annually since 1779, reported in his autobiography, "I was encouraged to continue my annual journey to Pyrmont because the royal ministry willingly granted me permission to do so each time, sometimes attesting that it was done with pleasure."[148]

On the one hand the spa as a heterochrony can be characterized as an opportunity to leave everyday life behind. On the other hand it also represented a multifunctional time that was connected to everyday life in various ways. A spa visit was described as an escape from everyday life because of its "important concomitants,"[149] which allowed members of the middle class to recover from strenuous work. In his prelude for the opening of the theater in Lauchstädt on 26 June 1802, Johann Wolfgang von Goethe put contemporary expectations about the spa as a heterochrony into verse:

> When bathing [being at a spa], one's first duty is to make sure
> That one does not rack one's brain
> And that one at the most studies
> How to lead the most cheerful life.[150]

And an article in the *Monthly for Germans (Monatsschrift für Deutsche)* argued in 1801, "The businessman, burdened with hard work that chains him to his desk all day long and often even several hours of the night, will certainly feel life's happiness twice if, free of his usual burden, he can live entirely according to his circumstances and his mood. He will certainly appreciate the place where he can meet like-minded people with the same needs, spend a few weeks here [at a spa] with them in cheerful familiarity, and see the rosy days of his happy youth revive."[151]

In order to avoid boredom, which was considered dangerous for mind and body, the spa had to provide sufficient amusements and "pleasures."[152] Knigge advised the spa visitor in his *Practical Philosophy of Social Life (Über den Umgang mit Menschen)*: "Drop all serious correspondence, shun all business which requires exertion, and provide yourself with as much money as will enable you to join in any innocent amusements."[153] The "innocent amusements" at the spa included the theater, balls, walks, and all kinds of social gatherings, but excluded gambling, which was strongly condemned in the published discourse.[154] This corresponds to the negative view of gambling as an aristocratic vice in contemporary bourgeois perception.[155]

Based on the dietetics of the soul[156] and the heterotopian ideal of the spa as a space for entertainment and recreation, the published discourse consistently condemned the pursuit of work at the spa.[157] The upper middle class – or, rather, men of the upper middle class – were supposed to rest, enjoy themselves, and strengthen their health. The exhausting mental labor, otherwise expected of them in everyday life, was frowned upon at the spa. In the published discourse, work is described as destroying the character of the spa as a heterochrony. As Marcard points out in his *Description of Pyrmont (Beschreibung von Pyrmont)*, a stay at the spa is "a time in which one abstains from all actual business with diligence."[158] Strikingly, Marcard uses the term "with diligence," usually reserved in the bourgeois discourse for mental labor,[159] to describe its opposite, namely leisure. In his advertising pamphlet for Doberan Vogel asserts, "Traveling to spas and watering places is often especially recommended to people by their physicians so that they can get into a freer, more pleasant, and quieter situation in order to avoid strenuous business, worries, and vexing circumstances, and to find amusements and diversions that are often not possible at home."[160]

At the same time, however, a stay at the spa served multiple purposes, not the least of which was work. As we have already seen in Chapter 2, people met with friends, made professional contacts, initiated marriages, and consumed luxury goods. And not only the fictional Dr. Katzenberger but also many real members of the educated elite took their work along to the spa. Scholars considered it almost absurd to follow the strict instructions of the spa physicians; rather, they clearly regarded a spa visit as an opportunity for work-related activities. Möser countered the stipulation to not work at the spa with an ironic comment: "Our great physician has forbidden me to think."[161] Giseke went even further in reducing the physicians' advice to absurdity: "Thinking here is medically a mortal sin, just as in some places it is politically a mortal sin to freely share one's thoughts."[162] We have already seen that Pütter and Strube used their annual Pyrmont visits to make professional contacts. Pütter described himself as a diligent worker who forsook opportunities for amusement to write his autobiography: "I used for this purpose such hours in Pyrmont and Rehburg that were spent by others at gaming tables or in theaters."[163]

Goethe's attitude toward work at the spa shows that he drew clear distinctions between spas. In the large, fashionable spas such as Karlsbad and Pyrmont he participated in social activities and amusements: "I live with many diversions, the whole day among people," he wrote to Christiane Vulpius from Karlsbad in 1795.[164] He remained uneasy, however, about not working and instead living this heterotopian lifestyle: "I haven't done much, by the way. The spring and the distraction of life here don't make you feel very composed," he wrote in 1806.[165] Goethe chose smaller spas, such as Tennstedt in Saxony, later Prussia,[166] to engage in intense work. He thus constructed a different kind of heterotopia where he could focus on writing. In a letter to Johann Heinrich Meyer in 1816, he commented, "And so you see here an exercise how I, as writing master of Tennstedt, lead a strange life, in the most absolute solitude."[167] In contrast to the ideal of abstaining from work propagated in the published spa discourse, contemporaries' experiences reflect the difficulties of navigating the relationship between work as a bourgeois virtue and times of recreation. Anticipating modern vacations, the educated elite engaged in recreation and diversion at the spa as a counterbalance to work, but at the same time, they found it difficult to find balance between work and leisure.[168] One might say that this is a dilemma still plaguing today's scholars on their vacations.

Second, in the published discourse and in personal narratives, everyday life at the spa is described as a daily routine. Be it Pyrmont or Karlsbad, Imnau or Teinach, from the most famous spas to small spas barely present in the published discourse, the course of a typical spa day was clearly defined by a succession of activities performed at certain times in certain spaces.[169] In his 1795 *Journey of a Livonian* (*Reise eines Liefländers*), Joachim Christoph Friedrich Schulz described the "order of the day in Karlsbad":

> One gets up between five and six o'clock and goes to the well, . . . Around eight o'clock, the various wells are completely empty of drinkers. It is a rule prescribed by the local physicians to stay at home for an hour and wait before looking for breakfast in one of the halls; . . . If one does not want to take part in it [breakfast], or if one is not invited to it, one goes for a walk or sits down at a gambling table, or plays billiards, or takes part in a conversation in the avenue. . . . This spectacle lasts until about twelve o'clock, when one hurries home to have a small bite. After this business, it is permitted to nap for a few minutes, . . . The ladies go to their dressing tables and dress for the ball, which is to start at four o'clock. . . . Others write letters, but they are on their guard against the spa physician, who has forbidden all thinking and writing during the spa visit. Others have arranged a walk, an outing into the countryside, and a communal dinner; . . . Around nine o'clock the ball is over, the walkers or carriage riders return to town, . . . and after nine o'clock everyone goes to bed.[170]

In his *Description of Pyrmont* (*Beschreibung von Pyrmont*), Marcard claims that a Pyrmont day has "its own course,"[171] but, notwithstanding Marcard's boast, the way a typical day unfolded in Pyrmont differed only marginally from what happened in Karlsbad. Baggesen's travelogue of 1789 highlights these similarities:

One generally gets up quite early. At six o'clock you can already see the genteel world [*feine Welt*] in full motion in the large avenue. . . . A pretty instrumental music entertains the ear during this time . . . One greets one's acquaintances, the friend seeks the friend, and the whole army gradually divides into larger and smaller groups, who drink the water together at the end of the avenue until around nine o'clock the movement flows into as many breakfast groups. . . . When breakfast is over, people walk up and down a couple of times, the crowd disperses, one now goes [horseback] riding, a second bathes, a third plays billiards, a fourth plays cards, a fifth goes on an outing: . . . After lunch, [the spa] society gathers again in the main avenue . . . At last, people divide into two main groups, the one that stays and the one that flees. The group that stays gathers in the assembly hall around the faro bank, or watches a comedy, and otherwise makes do with what the [main] avenue has to offer until the evening meal. The group that flees undertakes outings to the surrounding mountains in smaller groups, . . . Finally, one goes to bed in order to sleep, if one can, until the next morning when the same life begins again.[172]

Käppel's description of the daily routine in his *Pyrmont's Noteworthy Features* (*Pyrmonts Merkwürdigkeiten*) of 1800 speaks to the way the published discourse prepared spa visitors for the rhythm of this "everyday life outside of everyday life." He even provides a precise time of day for each activity:

At six o'clock the genteel world [*feinere Welt*] begins to show up and everyone hurries, glass in hand, to the pump room [*Brunnenhaus*]. . . . Precisely at 7 a.m. a band of hautbois starts playing a morning psalm. . . . Between 8 and 9 a.m. groups gather for breakfast, . . . After breakfast, the ladies make promenades either by carriage or on foot, in the avenues and garden areas on the sides [of the main avenue], or they also go to the bathhouse. . . . Echoes of "le jeu est fait!" ["the stakes are set," literally "the game is over"] can be heard from the ballroom [which also served as the casino]. . . . In this way, the morning lingers on until the lunch bell rings, when everyone hurries to the tables. At 3 o'clock, people are ready to leave the tables; . . . From 4 to 5 o'clock the main avenue is at its most glamorous. . . . At 5 o'clock the theater lovers hurry to see a play, and the nature lovers hurry into the surrounding area, . . . At 8 o'clock the play is over, the main avenue is full again. The faro bank pauses. The dinner bell rings. At 9 1/2 o'clock, dinner is over.[173]

While personal narratives generally mention only the "highlights" of a typical day at the spa, especially meetings with friends and acquaintances and outings, they often make direct or indirect references to the ubiquity of this daily routine. During her visit to Karlsbad in 1784, Sophie Becker remarked that she made only few entries into her diary "because here in this small world one day looks pretty much the same as the next."[174] In 1811 Christiane von Goethe summarized a day at the spa in a letter from Karlsbad: "We had breakfast on Thursday in the avenue where we met many acquaintances, . . . The Körners picked us up from there to go for a walk. Then we visited Frau von Flies and Oppenheimer. Privy councillor Meyer visited us. We had lunch at home. After lunch we both went on an outing; . . . We dressed beautifully for the ball."[175] And Goethe himself, who traveled to Pyrmont with his son in 1801, described the daily routine of father and son in his letter to Christiane: "We get up at 6 in the morning, drink from the well until 8, have breakfast at 9, walk around and talk until 11, then every other day we bathe until around 12, eat at home at 1, spend a few hours after lunch as we please, and in the evening we walk here and there in the surrounding area."[176]

The uniform nature of everyday life at the spa indicates how deeply embedded spas had become in the perception and practices of contemporaries. As participants in the circle of communication about spas identified in Chapter 2, spa guests learned about this everyday life outside of everyday life in various ways. They read about the daily ritual in spa guides, and the expectations raised were then fulfilled during spa visits and disseminated by spa guests' letters. The spa routine was further stabilized through ongoing repetition in the published discourse. As a result, this concept of a daily ritual at the spa became so firmly anchored in the minds of spa guests that spas could not deviate much from the established pattern.

Therefore, smaller spas like Imnau, in an attempt to establish themselves in the published discourse, imitated the daily routine of the larger spas, even if they lacked certain facilities and services, such as a theater:

> Early in the morning, woken by harmonious wind instruments, one got out of bed and went to the well, where a part [of the guests] drank the mineral water . . . and the other part that was only there for pleasure had breakfast in various groups, . . . and so it was 9 o'clock when one . . . got up, and one part [of the spa society] went to the bathhouse, the other part to get dressed. At 10 to half past 10 one searched for each other again, and found each other in the hallways of the building where the merchants offered their wares or in the assembly room where one could play . . . [or] began to talk, and so with general impatience awaited the stroke of 12 o'clock to be able to go to the tables . . . in the afternoon . . . one group walked, rode, and drove in one direction, the other in another direction; . . . In the evening . . . one sat down merrily at the table again, . . . After the meal, a walk followed, . . . or small games were played, and then one bid each other "good night!".[177]

Even in the emerging seaside resorts of the late eighteenth and early nineteenth centuries, the established pattern of daily life at the inland spas was followed closely. The daily routine in Doberan-Heiligendamm, for instance, differed from the daily routine in the inland spas in only one aspect: in the morning, drinking at the healing well in Doberan could be replaced by a carriage ride to Heiligendamm in order to bathe there. According to Vogel's spa guide, "the appropriate scheduling and use of time in Doberan" in the morning included activities such as "enjoying . . . a little rest" after returning from drinking the water or bathing, "grooming and dressing," "breakfast," "writing . . . a letter," "a walk, a visit, a game, etc. . . . and so on."[178] Spa guests listened to "the beautiful music" on the Kamp,[179] followed by lunch. "For many people, the time after the meal is the most boring, . . . But one should never be bored."[180] Vogel therefore recommends "writing a letter, pleasant, light reading, [or] an open conversation."[181] Notably, Vogel no longer tried to prevent spa visitors from letter-writing and reading, possibly because he knew that these activities were common. But his recommendation that the reading material be "pleasant" and "light" shows the enduring influence of the dietetics of the soul. As at inland spas, the collective activities in Doberan started again later in the afternoon: "Now comes the time for promenades by carriage, on horseback, and on foot, for which the beautiful region offers near and far excellent opportunities, or alternately for plays, balls, [or] gymnastic games of all kinds."[182]

By 1818, Princess Pauline of Lippe described the daily routine at the North Sea resort of Cuxhaven/Ritzebüttel as still similar to that of the inland spas. At the same time, however, new characteristics typical of seaside resorts emerged. The practice of sea bathing and other practices that were exclusive to seaside resorts made up a good part of the day: "The course of a weekday is that one drives, rides [on horseback], or walks to the baths [a bathhouse from which the bathing machines were launched into the water], where some chat, wait, work, have breakfast. The high tide determines and changes the hour. After the usual lunch one stays at home, drives around in the surrounding area, walks here and there, entertains oneself with outings on the water, drinks tea in the warm bathhouse [the bathhouse offering baths in warm sea water], climbs up the lighthouse, and usually ends the day in the 'Harmonie' [a restaurant and lodging house]."[183]

The daily routine established at the spas and seaside resorts had two important consequences. First, the structuring of time at the spas simultaneously resulted in a structuring of spaces and practices. At set times of the day the spa society came together in designated spaces and collectively pursued certain activities. These periods of time with fixed meeting places and practices alternated with other periods of the day when the spa guests could choose from a variety of activities and spaces. Everyone gathered at the healing well in the morning to drink water and meet friends and acquaintances. At the seaside resorts, the drinking of healing water was replaced by bathing in seawater. Breakfast, lunch, and dinner took place at fixed times, but spa guests were offered a choice between a communal and a more private setting. Before and after lunch there were periods of time that provided different options: shopping in the boutiques, walking in avenues and gardens, horseback riding, bathing in the bathhouse at spas, playing billiards, writing a letter, reading, and so forth. In the afternoon there again were common activities for the spa society or at least for smaller groups. Here, spa guests either chose activities within the interior spaces of the spa like various games, the theater, and the faro bank, or activities outside the spa. At the end of the eighteenth and the beginning of the nineteenth century, spas in mountainous regions and seaside resorts increasingly emphasized outings rather than internal activities during these afternoon hours. The heterochrony of the spa thus created a balance between communal practices that were repeated at fixed times and in defined spaces on the one hand, and periods of time with more individualized activities on the other.[184]

Second, the spa as a heterochrony was characterized by a high degree of social order and regulation coupled with a degree of personal freedom of choice. In 1785 Marcard noted, "A certain regularity that characterizes life in Pyrmont and that must prevail at a spa if one does not want to destroy the good effects of the water every day, is by no means a disadvantage for the spa society. It is a commendation for Pyrmont on the one hand, and on the other hand it has the advantage that one is always sure when and where one will find one's companions, without having to make special arrangements to meet."[185] Marcard describes the daily routine as part of dietetics and at the same time he defines it as an integral part of social life at the spa. The uniformity of everyday life effectively stabilized the spa as a heterotopia, which, as a space outside of everyday life, confronted spa visitors with many different activities and experiences. The daily routine created social cohesion through communal execution. In other words, the daily routine served to "tame" the exceptional situation in which spa visitors found themselves.

In sum, by the end of the eighteenth century, the spa visits of the bourgeoisie and the nobility had become an annual ritual. Friends and acquaintances arranged to meet at a spa or seaside resort, and people generally relied on these three to six weeks every year to find enjoyment and relaxation and to extend their social network. The published discourse about these summer resorts prepared guests for their visits in various ways. In addition to providing practical information about travel options, services, and facilities like lodging houses, guidebooks prepared visitors mentally for the experience of time and space. Thus, the published discourse introduced guests to the spa or the seaside resort as a spatial heterotopia and a heterochrony, a space and time separate from everyday life.

Notes

1. See, e.g., Weiss, *Entdeckung der Alpen*; Oppenheim, *Entdeckung der Alpen*; Faessler, *Bodensee und Alpen*; Woźniakowski, *Wildnis*, 213–275; Jost, *Landschaftsblick*; Raymond, *Von der Landschaft*; Boerlin-Brodbeck, "Die 'Entdeckung' der Alpen."
2. Ennen, "Residenzen," 194: "Die Residenzstadt . . . ist Mittelpunkt eines die Landschaft bewußt einbeziehenden Residenzraumes." See also Mintzker, *Defortification of the German City*. For Dresden, see Rosseaux, *Freiräume*, 259–274.
3. On the *Partie*, see Lempa, "The Spa," 61–63; Lempa, "Emotions." On walking and the *Partie*, see König, "Picknick."
4. On the development of walking and hiking, see Warneken, "Bürgerliche Gehkultur"; König, *Kulturgeschichte des Spazierganges*, 11–18, 186–204; Lempa, *Beyond the Gymnasium*, 163–193; Albrecht, Kertschner, *Wanderzwang*.
5. See Chapter 2.
6. See Kos, *Eroberung der Landschaft*, 23: "Tourism is, after all, a form of exploring and looking at views that no longer need to be defined with one's own eyes." ("Tourismus ist ja Begehung mit Blicken, die nicht mehr mit eigenen Augen definiert werden müssen.") See also Jost, *Landschaftsblick*, 126–138.
7. [Giseke], "Neue Briefe über Carlsbad, vom Jahre 1792, Erster Brief," 1793, 359 [i.e. 365]: "lauter gebirgigen Thälern zwischen entsetzlichen Steinen und Tiefen."
8. [Giseke], "Neue Briefe über Carlsbad, vom Jahre 1792, Erster Brief," 1793, 366: "Uebrigens ist die Gegend hier äusserst angenehm und romantisch." – "moosigen Klippen" – "dunklen Tannen" – "gütige Natur auch in ihrer schönen Wildheit" – "wenn wir nur Gefühl für sie haben, und vertraut mit ihr umzugehen verstehen!"
9. [Giseke], "Neue Briefe über Carlsbad, vom Jahre 1792, Erster Brief," 1793, 367: "Die ganze Gestalt der hiesigen Gegend ist sehr einnehmend. Man wird von dem ersten Anblick hingerissen, und freut sich, die Natur bei aller Wildheit, die sie hier hat, doch so freundlich zu finden."
10. See Raymond, *Von der Landschaft*, 52.
11. See Raymond, *Von der Landschaft*, 60–88.
12. [Giseke], "Fortsetzung der Briefe über Carlsbad," 1793, 809; "Eine kleine friedliche Wiese: die von allen Seiten, aber nicht ängstlich, eingeschlossen ist, gewährt gerade die Einschränkung, welche so wohlthätig für uns ist, weil sie nicht zertheilt, sondern zum wirklichen Genuß dessen, was die Wirklichkeit darbeut, einladet. Auf der einen Seite deckt Tannengebüsch die Höhen, auf der Anderen ragen Aecker, Wiesen, und komischgeformte Felsen schimmernd zwischen grünen Büschen hervor. Einzelne zerstreute Häuserchen benehmen der Gegend das Wilde."
13. [Giseke], "Fortsetzung der Briefe über Carlsbad," 1793, 806: "Wer noch nicht das Glück gehabt hat, Helvetien zu sehen, der kann hier einen Vorschmack davon bekommen."
14. [Giseke], "Fortsetzung der Briefe über Carlsbad," 1793, 807: "Hier erhebt sich ein hoher isolirter Felsen, der den einsamen Walker mit seiner pittoresken Form überrascht."
15. See [Giseke], "Neue Briefe über Carlsbad, vom Jahre 1792, Zweiter Brief," 1793, 383–400.
16. [Giseke], "Neue Briefe über Carlsbad, vom Jahre 1792, Zweiter Brief," 1793, 383: "Ohngeachtet nun die Stadt Carlsbad ihre Häuser, Strassen und

Plätze eben nicht für eine grosse Merkwürdigkeit ausgeben darf, so scheint es mir doch, als wenn ich wohlthäte, bei der gewöhnlichen Ordnung zu bleiben, und Sie, mein Freund, zuerst damit bekannt zu machen."

17. "Teutsche Badechronik," *JLM* (October 1796), 519–520: "Nenndorf. Nahe bei diesem Dörfchen hat der Landgraf von Hessen-Cassel im Jahr 1788 aus einer Wildniß einen reizenden Badeort machen lassen. . . . Die Berge rings umher sind in einer solchen Entfernung, daß der Ort, weit entfernt etwas ängstliches und eingeschlossenes zu haben, vielmehr die offensten, lachendsten Aussichten darbietet."

18. "Teutsche Badechronik," *JLM* (October 1796), 525: "einer Cellischen Gesellschaft von Adelichen."

19. "Teutsche Badechronik," *JLM* (October 1796), 525: "Die Badeanstalten liegen eine halbe Stunde vom Städtchen Rehburg in einem Thale, das wie ein Kessel von Berg und Wald eingeschlossen ist. Der Platz, wo die Badehäuser etc. liegen, ist nicht schön."

20. Deneken, "Bemerkungen bey dem Rehburger Gesundbrunnen," 1796, 195: "in einer überaus romantischen Gegend."

21. Deneken, "Bemerkungen bey dem Rehburger Gesundbrunnen," 1796, 198: "weit ausgebreitete, mahlerische Landschaft" – "die durch die Zeit schon halb verdunkelte[n] Bilder der Schweitzer Aussichten."

22. Deneken, "Bemerkungen bey dem Rehburger Gesundbrunnen," 1796, 198–199: "Ich glaubte in dem lieblichen Gemische der Waldungen . . . – vorzüglich aber in dem Anblicke des Steinhuder Meeres . . . und in den Bergen, welche in dämmernder Ferne diese reitzende Landschaft umschliessen, ein Miniatur-Gemälde irgend einer Schweitzer Gegend zu sehen."

23. Müller, *Welt des Baedeker*, 275: "Sehhilfen" – "als solche bilden sie Wahrnehmungsdispositive und werden zur Grundlage für eine die Realität überlagernde Seh- und Raumordnung."

24. Ficker, *Driburger Taschenbuch*, 1811, 109: "Die ehrwürdige Kette von Bergen, die Driburg umschließt, . . . geben der Gegend jene romantische Schönheit, die der Bewohner der Ebene so sehr bewundert, der Naturfreund besteigt sie gerne, . . . Doch sind auch die Spaziergänge in der Nähe des Driburger Mineralbrunnens ausgebreitet genug, um dem schwächern Kurgaste . . . einen Ersatz für den hohen Genuss zu geben, den der raschere Bergsteiger täglich haben kann."

25. Elise Bürger describes a typical outing (*Partie*) from Baden-Baden to Castle Eberstein and the Murgh valley in "Ein Sommermorgen in Baden-Baden. 1808." Bürger, *Lilien-Blätter*, 1826, 81–87. See also Reichard, *Passagier auf der Reise*, 1801, 351–393, where he provides extensive information for "excursions" ("Exkursionen") and "pleasure outings in the surrounding countryside" ("Lustpartien in der umliegenden Gegend").

26. Goethe, Vulpius, *Goethes Briefwechsel mit seiner Frau*, vol. 2, letter from Wiesbaden, 1 August 1814, 315: "Vier Chausseen, die von Hügeln und Bergen in die Tiefe führen, wo der Ort liegt, stieben den ganzen Tag von Zu- und Abfahrenden, von Lust- und Spazierfahrenden. Da solls nach Mainz, Biebrich, Elfeld, Schlangenbad, Schwalbach und wohin alles. Da liegen für Fußgänger verfallne Schlösser, mit Erfrischungs-Örtern, im nächsten Gebirg. Da, und so weiter! Zelter, ein furchtbarer Fußwanderer, hat das alles schon durchstrichen."

27. Pyrmont also provides an interesting case study in this regard. While Marcard, as we saw previously, focused on the depiction of the spa's interior spaces, the main avenue in Pyrmont lost some of its appeal in the late eighteenth century. Frankenau commented, "So I can boast to have seen many

avenues which are more beautiful than this one." ("So kann ich doch rüh-
men, viele Alleen gesehen zu haben, welche schöner sind als diese.") Frankenau, *Pyrmont*, 1799, 22. Menke, in his *Pÿrmont und seine Umgebungen*
of 1818, then dedicates a lot of space to the representation of Pyrmont's
surroundings rather than its interior spaces.

28. "Teutsche Badechronik," *JLM* (December 1796), 602–603: "Sie werden,
    lieber Freund, das Detail der Promenaden von Karlsbad nicht zu lang fin-
    den, wenn Sie wissen, daß sie eine von den Haupt-Annehmlichkeiten dieses
    schönen Bades ausmachen, und deren sich kein andres rühmen kann. Künst-
    liche Anlagen hat Karlsbad nicht, aber die Natur hat dafür rings umher
    einen großen Park von schönen Berg-Wäldern, reichen Aussichten und
    Thälern geschaffen, wo sie sich in einer so reitzenden, freyen und unver-
    stellten Anmuth zeigt."

29. "Teutsche Badechronik," *JLM* (December 1796), 598: "schöne, schmale
    Töpel-Thal."

30. See "Teutsche Badechronik," *JLM* (December 1796), 600.

31. "Teutsche Badechronik," *JLM* (December 1796), 601: "Bergsteigen." In
    contrast, the 1798 travelogue *Reise nach den Badeörtern* still aligned with
    the older landscape perception. The author maintains that the best part of a
    walk in the area surrounding Karlsbad was the view into the town below. He
    also compares Karlsbad's surroundings with the Alps, but in an unexpected
    way, arguing: "I do believe that there are equally bad areas [with rugged
    rocks and outcrops] in the Alps, but one does not go for walks there."("Ich
    glaube schon, daß es auf den Alpen eben so arge Stellen geben mag: nur geht
    man dort darauf nicht spatzieren.") *Reise nach den Badeörtern*, 1798, 157,
    see 141–157.

32. Harrer, *Karlsbad und die umliegende Gegend*, 1801, 9: "Die natürliche Lage
    des Orts ist schon ganz zum Kurorte geschaffen. Ein enges romantisches Tal,
    von dem Töplflusse durchschnitten, mit Gebürgen umgeben."

33. "Bade-Chronik," *JLM* (November 1815), 655: "darf Carlsbad auch in
    Hinsicht seiner Lage jedem andern Brunnenorte den Rang streitig machen"
    – "fast wie eingeklemmt in dem lieblichen Thale, welches die Töpel durch-
    strömt, umgeben von herrlichen waldgekrönten Felsen, bietet es eine
    unendliche Abwechselung der freundlichsten und erhabensten Scenen." See
    also Schopenhauer, "Das Badeleben in Karlsbad während der Monate Julius
    und August im Jahre 1815," 286.

34. Schopenhauer, "Brief aus Karlsbad 1821," 314: "In der Stadt selbst ist jeder
    dazu einigermaßen schickliche Platz bebaut, fast jedes grüne Gartenfleck-
    chen, und zwar mit zwei oder drei Stock hohen Häusern, wodurch man gar
    viel vom Anblick der prächtigen Felsen verliert, die Karlsbad so herrlich
    umfrieden, und die, wenn das so fortgeht, bald nur noch mit den Spitzen
    über die Masse von Häusern hervorragen werden."

35. Baggesen, *Labyrinth*, 168: "langweilig."

36. See Baggesen, *Labyrinth*, 169–188.

37. Recke, *Tagebücher und Selbstzeugnisse*, 123: "Diese Bergformen sind sehr
    gleichförmig und haben keine romantische Schönheit. Einem an die Fläche
    gewöhnten Auge wird diese Gegend . . . angenehme Abwechslung darbieten,
    aber wer die böhmischen Gebirg kürzlich gesehen hat, von Dresden kommt,
    der findet diese Gegend unbedeutend."

38. Recke, *Tagebücher und Selbstzeugnisse*, 321: "schönen Felsenmassen."

39. Recke, *Tagebücher und Selbstzeugnisse*, 322: "romantischen Tälern."

40. Recke, *Tagebücher und Selbstzeugnisse*, 324: "unschuldigen Naturfreuden."
    See also Luise von Preussen, *Fünfundvierzig Jahre aus meinem Leben*, 135,

about her visit to Karlsbad in 1800. Luise von Preußen shared Recke's perception of the landscape around Karlsbad as "romantic" and "enchanting" ("romantisch" – "bezaubernd").

41. Recke, *Tagebücher und Selbstzeugnisse*, 327: "Der junge Mitterbacher hatte uns einen Führer besorgt, dem er es zutraute, daß er uns die schönsten Gegenden um Ellenbogen zeigen würde. Aber dieser Mann hatte durchaus keinen Sinn für schöne Landschaften und Felsenpartien – er führte uns . . . auf einen steilen schattenlosen Berg hinan, auf welchem man die Stadt übersehen konnte, und da sagte er mit selbstgenügender Einfalt: 'Sehen Sie hier, da sieht man so recht unser Stadttor, . . .' Der gute Mitterbacher war ganz beschämt, daß uns statt malerischer Felsenpartien nur dies elende Tor nach einem solchen mühsamen Spaziergange gezeigt wurde."

42. Reuß, "Tagebuch einer Reise nach Karlsbad, 1768," 222: "der schöne prospect herunter in die Stadt beschauet."

43. Recke, *Tagebücher und Selbstzeugnisse*, 329–330: "Dann gingen wir einen steilen, hohen Berg hinan, der dicht mit dunklen Tannen besetzt ist und auf dem sich übereinandergestürzte Felsenmassen schauerlich zusammentürmen. Nieuport sagte mir, daß solche wilde, schauerliche Gegenden ihn mehr als sanft lächelnde Landschaften anziehen. Auch für mich haben die rauhesten Felsenpartien den größten Reiz – warum schroffe Felsen meine Seele mit größeren Ideen erfüllen als schöne, lachende Gegenden, *darüber weiß ich mir keine Rechenschaft zu geben*." (Italics by ULH.)

44. Schopenhauer, *Tagebücher der Adele Schopenhauer*, vol. 1, 33: "Mir ist sehr wohl hier, *ich weiß nicht*, was mir an dieser stillen grünen Waldgegend so gut gefällt." (Italics by ULH.) In contrast, see the 1747 description of Schlangenbad in Chapter 3.

45. See Raymond, *Von der Landschaft*, 88.

46. Augustusbad near Radeberg, Berggießhübel, Buschbad near Meißen, Schandau, Tharand, Wiesenbad, and Wolkenstein. See Götzinger, *Schandau und seine Umgebungen*, 1812.

47. The Renchtal spas are Antogast, Freiersbach, Griesbach, Peterstal, and Sulzbach. See, e.g., "Schwäbische Bade-Chronik," 1814; "Nachtrag zur Bade-Chronik (Schwäbischen)," 1815.

48. In addition to the inland spas, seaside resorts also expanded this map in the early nineteenth century.

49. Altwasser, Charlottenbrunn, Cudowa, Flinsberg, Landeck, Reinerz, Salzbrunn, and Warmbrunn. See, e.g., Mosch, *Heilquellen Schlesiens*, 1821; see also Chapter 1.

50. [Zahn], *Deinach*, 1789, 11–12: "Für Deinach selbst hat die Natur sehr viel, die Kunst aber gerade nur so viel getan, als nöthig ist, um mit Bequemlichkeit sich hier aufhalten zu können. . . . Wahr ist es, in Vergleichung mit Pyrmont, Spaa, und wann man diese Orte als Maaßstab nimmt, ist Deinach freylich arm an Vergnügungen." – [Zahn], *Deinach*, 1789, 13–14: "Wer aber Vergnügen findet an Betrachtung der Natur, die man in der Nähe der Städte nie in ihrer Reinheit erblickt, wo sie höchstens in Englischen Gärten nachgekünstelt wird: . . . wer seinen Geist dem Geräusch entziehen will, . . . der komme hierher, und geniesse der Natur."

51. See Kehn, "Gartenkunst," 213.

52. Mezler, *Vorläufige Nachrichten über den Kurort zu Imnau*, 1795, 9: "Es liegt in einem, durch seine natürlichen Schönheiten sehr reizenden, und durch die anscheinende Abgeschiedenheit sehr anmuthigen Wiesenthal, . . . Die Berge, welche dasselbe umgeben, sind zimlich nahe, . . . und verbinden ihr schwarzes Thannengrün in verschiednen Busen, und Biegungen mit dem schönen Hellgrün der im Thale befindlichen Wiesen."

53. Mezler, *Vorläufige Nachrichten über den Kurort zu Imnau*, 1795, 11–12: "die Kurgäste . . . [haben] den Vortheil, daß sie durch kleine Excursionen mit vortrefflichen Leuten, mit schönen Naturscenen, und verschiedenen Merkwürdigkeiten bekannt werden."

54. See, e.g., Mezler, *Vorläufige Nachrichten über den Kurort zu Imnau*, 1795, 16–21.

55. Mezler, *Vorläufige Nachrichten über den Kurort zu Imnau*, 1795, 51: "Nachmittag, wo sonst in andern Kurorten die eigentlichen langweiligen Stunden sind, da geht, reitet und fahrt eine Parthie dahinaus, die andere dorthinaus."

56. See Lempa, "The Spa."

57. Götzinger, *Schandau und seine Umgebungen*, 1812, 361–362: "Vorschläge für Schandauer Badegäste, die sächs[ische] Schw[eiz] während ihrer Badezeit in kleinen Partieen zu bereisen."

58. Krieger, *Alexis-Bad*, 1812, 151–328. See also Harleß, *Bad zu Bertrich*, 1827.

59. Krieger, *Alexis-Bad*, 1812, 153–154: "Eine gute Nachbarschaft, sie beziehe sich auf die todte oder lebendige Natur, wer zählt sie nicht zu den größten Annehmlichkeiten des Lebens, zur Schöpferin der reinen Freuden? . . . Solcher Nachbarn, zu jeder Tagszeit besuchbar, jeder Neigung ansprechend, zwar oft ohne Haus und Dach, dennoch aber das schönste Haus machend, erfreut sich allen Himmelsgegenden hin, das Alexisbad. Will man also zur frohern Rückerinnerung, – ein reicher Stoff zur Unterhaltung in der Heimath – nur die nähern und anziehendern kennen lernen, und jeden Tag sich nur auf eine Bekanntschaft beschränken, so kann man leicht die ganze Badezeit mit solchen Tags-Excursionen ausfüllen."

60. Hoser, *Beschreibung von Franzensbrunn*, 1799, 120–121: "Ungeachtet die nächste Gegend um Franzensbrunn, bis itzt noch nicht malerisch genannt zu werden verdient, und auf diese Benennung erst in einigen Jahren Ansprüche haben wird; so sind doch die Lage entfernterer Dorfschaften, und der ganze Kreis der, dieses fruchtbare Ländchen umschlissenden Gebürge in jeder Hinsicht voll pittoresker Schönheiten, und werden sicher in mehr als einer Rücksicht, jeden Menschen dessen Gefühl für Natur noch nicht erloschen ist, ächtes Vergnügen und reinen Genuss aus seinen Wanderungen durch dieselben gewähren." In 1815, Elise Bürger complained that – compared to Karlsbad – Franzensbad was "sandy and colorless" – "sandig und farblos." Bürger, *Lilien-Blätter*, 1826, 140.

61. Götzinger, *Schandau und seine Umgebungen*, 1812.

62. Krieger, *Alexis-Bad*, 1812.

63. Pienitz, *Beschreibung des Augustusbades*, 1814.

64. [Eichler], *Beschreibung von Teplitz und seinen pitoreskischen Umgebungen*, 1811. This work was reprinted many times. See, e.g., Eichler, *Beschreibung von Teplitz und seinen mahlerischen Umgebungen*, 1823.

65. Harrer, *Karlsbad und die umliegende Gegend*, 1801.

66. Klüber, *Beschreibung von Baden*, 1810.

67. Mosch, *Bäder und Heilbrunnen*, 1819.

68. Soden is not on the map at the end of this book because it remained a spa with only local significance during the period covered in this study.

69. See Gerning, *Die Heilquellen am Taunus*, 1814.

70. See Gerning, *Die Heilquellen am Taunus*, 1814, fold-out map at end of volume.

71. See Mosch, *Bäder und Heilbrunnen*, 1819, vol. 2, fold-out map at end of volume.

72. Klüber, *Beschreibung von Baden*, 1810.

73. "Badechronik," *JLM* (October 1805), 678: "Wo nur die Natur hie und da einigen Mineralgehalt in hervorbrechenden Quellen verrieth, wo man hoffen durfte, daß die reizende Gegend, mehr noch als die Kräfte der Quelle, . . . Besuchende anziehen würde, entstand ein neues Bad, und ihr haben wir die so schnell gediehenen Schöpfungen von Tharand und Schandau zu danken."
74. See Raymond, *Von der Landschaft*, 120–165.
75. See, e.g., Hufeland, *Praktische Uebersicht der vorzüglichsten Heilquellen Teutschlands*, 1831, 74 (Pyrmont), 78 (Driburg), 109 (Freienwalde in the plains north of Berlin, which allegedly is situated in a "charming mountain-ous-romantic" ["reizende bergigt-romantische"] area), 150 (Nenndorf).
76. See Lichtenberg, "Warum hat Deutschland noch kein großes öffentliches Seebad? [1793]."
77. See Luz, *Büchlein vom Bade*, 143; Corbin, *Lure of the Sea*, 257.
78. Wurst argues that Lichtenberg spoke within the framework of an established discourse. This is only correct in so far as Lichtenberg took the discourse that was established in England as his model. In Germany, seaside resorts were not part of the dominant discourse when Lichtenberg published his article. See Wurst, *Fabricating Pleasure*, 255.
79. Hirschfeld, *Theory of Garden Art*, 232. See also Hirschfeld, *Theorie der Gartenkunst*, vol. 2, 85.
80. Lichtenberg, "Warum hat Deutschland noch kein großes öffentliches Seebad? [1793]," 95: "fast in jedem Dezennium."
81. Lichtenberg, "Warum hat Deutschland noch kein großes öffentliches Seebad? [1793]," 95: "Warum findet sich bei dieser Bereitwilligkeit unsrer Landleute, sich nicht bloß neue Bäder empfehlen, sondern sich auch wirklich dadurch heilen zu lassen, kein spekulierender Kopf, der an die Einrichtung eines Seebades denkt?"
82. Lichtenberg, "Warum hat Deutschland noch kein großes öffentliches Seebad? [1793]," 96: "der unbeschreibliche Reiz[,] den ein Aufenthalt am Gestade des Weltmeeres in den Sommermonaten, zumal für den Mittelländer hat."
83. Lichtenberg, "Warum hat Deutschland noch kein großes öffentliches Seebad? [1793]," 96: "Waschbecken-Tumult."
84. Lichtenberg, "Warum hat Deutschland noch kein großes öffentliches Seebad? [1793]," 96: "unbeschreiblich große Schauspiel der Ebbe und Flut."
85. Lichtenberg, "Warum hat Deutschland noch kein großes öffentliches Seebad? [1793]," 96: "gefühlvollen Menschen mit einer Macht, mit der sich nichts in der Natur vergleichen läßt."
86. Lichtenberg, "Warum hat Deutschland noch kein großes öffentliches Seebad? [1793]," 96: "ein Spaziergang am Ufer des Meeres" – "dumpfigen Alleen der einländischen Kurplätze."
87. Lichtenberg, "Warum hat Deutschland noch kein großes öffentliches Seebad? [1793]," 98: "Vergnügen."
88. Lichtenberg, "Warum hat Deutschland noch kein großes öffentliches Seebad? [1793]," 100: "Ball und Pharao."
89. Lichtenberg, "Warum hat Deutschland noch kein großes öffentliches Seebad? [1793]," 102: "Die Fische, die einen Propheten fressen könnten, sind da so selten als die Propheten. Eher könnte man die dortigen Fische vor den Badegästen warnen. Seit jeher sind zwar die Fische dort, zumal von Fremden, mit großer Prädilektion gespeiset worden, es ist mir aber nicht bekannt, daß je einer von ihnen das Kompliment erwidert hätte."
90. See Günzel, *Bäder-Residenzen*, 122; Heuvel, "Warum hat Deutschland," 142.
91. See Heuvel, "Warum hat Deutschland," 143.

92. See the 1783 letter by Gerhard Otto Janus to King Frederick II of Prussia, reprinted in Kurverwaltung Nordseeheilbad Juist, *150 Jahre Seebad Juist*, 48–51. See also Hedinger, *Saison am Strand*, 14–17.

93. See Günzel, *Bäder-Residenzen*, 121.

94. See Chapter 1.

95. See Günzel, *Bäder-Residenzen*, 121; Prignitz, *Vom Badekarren zum Strandkorb*, 16–21; Vogel, *Entstehung des ersten deutschen Seebades*, 15.

96. See Vogel, *Entstehung des ersten deutschen Seebades*, 16: "Since I care about making some sick people happy, and not to forget that the money will be spent in the territory, which otherwise spas in other territories would take away from it." ("Da es mir nicht gleichgültig seyn kann, manchen kranken Menschen dadurch glücklich zu machen, nicht zu gedenken, daß das Geld im Lande verzehrt wird, was auswärtige Bäder demselben entziehen.") See also Prignitz, *Vom Badekarren zum Strandkorb*, 19; Günzel, *Bäder-Residenzen*, 121–122.

97. See Günzel, *Bäder-Residenzen*, 122; Prignitz, *Vom Badekarren zum Strandkorb*, 22.

98. See Günzel, *Bäder-Residenzen*, 122; Nizze, *Doberan-Heiligendamm*, 18.

99. See Vogel, *Entstehung des ersten deutschen Seebades*, esp. 116–130.

100. See Vogel, *Entstehung des ersten deutschen Seebades*, 34–38; Mosch, *Bäder und Heilbrunnen*, 1819, vol. 1, article "Doberan," [unpaginated]; *Dehio – Handbuch der deutschen Kunstdenkmäler: Mecklenburg-Vorpommern*, article "Doberan," 38–39; Thielcke, *Bauten des Seebades Doberan-Heiligendamm*, 13–18; Günzel, *Bäder-Residenzen*, 125; Prignitz, *Vom Badekarren zum Strandkorb*, 24–26; Luz, *Büchlein vom Bade*, 151–152.

101. See Corbin, *Lure of the Sea*, 254–255, about England: "The model of bathing holidays at inland spas weighed heavily on the invention of the beach. . . . Seaside resorts, like inland ones, had bathing establishments and bookshops with reading-rooms; the simplest ones offered mobile libraries. Each spa offered a network of walks and a range of excursions. . . . Balls, conversation rooms, and gaming rooms made for pleasant evenings."

102. See the article about Doberan in the 1809 *Journal des Luxus und der Moden*, which does not mention the seaside at all. "Bade-Chronik," *JLM* (November 1809).

103. Röper, *Geschichte und Anekdoten von Dobberan*, 1808, 49–61 (on spa practices in Doberan including games), 61–70 (on outings): "Lustpartien über Land."

104. See Vogel, *Zur Nachricht und Belehrung für die Badegäste in Doberan*, 1798.

105. Vogel, *Zur Nachricht und Belehrung für die Badegäste in Doberan*, 1798, 3: "diese schöne Heilquelle." – "Von allen Seiten eilt die Kunst der Natur zu Hülfe."

106. Lichtenberg, "Warum hat Deutschland noch kein großes öffentliches Seebad? [1793]," 198: "dumpfigen Alleen der einländischen Kurplätze."

107. Vogel, *Zur Nachricht und Belehrung für die Badegäste in Doberan*, 1798: "die Menge und Mannigfaltigkeit beschatteter Promenaden."

108. See Günzel, *Bäder-Residenzen*, 122.

109. See *Dehio – Handbuch der deutschen Kunstdenkmäler: Mecklenburg-Vorpommern*, article "Doberan," 40; Thielcke, *Bauten des Seebades Doberan-Heiligendamm*, 9, 37.

110. Vogel, *Zur Nachricht und Belehrung für die Badegäste in Doberan*, 1798, 70: "Auch ist in den Badeschaluppen irgend ein Unglück nicht zu fürchten."

111. See Prignitz, *Vom Badekarren zum Strandkorb*, 23.

112. See Vogel, *Zur Nachricht und Belehrung für die Badegäste in Doberan*, 1798, 7. The fact that Vogel quotes these figures at the beginning of his advertising pamphlet indicates that, in view of the obvious reservations about the sea and sea bathing that continued to prevail, he considered it a success that 20 percent of the guests bathed in seawater. In 1805, 650 out of 1200 guests bathed in seawater, i.e. the percentage of guests had risen to 50 percent. See Prignitz, *Vom Badekarren zum Strandkorb*, 30.

113. Vogel, *Zur Nachricht und Belehrung für die Badegäste in Doberan*, 1798, 45: "Bangigkeit"; 44: "Je froher und furchtfreyer man ins Bad steigt, desto besser."

114. Somewhat ironically, and similar to Doberan, the first health resort on the island of Rügen was the spa of Sagard, which was founded in 1795. See Willich, *Vorläufer einer künftigen ausführlichen Beschreibung des Gesundbrunnens zu Sagard*, 1795.

115. See Mosch, *Bäder und Heilbrunnen*, 1819, vol. 1, article "Doberan," [unpaginated].

116. Mosch, *Bäder und Heilbrunnen*, 1819, vol. 1, article "Doberan," [unpaginated]: "Wasserpartien."

117. Mosch, *Bäder und Heilbrunnen*, 1819, vol. 1, article "Doberan," [unpaginated]: "eine schöne Aussicht auf die Spiegelfläche des Meeres."

118. Mosch, *Bäder und Heilbrunnen*, 1819, vol. 1, article "Doberan," [unpaginated]: "mit Schiffen bedeckt" – "die reine See-Morgenluft."

119. Mosch, *Bäder und Heilbrunnen*, 1819, vol. 1, article "Doberan," [unpaginated]: "am Strande" – "das Volk entdecken, welchem das Schiff gehört."

120. Mosch, *Bäder und Heilbrunnen*, 1819, vol. 2, article "Travemünde," [unpaginated]: "Aehrenwogen" – "Wogen der See."

121. Mosch, *Bäder und Heilbrunnen*, 1819, vol. 2, article "Travemünde," [unpaginated]: "interessant" – "Bewohner des inneren Landes."

122. For example, right at the beginning of the article about Travemünde it says, "Its location is very interesting. You always have the sight of the sea and the spectacle of arriving and departing ships." ("Seine Lage ist sehr interessant. Stets hat man den Anblick des Meeres und das Schauspiel ankommender und abgehender Schiffe.") Mosch, *Bäder und Heilbrunnen*, 1819, vol. 2, article "Travemünde," [unpaginated].

123. Mosch, *Bäder und Heilbrunnen*, 1819, vol. 1, article "Doberan," [unpaginated]: "Eine der nächsten und schattenreichsten [Promenaden] ist die auf dem Kamp, mit welcher eine englische Anlage verbunden ist. Sehr angenehm ist der nahe Park mit seinem Wasserbecken, und der Jungfernberg mit seinem trefflichen Holze und den schönen Spaziergängen. Malerisch zieht sich an des letztern Fuße Doberan hin und verschönert durch seine Lage die sonst so wenig reizvolle Küstengegend. . . . seewärts verliert sich das Auge in der mit Schiffen bedeckten unabsehbaren Meereswüste."

124. Mosch, *Bäder und Heilbrunnen*, 1819, vol. 1, article "Cuxhaven," [unpaginated]: "auf einem Damme zwischen zwei kleinen Landseen, die mit dem Hafen von Hamburg in Verbindung stehen" – "Wirkung des Badens im offenen Meere genießen, ohne sich selbst ihm auszusetzen."

125. Lichtenberg, "Warum hat Deutschland noch kein großes öffentliches Seebad? [1793]," 198: "Alleen der einländischen Kurplätze."

126. Mosch, *Bäder und Heilbrunnen*, 1819, vol. 2, article "Norderney," [unpaginated]: "merkwürdiges Schauspiel" – "besonders interessant."

127. Mosch, *Bäder und Heilbrunnen*, 1819, vol. 2, article "Norderney," [unpaginated]: "An Spaziergängen herrscht keine große Abwechselung; man wandert gemeiniglich an dem Meeresufer, oder im Gehölz, dem einzigen der Insel. Die Dünen zu ersteigen, hindert gemeiniglich das beschwerliche

Sandwaden, obschon die weite Aussicht aufs Meer und der Blick in die inneren bewachsenen Schluchten der Dünen der Mühe lohnt."

128. Halem, *Die Insel Norderney*, 1822, 195: "große helle Speise- und Tanzsäle, Billard und Spielzimmer, ein Zimmer worin Zeitungen und Tageblätter bereit liegen."

129. Halem, *Die Insel Norderney*, 1822, 73: "wenn sie mit Geduld und der Individualität der Inseln angeeignet vorgenommen werden."

130. Halem, *Die Insel Norderney*, 1822, 171: "Grosse Logierhäuser geben allerdings ein mehr imposantes Aussehen, als die kleinen bloss ein Stockwerk haltenden Häuserchen unserer Insel. Wer aber einmahl die Unruhe und Ungemächlichkeit solcher grossen Anstalten erprobt hat, wird sich bei der gutmüthig freundlichen Bedienung der Einwohner, sehr bald von den scheinbaren Vorzügen moderner Gestaltungen entwöhnen."

131. Halem, *Die Insel Norderney*, 1822, 73–74: "Ein so öder Sandhaufen, als die Unkunde sich wohl denken möchte, ist unsere kleine Insel daher gar nicht, und wenn ihr auch die schattigten Alleen vieler Land-Bäder fehlen, so fehlt ja diesen die belebende Seeluft."

132. Halem, *Die Insel Norderney*, 1822, 212: "Es ist der Genuss, den die einfach erhabene Natur hier am Strande in der höchsten Vollkommenheit ihren Verehrern bietet."

133. Warnstedt, *Die Insel Föhr*, 12: "rauschende Vergnügungen" – "glänzenden Badeanstalten."

134. See Warnstedt, *Die Insel Föhr*, 1824, 141–142.

135. Warnstedt, *Die Insel Föhr*, 1824, 145: "ein fast immer trockener Sandweg." For Pyrmont, see Marcard, *Beschreibung von Pyrmont*, vol. 1, 1784, 14, 181–182.

136. Warnstedt, *Die Insel Föhr*, 1824, 146: "Wanderung."

137. Warnstedt, *Die Insel Föhr*, 1824, 146: "Die Natur in ihrer unendlichen Größe erfaßt den einsamen Wanderer, das gleichförmig unter ihm hertönende Brausen und Rollen der Wogen aus tiefer dunkler Ferne bezaubert ihn wunderbar, versenkt ihn ins Unendliche des ernsten Gedankens und in unaussprechlicher Wonne fühlt er sich dem kleinlichen Gewirre des Lebens entwunden, freier, und dem großen unendlichen All näher gestellt!"

138. Warnstedt, *Die Insel Föhr*, 1824, 147: "Gehen, Reiten, Fahren am Strande selbst" – "zu den einladendsten und wohlthätigsten Vergnügungen."

139. Warnstedt, *Die Insel Föhr*, 1824, 3: "Diese beiden . . . Inseln schützen besonders Föhr durch ihre hohen Sand-Dünen, die in ihrer Formung und ihren mit Sandhafer blasgrün bewachsenen Kuppen und . . . schroffen, weißen Sand-Abhängen die auffallendste Aehnlichkeit mit Schweizerischen Gebirgsgegenden en miniature darbieten."

140. Mosch, *Bäder und Heilbrunnen*, 1819, includes articles for the seaside resorts of Cuxhaven, Doberan, Norderney, Putbus, and Travemünde among a long list of inland spas. Only Doberan receives unreserved praise, however, for its "manifold diversions and entertainments, and several conveniences" ("mannigfaltigen Zerstreuungen und Unterhaltungen, und mehrer Bequemlichkeiten"), all of which are derived from the inland spas. See Mosch, *Bäder und Heilbrunnen*, 1819, vol. 1, article "Doberan," [unpaginated].

141. Humboldt, *Briefe an eine Freundin*, vol. 2, 300: "Dabei ist das Meer und sein beständiger Anblick, so öde auch Strand und Insel sind, eine schöne Zugabe."

142. See also Chapter 2.

143. See on summer retreats: Rosseaux, *Freiräume*, 225–234. Rosseaux argues that the summer retreat was parallel to spa visits, but that was clearly not the case.

144. See the travel diary by Friedrich Wilhelm von Ketelhodt who remarks about the arrival of the entourage of the princes of Schwarzburg-Rudolstadt in Pyrmont on 20 May 1790: "and [the entourage] came . . . to the famous spa Pyrmont, where, however, due to it being early in the season, there were no spa guests except one English family, and the necessary preparations for their [the spa guests'] reception in the bathhouse . . . had not yet been made" ("und kamen . . . in dem berühmten Bad- und Brunnen-Ort Pyrmont an, wo aber der zu frühen Jahreszeit wegen außer einer Englischen Familie noch keine Brunnen-Gäste vorhanden, auch die zu deren Empfang erforderlichen Anstalten im Badhaus . . . noch nicht gemacht waren"). Ketelhodt, *Tagebuch einer Reise*, 259.

145. Pütter described Pyrmont at the beginning of the 1790s thus: "Especially in the years since 1778 the spa season in Pyrmont, mainly in the month of July, became more and more glamorous." ("Wie vorzüglich in den seit 1778 verflossenen Jahren die Brunnenzeit zu Pyrmont, hauptsächlich im Monathe Julius, immer glänzender wurde.") Pütter, *Selbstbiographie*, vol. 2, 557.

146. [Schulz], *Reise eines Liefländers*, 1795, 78: "Dieses Geräusch dauert von den ersten Tagen des Junius bis ungefähr zu den letzten des Julius, wo es sich auf einmal, meist immer in drey Tagen, verliert, weil die Gesellschaft, die es machte, sich gleichsam das Wort gegeben hatte, zu gleicher Zeit zu kommen und zu gehen. Jetzt schöpfen die übrigen Brunnengäste wieder Athem, und ihre Anzahl wird durch solche Geschäftsleute vermehrt, die nun – in den Hundstagen – ihre Gesundheit wahrnehmen können; . . . Dieser Zeitraum dauert bis zum Anfange des Septembers, wo noch Landwirte, Prediger aus der Nachbarschaft, Krämer mit ihren Frauen und Kindern und Landleute nach Karlsbad kommen."

147. See, e.g., Voigts, *Im Geist der Empfindsamkeit*, 218; August von Sachsen-Gotha-Altenburg, "Reisetagebuch"; Becker, *Vor hundert Jahren*, 32–53, 142–157.

148. Pütter, *Selbstbiographie*, vol. 2, 550: "bestärkte mich in der nunmehr jährlichen Fortsetzung der Pyrmonter Reise die Art, wie das königliche Ministerium mir jedesmal die Erlaubniß dazu höchstwillfährig, zum Theil mit selbst darüber bezeugtem Wohlgefallen, ausfertigen ließ."

149. [Mende], "Ueber den Besuch der Bäder," 1801, 116: "wichtigen Nebenumstände."

150. Quoted in Zeman, "Vom Badreisen und vom Dichten," 266: "Beim Baden sei die erste Pflicht, | Daß man sich nicht den Kopf zerbricht | Und daß man höchstens nur studiere | Wie man das lustigste Leben führe."

151. [Mende], "Ueber den Besuch der Bäder," 1801, 116–117: "Der Geschäftsmann, mit schweren Arbeiten belastet, die ihn den ganzen Tag und oft sogar mehrere Stunden der Nacht an sein Schreibpult anketten, wird gewiß des Lebens Glück doppelt fühlen, wenn er seiner gewohnten Bürde entladen, ganz seinen Umständen und seiner Laune gemäß leben kann. Er wird gewiß den Aufenthaltsort für sehr schätzbar halten, wo er gleichgesinnte Menschen mit gleichen Bedürfnissen antrifft, hier einige Wochen mit ihnen in heiterer Traulichkeit verleben, und seiner frohen Jugend Rosentag wieder aufleben sehen kann."

152. Marcard, *Beschreibung von Pyrmont*, vol. 1, 1784, 45: "Ergötzungen."

153. Knigge, *Practical Philosophy of Social Life*, 226–227. See also Knigge, *Ueber den Umgang mit Menschen*, part 2, 249.

154. See, e.g., "Badechronik," *JLM* (May 1798), 293; "Badechronik," *JLM* (February 1800), 78; Chun, *Reise der Chunischen Zöglinge*, 1791, 58; Piepenbring, *Bemerkungen über die Schrift des Herrn Doctor Frankenau*, 1801,

25–26. See also [Hesler], *Das Leben eines Farospielers*, 1794, a story with a narrative arc appealing to bourgeois values: a faro player who visits several spas and goes deeper and deeper into debt is at the end saved and forgiven by his wife and parents.

155. See Maurer, *Biographie des Bürgers*, 421–424.

156. See Chapter 2.

157. See, e.g., Hufeland, *Praktische Uebersicht der vorzüglichsten Heilquellen Teutschlands*, 1831, 34.

158. Marcard, *Beschreibung von Pyrmont*, vol. 1, 1784, 45: "eine Zeit, in welcher man sich aller eigentlichen Geschäfte mit Fleiß enthält."

159. See Introduction to Part III.

160. Vogel, *Zur Nachricht und Belehrung für die Badegäste in Doberan*, 1798, 23: "Nach Bädern und Brunnen zu reisen wird vielen Menschen von ihren Ärzten oft vorzüglich mit darum gerathen, um da in eine ungebundenere, angenehmere und ruhigere Lage zu kommen, um anstrengenden Geschäften, Sorgen und verdrießlichen Verhältnissen aus dem Wege zu gehen, und Ergötzungen und Zerstreuungen zu finden, welche zu Hause oft nicht möglich sind."

161. [Möser], *Schreiben des Verfassers*, 1746, 27: "unser grosser Medicus hat mir das Denken verboten."

162. [Gieseke], "Neue Briefe über Carlsbad, vom Jahre 1792, Erster Brief," 1793, 367–368: "Das Denken ist hier eine medizinische Todsünde, so wie es an manchen Orten eine politische Todsünde ist, seine Gedanken frei mitzutheilen."

163. Pütter, *Selbstbiographie*, vol. 1, Vorrede, 3r: "wandte ich auch zu Pyrmont und zu Rehburg solche Stunden dazu an, die von anderen an Spieltischen oder in Schauspielhäusern zugebracht wurden."

164. Goethe, Vulpius, *Goethes Briefwechsel mit seiner Frau*, vol. 1, letter from Karlsbad, 25 July 1795, 52: "Ich lebe sehr zertreut, den ganzen Tag unter Menschen."

165. Goethe, Vulpius, *Goethes Briefwechsel mit seiner Frau*, vol. 1, letter from Karlsbad, 28 July 1806, 471: "Gethan habe ich übrigens nicht viel: denn der Brunnen und die Zerstreuung des hiesigen Lebens lassen einen nicht recht zur Fassung kommen." See also Goethe, Vulpius, *Goethes Briefwechsel mit seiner Frau*, vol. 1, letter from Pyrmont, 3 July 1801, 318.

166. Tennstedt is not on the map at the end of this book because it remained a spa with only local significance during the period covered in this study.

167. Goethe, *Briefe – Tagebücher – Gespräche*, 13583 (i.e. Goethe-WA-IV, vol. 27, 124), letter from Tennstedt, 29 July 1816: "Und so sehen Sie hier ein Exerzitium wie ich, als Schreibemeister zu Tenstet, ein sonderbares Leben, in der absolutesten Einsamkeit führe."

168. On this question in general, see Maurer, *Biographie des Bürgers*, 424.

169. See, e.g., [Weikard], *Neueste Nachricht von den Mineralwässern bei Brückenau*, 1780, 26–28.

170. [Schulz], *Reise eines Liefländers*, 1795, 92–97: "Tagesordnung in Karlsbad" – "Man steht zwischen fünf und sechs Uhr auf und verfügt sich zu dem Brunnen, . . . Gegen acht Uhr wird es an den verschiedenen Quellen von Trinkern ganz leer. Es ist eine von den hiesigen Aerzten vorgeschriebene Regel, eine Stunde zu Hause zu bleiben und sich abzuwarten, ehe man sich in einem der Säle ein Frühstück sucht; . . . Will man nicht Theil daran nehmen, oder ist man nicht dazu eingeladen, so geht man spatzieren oder setzt sich an einen Spieltisch, oder spielt Billard, oder nimmt Theil an einer Unterhaltung in der Allee. . . . Dieß Schauspiel dauert bis gegen zwölf Uhr, wo man nach

Hause eilt, um seinen schmalen Bissen zu essen. Nach diesem Geschäft ist es erlaubt, einige Minuten zu schlummern, . . . Die Damen gehen an den Putztisch und kleiden sich zum Ball, der um vier Uhr seinen Anfang nehmen soll. . . . Andere schreiben Briefe, doch sind sie auf der Huth gegen den Brunnenarzt, der alles Denken und Schreiben während der Kur untersagt hat; andere haben einen Spaziergang, eine Landfahrt und ein gemeinschaftliches Abendessen verabredet; . . . Gegen neun Uhr ist der Ball zu Ende, die Spaziergänger oder Spatzierfahrer kommen in die Stadt zurück, . . . und nach neun Uhr endlich sucht jedermann sein Bette."

171. Marcard, *Beschreibung von Pyrmont*, vol. 1, 1784, 55: "seinen eigenen Gang." For Marcard's description of the daily routine in Pyrmont, see 56–63. See also Chapter 2.

172. Baggesen, *Labyrinth*, 163–164: "Man steht im allgemeinen ziemlich früh auf. Um sechs Uhr sieht man die feine Welt schon in voller Bewegung in der großen Allee . . . Eine hübsche Instrumentalmusik unterhält derweilen das Ohr . . . Man grüßt seine Bekannten, der Freund sucht den Freund, und das ganze Heer teilt sich nach und nach in größere und kleinere Gruppen auf, die am Ende der Allee gemeinsam Brunnen trinken, bis die Bewegung gegen neun Uhr in ebenso viele Frühstücksgruppen mündet. . . . Wenn das Frühstück vorbei ist, wird ein paarmal auf und ab spaziert, die Menge zerstreut sich, der eine reitet jetzt, der zweite badet, der dritte spielt Billard, der vierte Karten, der fünfte fährt aus: . . . Nach der Mittagsmahlzeit versammelt sich die Gesellschaft wiederum in der großen Allee . . . Endlich teilt man sich in zwei Hauptpartien ein, die bleibende und die fliehende. Die bleibende schart sich im Versammlungssaal um die Pharao-Bank oder besucht die Komödie und nimmt ansonsten mit dem vorlieb, was die Allee bis zur Abendmahlzeit zu bieten hat. Die fliehende unternimmt in einzelnen Gruppen Landpartien zu den umliegenden Bergeshöhen, . . . Endlich geht man ins Bett, um, falls man kann, zu schlafen, bis man am nächsten Morgen dasselbe Leben von vorn beginnt."

173. [Käppel], *Pyrmonts Merkwürdigkeiten*, 1800, 47–50: "Um sechs Uhr fängt die feinere Welt an sich sehen zu lassen und alle eilen, mit ihrem Glase in der Hand, dem Brunnenhause zu. . . . Präcise um 7 Uhr stimmt ein Corps Hautboisten einen Morgenpsalm an. . . . Zwischen 8 und 9 Uhr nehmen die Frühstückspartien ihren Anfang, . . . Nach dem Frühstück promenieren die Damen entweder zu Wagen, oder zu Fuß, in den Seitenanlagen, oder sie gehen auch ins Bad. . . . Der Ballsaal widerhallt von: le jeu est fait! . . . Auf diese Weise schleicht der Vormittag hin, bis die Mittagsglocke tönt, worauf Alle zu den Speisetischen eilen. Um 3 Uhr hebt man gerne die Tafeln auf; . . . Von 4 bis 5 Uhr ist die Allee in ihrem glänzendsten Flor. . . . Um 5 Uhr eilen die Schauspielliebhaber ins Theater, und die Verehrer der Natur in die umliegende Gegend, . . . Um 8 Uhr ist das Schauspiel zu Ende; die Allee wird wieder voll. Die Pharobank pausiert. Die Essklocke schlägt an. Um 9 1/2 Uhr ist die Abendtafel vorbei."

174. Becker, *Vor hundert Jahren*, entry of 31 August 1784, 34: "weil hier in dieser kleinen Welt ein Tag dem andern ziemlich gleich sieht."

175. Goethe, Vulpius, *Goethes Briefwechsel mit seiner Frau*, vol. 2, letter-diary from Karlsbad, 10–12 July 1811, 214: "Donnerstag in der Allee gefrühstückt, wo wir viel Bekannte antrafen, . . . Körners holten uns von da zum spaziergehen ab; alsdann besuchten wir Frau von Flies und Oppenheimer. Der Hofrath Meyer besuchte uns. Den Mittag speisten wir zu Hause. Nach Tische fuhren wir beide spazieren; . . . Wir putzten uns sehr schön zum Ball."

176. Goethe, Vulpius, *Goethes Briefwechsel mit seiner Frau*, vol. 1, letter from Pyrmont, 26 June 1801, 317: "Früh um 6 Uhr wird aufgestanden, bis 8 Uhr

Brunnen getrunken, um 9 Uhr gefrühstückt, bis 11 Uhr herumgeschlichen und discurrirt, dann über den andern Tag bis gegen 12 Uhr gebadet, um 1 Uhr zu Hause gegessen, ein paar Stunden nach Tische zugebracht, wie es gehen will, und des Abends in der Gegend bald da-, bald dorthin spazieren gegangen." See for another example, Goethe, Vulpius, *Goethes Briefwechsel mit seiner Frau*, vol. 2, 11, letter from Karlsbad, 2 June 1807.

177. Mezler, *Vorläufige Nachrichten über den Kurort zu Imnau*, 1795, 48–52: "Morgen frühe stand man, von einer Harmonie blasender Instrumenten geweckt, vom Bette auf, und begab sich an den Brunnen, wo ein Theil die Mineralquelle ... trank, und der andere Theil, der nur des Vergnügens wegen da war, in verschiedenen Parthien frühestükte, ... und so wards 9 Uhr, wo man ... aufstand, und ein Theil ins Bade, der andere zum Anziehen ging. Um 10-halb elf Uhr suchte man sich schon wieder, und fand sich auf den Gängen des Hauses, wo die Kaufleute ihre Waaren darbothen, oder auf dem Gesellschaftszimmer, wo man zu spielen ... sich zu unterhalten anfing, und so mit allgemeiner Ungeduld den Schlag 12 Uhr erwartete, um zu Tische gehen zu können. ... Nachmittag[s] ... geht, reitet, und fahrt eine Parthie dahinaus, die andere dorthinaus; ... Abends ... hat man sich wieder fröhlich zu Tische gesetzt, ... Nach Tisch kam dann ein Spaziergang aus, ... oder es wurden kleine Spiele gemacht, und sich dann gute Nacht! gesagt." See also Krieger, *Alexis-Bad*, 1811, 48–67: "The general order of the day." – "Gewöhnliche Tagesordnung."

178. Vogel, *Zur Nachricht und Belehrung für die Badegäste in Doberan*, 1798, 29–30: "die zweckmäßige Eintheilung und Benutzung der Tageszeit in Doberan" – "etwas Ruhe ... genießen" – "Toilette ... machen" – "frühstücken" – "einen Brief ... schreiben" – "eine Promenade, einen Besuch, ein Spiel u.d.g."

179. Vogel, *Zur Nachricht und Belehrung für die Badegäste in Doberan*, 1798, 30: "der schönen Musik."

180. Vogel, *Zur Nachricht und Belehrung für die Badegäste in Doberan*, 1798, 30: "Die Zeit nach Tische ist für viele die langweiligste, ... Aber Langeweile sollte man nie haben."

181. Vogel, *Zur Nachricht und Belehrung für die Badegäste in Doberan*, 1798, 31: "das Schreiben eines Briefs, eine angenehme, leichte Lektüre, eine ungenirte Conversation."

182. Vogel, *Zur Nachricht und Belehrung für die Badegäste in Doberan*, 1798, 32: "kommt nun die Zeit zu Promenaden zu Wagen, zu Pferd und zu Fuße, wozu die schöne Gegend nähere und entferntere vertrefliche Gelegenheiten darbietet, oder abwechselnd zum Schauspiele, zu Bällen, zu gymnastischen Spielen allerley Art."

183. Pauline zur Lippe, *Eine Fürstin unterwegs*, 278–279: "Der Lauf der ... Wochentage ist, daß am Morgen nach den Bäädern gefahren, geritten, gegangen wird, wo einige plaudern, warten, arbeiten, frühstücken. Die Flut gebietet und ändert die Stunde. Nach dem gewohnten Mittagessen verweilt man zu Hause, fährt in der Gegend herum, spaziert dort und da, belustigt sich mit Spazierfarthen zu Wasser, trinkt Thee auf der warmen Baadeanstalt, besteigt den Leuchtthurm und endigt den Tag gewöhnlich in der 'Harmonie'."

184. Johanna Schopenhauer, who visited Bath and other English spas with her husband, remarked that "life in the English spa is much more regulated than in Germany. One knows to the last detail how every day is to be spent and there is no aimless drifting about here and there as in Pyrmont and Karlsbad." Although Schopenhauer records this in a neutral way and without providing an indication of her own preference, she confirms that the daily

routine at German spas provided visitors with unregulated periods of time.
Schopenhauer, *A Lady Travels*, 120.

185. Marcard, *Beschreibung von Pyrmont*, vol. 1, 1784, 55: "Eine gewisse
Regelmäßigkeit, welche das Leben in Pyrmont hat, und die an einem Bade
herrschen muß, wenn man nicht täglich die guten Würckungen des Wassers
zerstören will, gereicht der Gesellschaft keineswegs zum Nachtheil. Sie ist
ein Lob für Pyrmont auf der einen Seite, und hat auf der andern den Nutzen,
daß man allemal gewiß ist, wann und wo man seine Gesellschaft finden
wird, ohne deswegen besondere Verabredungen zu treffen." Vogel wrote in
1798: "A very important point are the activities during the day for the spa
guests. A good arrangement of these certainly contributes immensely to the
promotion of well-being and of the cure." ("Ein sehr wichtiger Punkt sind
die Beschäftigungen des Tages für die Badegäste. Ungemein viel trägt gewiß
eine gute Anordnung derselben zur Beförderung des Wohlseyns und der Cur
bei.") Vogel, *Zur Nachricht und Belehrung für die Badegäste in Doberan*,
1798, 29.

Part III
Meeting Place

Introduction to Part III

In the eighteenth century, Enlightenment societies and "other institutions of the Enlightenment public sphere"[1] were important zones of contact for the nobility and the upper middle class, in particular the educated bourgeoisie. Historiography has analyzed a broad range of associations of eighteenth-century sociability, from reading societies as well as patriotic and charitable societies to secret societies, especially Masonic lodges.[2] Furthermore, historians have focused on coffeehouses and salons as important institutions of Enlightenment sociability.[3] This field of research has a long tradition. In his study *Critique and Crisis*, originally published in 1959, Reinhart Koselleck emphasized the close connection between the political and the social role of Freemasonry in the eighteenth-century absolutist state.[4] In recent decades, the focus in historiography has shifted to the social and cultural aspects of Enlightenment associations.[5] In spite of this broader approach, we still lack studies that examine noble-bourgeois meeting places beyond Enlightenment societies, Masonic lodges, salons, and coffeehouses. As we have already seen in Chapter 2, the spa constituted such a zone of contact. Its function as a social heterotopia, a space where noble and bourgeois elites could transcend social boundaries in the late eighteenth and early nineteenth centuries, will be discussed in the following two chapters.

Studies on Enlightenment societies and institutions agree that contemporaries practiced new, more egalitarian forms of interaction within these different spaces of sociability.[6] In principle, these associations were supposed to overcome the social restrictions of early modern society: "As places where individuals from diverse social and occupational backgrounds intermingled, [they] tended to dissolve distinctions of rank and foster the more egalitarian style of sociability characteristic of the Enlightenment public sphere."[7] Members of Enlightenment associations expressed the ideals of equality and friendship in various ways. Freemasons, for example, addressed each other as "brothers," and reading societies held votes on purchases and the admission of new members.[8]

However, historiography has also pointed to the limits of this ideal in the eighteenth century. Many Enlightenment associations restricted their membership to the upper middle class and the nobility and excluded vast swaths of the population. James Van Horn Melton has described this as "a fundamental paradox" of the Enlightenment public sphere: "While bridging the social and cultural divide separating noble and non-noble, it simultaneously widened the distance between propertied and plebeian."[9] For example, Enlightenment societies charged admission and membership fees. As a result, these societies remained open to the nobility but in effect were closed to many members of the middle and especially lower middle class.[10] In addition, some Enlightenment associations kept their inner space, where only members were admitted, separated from the rest of society. This holds especially true for the Masonic lodges and other societies like the Illuminati that conducted their meetings in secret.[11] And salons, such as the salons of Jewish women like Rahel Levin and Henriette Herz in Berlin, were held in private homes.[12] As Lucian Hölscher has argued, the "public sphere" in the eighteenth century meant a limited public sphere: "A society, such as a salon, a club, or an open-air assembly was called 'public' not because everyone could or did participate, but because specific groups were not excluded from it. A concert, a dance, or theater performance could be called 'public' if it was a meeting place for the nobility and the upper middle class. . . . The labeling of an assembly as 'public' . . . signaled the leveling of certain, not all, social differences."[13]

Notwithstanding these limitations, Enlightenment associations served important functions in the late eighteenth and early nineteenth centuries. Historians have pointed out that the various connections between members of and participants in the societies and institutions of Enlightenment sociability led to the creation of wide-ranging communication networks.[14] And due to the high degree of exchange and integration fostered by these Enlightenment associations, a new social formation, an enlightened educated elite (*gebildete Stände, Stand der Gebildeten*), emerged. This new educated elite consisted of members of the nobility and the educated bourgeoisie. It was neither an estate in the early modern sense of the word nor a social class in the modern sense. Rather, its members regarded themselves as connected by principles of humanity and education. The educated elite also formed the core of the emerging public sphere.[15] Historians like Ute Daniel and James Van Horn Melton have argued that the "bourgeois public sphere," a term originally introduced by Jürgen Habermas in 1962,[16] actually included many educated nobles who considered themselves enlightened. Thus, Daniel and Melton have asserted that it is more appropriate to speak of an "enlightened public sphere."[17]

Still, underlying questions about the definition of social groups during the Enlightenment era and beyond remain. Research into the social history of the nobility and the middle class has to contend with the fact that both groups were very diverse in socioeconomic terms. Both groups were so amorphous that recent research has turned to cultural historical approaches, namely identity formation and markers of difference, in an attempt to define them. Historiography has thus moved away from the social history, especially the so-called middle class research (*Bürgertumsforschung*) of the second half of the twentieth century, which in Germany had been dominated by Hans-Ulrich Wehler and Jürgen Kocka in Bielefeld and Lothar Gall in Frankfurt am Main and their respective schools of thought.[18]

By the eighteenth century, the middle class or bourgeoisie (*Bürgertum*) in Germany included not only the burghers (*Stadtbürgertum*), ranging from artisans to urban elites like patricians, but also the educated bourgeoisie (*gebildetes Bürgertum*), above all princely officials, lawyers, professors, and the clergy, as well as the so-called economic bourgeoisie (*Wirtschaftsbürgertum*) like entrepreneurs involved in, for example, the putting-out system and manufactures.[19] The disparate nature of the *Bürgertum* thus made it impossible to define it in socioeconomic terms. As Jürgen Kocka has remarked, the *Bürgertum* was a "very heterogeneous conglomerate of social categories"[20] and can be described above all by social demarcations – vis-à-vis the nobility, the lower classes, the peasants, and increasingly also the petty bourgeoisie (*Kleinbürgertum*).[21] In 1981, Rudolf Vierhaus described the *Bürgertum* of the eighteenth century in terms of the "characteristics of being bourgeois" (*Bürgerlichkeit*), namely "conduct and mentality."[22] He thus shifted the definition of *Bürgertum* from a social to a cultural category.

Jürgen Kocka's proposal to define the *Bürgertum* of the nineteenth century on the basis of its "bourgeois culture," encompassing specific "norms, attitudes, and lifestyles" that fostered "cohesion," was highly influential in historiography.[23] As a result, research focusing on the late eighteenth and early nineteenth centuries explored different aspects of this bourgeois culture. In addition to studies about gender and gender relations,[24] historians have, among other topics, researched cleanliness as a bourgeois virtue, walking as a part of bourgeois culture, bourgeois travel and the summer retreat, biography-writing as an expression of bourgeois mentality, as well as etiquette books and other normative writings as indicators of bourgeois values.[25]

Categories like *Bürgerlichkeit* and bourgeois culture, however, are just as vague as any socioeconomic definition of the *Bürgertum*.[26] Different definitions of bourgeois culture have been put forward in recent decades. Some of these definitions use Bourdieu's concept of "habitus" to define bourgeois culture as "a cultural model that is multi-layered and varied, but also binding in its basic features, and that contains decisive elements of social identity."[27] Others view bourgeois culture as a "cultural everyday practice"[28] and a "process of communication and conflict about values, attitudes, and binding norms for everyday actions."[29] Finally, some interpretations emphasize a "canon of values," especially values like education, work, and diligence.[30] This bourgeois "value system,"[31] these historians contend, was sustained through "a process of individual appropriation, the internalization of values, [and] the learning of social practices by individuals."[32] All in all, Thomas Mergel has argued, "The answers were manifold, but they all pointed to the fact that a background of shared values, a shared way of life, and a similar view of the world glued the bourgeoisie together in a way that socioeconomic factors did not."[33]

The nobility (*Adel*) of the long eighteenth century was also no longer reliably "glued together" by social and economic factors.[34] In the eighteenth century, nobility was a broad social category, ranging from impoverished local nobles to imperial princes and electors, and from recently ennobled members of the bourgeoisie to imperial knights from old noble families. The nobility was thus an equally broad social group as the *Bürgertum*, defying socioeconomic definition.[35] Therefore, similarly to the historiography of the bourgeoisie, in recent decades research on the nobility has increasingly taken a cultural turn, focusing on noble lifestyle, habitus, and ways of expressing social distinction.[36]

In the early modern and eighteenth-century empire, the nobility was, above all, defined by its legal status.[37] Therefore, "as long as at least the appearance of a noble lifestyle could be maintained, . . . one [was] in a position to claim all the privileges of one's social standing."[38] Despite the gradual dismantling of this legal status in the nineteenth century, the nobility remained the "first estate in the state," partially through new legal codification, for example in the General Prussian Land Law (*Allgemeines Preußisches Landrecht*) of 1794, and partially through long-term social standing.[39] Researchers agree that the nobility succeeded in maintaining their status by flexibly employing the different elements of their social position – tradition, family, connubium, landed estates, participation in government, lifestyle, and habitus.[40]

At the same time, however, historiography has also identified definite limits to the nobility's flexibility. Nobles embraced certain bourgeois ideals, such as the new ideal of marriage and the family, but they neither adopted bourgeois values in their entirety nor responded to change in a uniform way. While some nobles became part of the new enlightened educated elite, degraded nobles turned against the bourgeoisie.[41] The bourgeoisie's attitude toward the nobility followed a similar pattern. Michael Maurer has argued that "the self-image of the bourgeoisie . . . is partially constructed through confrontation with the nobility as the leading social group."[42] Thus, members of the bourgeoisie could either criticize nobles and cast a negative light on them or depict them as "bourgeois" and therefore as deserving of their noble status because of their virtuous conduct.[43] Overall, as Heinz Reif has emphasized, "the boundary between nobility and bourgeoisie [remained] conspicuously inflexible in Germany."[44]

While Reif's conclusion is certainly valid in a European comparative context, there is still a need for studies that examine this boundary more closely in the German lands of the late eighteenth and early nineteenth centuries. Most historians have focused on either the nobility or the bourgeoisie, while far fewer studies analyze the interactions of these two groups in shared spaces. As Elisabeth Fehrenbach already remarked in 1994, we need to look at "the zones of social contact and social blending where the dividing lines between the nobility and the bourgeoisie became blurred or entrenched."[45] In addition, the existing research indicates that the formation of bourgeois identity depended to a considerable degree on defining the bourgeoisie's relationship to the nobility. Therefore, we need more case studies that examine how bourgeois identity was constructed in relation to the nobility.[46]

In the following two chapters, I will analyze the dual function of the spa as a social heterotopia during the late eighteenth and early nineteenth centuries. On the one hand, spas – as *actual* spaces of leisure – were important meeting places for the nobility and the upper middle class, especially the educated bourgeoisie. Thus, spas were spaces that fostered the creation of the enlightened educated elite as a new social formation. On the other hand, the published discourse gave voice to bourgeois expectations and demands associated with the spa as a social heterotopia. This was, in many ways, a remarkable process. At the end of the eighteenth century, when the middle class frequented spas in growing numbers, a process of "discursive occupation" took place: in the publications of the spa discourse, the bourgeoisie figuratively claimed a space that had been created by princes and was dominated by the nobility. The bourgeoisie projected its demands for social equality onto the spa, defining the spa as a heterotopia where the nobility and the middle class should be able to interact without the constraints of rank imposed by the early modern social order. Consequently, the published spa discourse was, as we will see later, infused with Enlightenment ideas. As a "bourgeois discourse," the spa discourse addressed the members of the middle class, articulated their demands vis-à-vis the nobility, and thereby actively shaped the creation of bourgeois identity. At the same time, as an "enlightened discourse," it attempted to broaden its appeal with the objective of including enlightened members of the nobility. Overall, however, the spa as an *actual* meeting place – as a lived heterotopia if you will – was never able to fulfill the demands articulated in the published discourse, and frustration about this shortfall was expressed both in personal narratives and in the spa discourse.

Notes

1. Melton, *Rise of the Public*, 197.
2. See Tilgner, *Lesegesellschaften*; Dann, "Lesegesellschaften"; Puschner, "Lesegesellschaften"; Stützel-Prüsener, "Lesegesellschaften"; Hardtwig,

Genossenschaft; Agethen, *Geheimbund*; Vierhaus, *Deutsche patriotische und gemeinnützige Gesellschaften*; Im Hof, *Das gesellige Jahrhundert*; Ludz, *Geheime Gesellschaften*; Reinalter, *Aufklärungsgesellschaften*; Reinalter, *Freimaurer und Geheimbünde*; Dülmen, *Gesellschaft der Aufklärer*; Zaunstöck, *Sozietätslandschaft*; Zaunstöck, Meumann, *Sozietäten*; Melton, *Rise of the Public*, 252–272. For a brief overview, see also Müller, *Aufklärung*, 15–25.

3. See Melton, *Rise of the Public*, 197–251; Seibert, *Der literarische Salon*; Wilhelmy-Dollinger, "Emanzipation durch Geselligkeit"; Bödeker, "Kaffeehaus." See also Zaunstöck, *Sozietätslandschaft*, 34–35.
4. See Koselleck, *Kritik und Krise*. For more recent studies on the political function of Freemasonry, see Neugebauer-Wölk, "Arkanwelten." For Goethe's Freemasonry, see Wilson, *Unterirdische Gänge*; Bauer, Müller, *"Des Maurers Wandeln"*.
5. For a concise summary of the historiography of Enlightenment associations and institutions, see Borgstedt, *Zeitalter der Aufklärung*, 62–70.
6. See Hardtwig, *Genossenschaft*, 309; Hardtwig, "Eliteanspruch," 73–78; Nipperdey, "Verein"; Agethen, "Aufklärungsgesellschaften," 452; Reinalter, "Freimaurerei," 86–88; Maurice, "'Staat im Staate'," 10; Maurice, *Freimaurerei*, 7; Hettling, "Soziale Figurationen," 265; Schindler, "Freimaurerkultur," 245; Wilhelmy-Dollinger, "Emanzipation durch Geselligkeit," 121–122; Neugebauer-Wölk, *Esoterische Bünde*.
7. Melton, *Rise of the Public*, 252.
8. See Tilgner, *Lesegesellschaften*, 385; Stützel-Prüsener, "Lesegesellschaften," 47; Schlögl, "Die patriotisch-gemeinnützigen Gesellschaften," 75; Zaunstöck, *Sozietätslandschaft*, 35–36.
9. Melton, *Rise of the Public*, 12.
10. See Stützel-Prüsener, "Lesegesellschaften," 48; Tilgner, *Lesegesellschaften*, 384; Wehler, *Deutsche Gesellschaftsgeschichte*, 328.
11. See Hardtwig, "Eliteanspruch," 67. On the role of Masonic lodges in communication circles at spas, see Chapter 2.
12. See Möller, *Fürstenstaat*, 480; Frevert, "Ausdrucksformen bürgerlicher Öffentlichkeit."
13. Hölscher, "Die Öffentlichkeit begegnet sich selbst," 30: "'Öffentlich' hieß eine Gesellschaft, etwa ein Salon, ein Klub oder eine Versammlung unter freiem Himmel nicht deshalb, weil alle daran teilnahmen oder auch nur teilnehmen konnten, sondern weil davon ganz bestimmte Gruppen nicht ausgeschlossen waren. 'Öffentlich' konnte etwa ein Konzert, eine Tanz- und Theaterveranstaltung dann heißen, wenn sich dort Adel und gehobenes Bürgertum begegneten. . . . Die Etikettierung einer Versammlung als 'öffentlich' . . . signalisierte die Einebnung bestimmter, nicht aller gesellschaftlichen Unterschiede."
14. See Bödeker, "Aufklärung." See also Hardtwig, *Genossenschaft*, 297–298; Zaunstöck, "Die vernetzte Gesellschaft"; Zaunstöck, "Zur Einleitung"; Zaunstöck, *Sozietätslandschaft*; Löffler, "Aufklärerische Kommunikationsformen." On the spas a centers of communication, see Chapter 2.
15. See Vierhaus, "Umrisse einer Sozialgeschichte"; Bödeker, "Die 'gebildeten Stände'"; Fehrenbach, *Adel und Bürgertum in Deutschland*, XI; Fehrenbach, *Adel und Bürgertum im deutschen Vormärz*, 24; Rees, Siebers, *Erfahrungsraum*, 58.
16. Habermas, *Strukturwandel der Öffentlichkeit*; English translation: Habermas, *Structural Transformation of the Public Sphere*.
17. See Daniel, "How Bourgeois Was the Public Sphere"; Melton, *Rise of the Public*, 11.
18. While the Bielefeld school argued that the emergence of the "bourgeois society" of the nineteenth century was primarily driven by the "new" bourgeoisie,

i.e. the educated upper middle class and rising entrepreneurs, the Frankfurt school focused its research on the burghers (*Stadtbürger*) and emphasized their contribution to social change and the emergence of nineteenth-century bourgeois society. See, e.g., Gall, *Von der ständischen zur bürgerlichen Gesellschaft*; Gall, *Vom alten zum neuen Bürgertum*; Kocka, *Bürger und Bürgerlichkeit im 19. Jahrhundert*; Wehler, *Deutsche Gesellschaftsgeschichte*; Haltern, "Gesellschaft der Bürger"; Mergel, "Bürgertumsforschung"; Lundgreen, *Sozial- und Kulturgeschichte des Bürgertums*.

19. See Schilling, "Wandlungs- und Differenzierungsprozesse"; Mörke, "Social Structure"; Friedeburg, Mager, "Learned Men and Merchants."

20. Kocka, "Bürgertum und Bürgerlichkeit," 27: "sehr heterogenes Konglomerat sozialer Kategorien."

21. See Kocka, "Bürgertum und Bürgerlichkeit," 35; Nipperdey, "Kommentar: 'Bürgerlich' als Kultur," 145.

22. Vierhaus, *Bürger und Bürgerlichkeit*: "Verhaltensweise und Mentalität."

23. Kocka, "Bürgertum und Bürgerlichkeit," 44: "bürgerliche Kultur" – "gewisse Normen, Einstellungen und Lebensweisen" – "Zusammenhalt."

24. See, e.g., Habermas, *Frauen und Männer des Bürgertums*; Trepp, *Sanfte Männlichkeit*.

25. See, e.g., Frey, *Der reinliche Bürger*; König, *Kulturgeschichte des Spazierganges*; König, "Frei vom Gängelband?"; Warneken, "Bürgerliche Gehkultur"; Kaschuba, "Erkundung der Moderne"; Mai, "Touristische Räume"; Maurer, *Biographie des Bürgers*; Döcker, *Ordnung der bürgerlichen Welt*; Döcker, "Zur Konstruktion"; Frieling, *Ausdruck macht Eindruck*.

26. See Hein, Schulz, *Bürgerkultur*, 12–13; Hettling, "Bürgerliche Kultur," 321.

27. Kaschuba, "Deutsche Bürgerlichkeit," 101: "ein in sich zwar vielfach abgestuftes und variiertes, in seinen Grundzügen jedoch verbindliches Kulturmodell, das entscheidende Momente sozialer Identität in sich birgt."

28. Hein, Schulz, *Bürgerkultur*, 13: "kulturellen Alltagspraxis."

29. Hein, Schulz, *Bürgerkultur*, 15: "Prozeß der Verständigung und Auseinandersetzung über Werte, Lebenshaltungen und verbindliche Normen für das Alltagshandeln."

30. Hahn, Hein, "Bürgerliche Werte," 12: "Wertekanon."

31. Hettling, Hoffmann, "Zur Historisierung bürgerlicher Werte," 18: "Wertehimmel." See also Hettling, Hoffmann, "Der bürgerliche Wertehimmel."

32. Hettling, "Bürgerliche Kultur," 320: "den Prozeß der individuellen Aneignung, der Internalisierung von Werten, des individuellen Lernens von sozialen Praktiken."

33. Mergel, "Bürgertumsforschung," 524: "Die Antworten waren vielgestaltig; sie deuteten aber alle darauf hin, dass ein gemeinsamer Wertehintergrund, eine geteilte Lebensweise und eine ähnliche Sicht auf die Welt dem Bürgertum den Kitt verlieh, den es ökonomisch und sozial nicht hatte."

34. See Demel, *Der europäische Adel*, 412: "In the eighteenth century the European nobility was more heterogeneous than ever before." ("Der europäische Adel war im 18. Jahrhundert so heterogen wie nie zuvor.")

35. See Frie, "Adel und bürgerliche Werte," 407.

36. See, e.g., Asch, *Der europäische Adel*; Demel, *Der europäische Adel*; Wieland, "Selbstzivilisierung."

37. See Demel, *Der europäische Adel*, 412.

38. Asch, "Staatsbildung und adlige Führungsschichten," 395: "solange zumindest der Anschein einer standesgemäßen Lebensführung aufrechterhalten werden konnte, . . . man durchaus dazu in der Lage [war], auch alle Standesprivilegien für sich in Anspruch zu nehmen."

39. Kunisch, "Die deutschen Führungsschichten," 117: "erster Stand im Staate."

40. See Frie, "Adel und bürgerliche Werte"; Braun, "Konzeptionelle Bemerkungen zum Obenbleiben"; Asch, "Zwischen defensiver Legitimation und kultureller Hegemonie."
41. See Frie, "Adel und bürgerliche Werte"; Fehrenbach, *Adel und Bürgertum in Deutschland*; Kreutzmann, *Zwischen ständischer und bürgerlicher Lebenswelt.*
42. Maurer, *Biographie des Bürgers*, 123: "die Selbstverständigung des Bürgertums . . . zum Teil als Auseinandersetzung mit dem sozial führenden Adel statt[findet]."
43. See Maurer, *Biographie des Bürgers*, 122–123, 135–144.
44. Reif, *Adel*, 61: "die Grenze zwischen Adel und Bürgertum [blieb] in Deutschland auffällig hart." See 61–62.
45. Fehrenbach, *Adel und Bürgertum in Deutschland*, X: "den gesellschaftlichen Misch- und Kontaktzonen, in denen sich die Trennlinien zwischen Adel und Bürgertum verwischten oder verfestigten." See also Fehrenbach, *Adel und Bürgertum im deutschen Vormärz*, 7.
46. See Langewiesche, "Bürgerliche Adelskritik"; Frey, "'Offene Gesellschaft'." See also the older study by Schultze, *Die Auseinandersetzung zwischen Adel und Bürgertum.*

5 The Spa in the Eighteenth Century
From Social Hierarchy to New Demands for Equality

The Spa Until 1750: A Society of Estates

The early modern published discourse often described spas as spaces for all social classes. The healing power of the spring water was considered a gift from God, and therefore spas were supposed to be open to all estates (*Stände*). To illustrate this claim, spa publications used the idea of the "world in miniature."[1] *The Schwalbach Perpetuum Mobile Lasting All Summer* (*Das Schwalbacher Sommer-wehrende Perpetuum mobile*) of 1690 presents an ironic panorama of early modern spa society to the reader from the perspective of the god Mercury looking down from above:

> The princes, counts, lords, the nobility, and priests,
> Canons, nuns, monks, and many unnoble monkeys,
> Lawyers, physicians, innumerable doctors
> . . .
> The ladies and the maids confess in the doctor's ear
> . . .
> Many men, women, servants, many virgins . . .
> Wet nurses, whores also, and little children,
> Lackeys, coachmen, and many burghers, also many peasants,
> Many swindlers and many prowling evil crooks,
> Also high- and low-ranking officers there,
> Foot-servant[s] and riders he [Mercury] saw together with
>   merchants.
> Learned and unlearned, landlord[s], innkeeper[s], and chandlers,
> . . .
> The whole guild of beggars, many lame, stooped people.[2]

Balthasar Ludwig Tralles in his *Ode* to Karlsbad of 1756 summarized: "In a small space I see the game of the world."[3]

In the context of the early modern social hierarchy, the presence of a diverse group of social classes at the spa did not mean, however, that the different social groups also shared spaces and activities. Rather, the social groups frequenting the spa mostly occupied separate spaces and interacted within their own circles. In Wildbad in Württemberg, for example, different baths were reserved for different social ranks and sexes during the sixteenth century. Wildbad had a princes' bath (*Fürstenbad*), a so-called lords' bath (*Herrenbad*), a bath for the burghers and the peasants (*Bürger- und Bauernbad*) as well as baths for women and for the poor.[4] The early modern social hierarchy was also reflected in Wildbad's bathing ordinance (*Badeordnung*) of 1549: "Fifthly, no one shall sit in another person's rightful place, but if a person is of a higher estate [*Stands*] than the other, the person of the lower estate shall equitably grant him his place and yield to him."[5]

Personal narratives confirm this picture. When the Augsburg merchant Lucas Rem visited Wildbad in 1521, he first used the lords' bath, but then moved to the largest bath, the bath for the burghers and the peasants, because, as he put it, "it was warmer and there was more company."[6] Rem, in fact, belonged to a small minority of people in the early modern era who effectively straddled two social estates, and his bathing practices were a direct reflection of this. He was a rich Augsburg merchant and a patrician and thus a member of the imperial city's ruling elite (*Geschlechter*). Rem was granted access to the lords' bath on account of his elevated status as a member of the highest urban rank. He did, however, prefer to use the larger and more diverse bath for the burghers and the peasants, perhaps because he felt more comfortable among townspeople. Michel de Montaigne's travel diary tells of similar forms of social separation in central European spas. He reports in detail about the large main bath in Plombières (Figure 1.1), but as a nobleman he used other, smaller baths reserved for the higher-ranking estates, which he does not describe further.[7] In Baden in Switzerland Montaigne encountered a similar set-up: "There are two or three uncovered public baths, which are frequented only by poor folk. Of the other kind there are great number within the houses, divided into small private rooms, both closed and open, which are let with the lodgings."[8]

Before 1750, personal narratives, travelogues, and spa publications about fashionable European spas leave no doubt that these spaces were dominated by the nobility and that spa offerings and amusements were primarily geared toward noble guests. A comparison between the experiences of Montaigne and the Nuremberg merchant Balthasar Paumgartner illustrates the different entertainment activities of a nobleman and a burgher. Paumgartner's activities at the spa were limited; in Schwalbach he took walks, and in Bagni di Lucca he watched other spa guests gamble.[9] In a letter to his wife, Paumgartner stated that he had felt compelled to go to Bagni di Lucca for health reasons, although he "had enough to do and his hands full" as a merchant in the city of Lucca. He went to the spa, which he ironically calls a "paradise," "to make a virtue out of necessity" and "to live well completely against my will."[10] In other words, Paumgartner acted like the thrifty merchant and housefather he was, even when visiting a spa.

In contrast, Montaigne's spa activities are characterized by practices of noble self-representation. He socialized with other nobles and they sent each other spa gifts and invited each other to balls.[11] Montaigne's interactions with other social groups either were brief or they served to express his noble status. For example, Montaigne was eager to hold the first ball of the season in Bagni di Lucca, both to display his generosity toward his peers and his status toward the lower orders. The ball was a large affair with more than a hundred people, ranging from the local peasants to his fellow noble spa guests, with Montaigne giving gifts and providing a lavish dinner for the nobility.[12] In contrast to Paumgartner's walks at the spa, Montaigne was on horseback most of the time, in keeping with his noble status.[13]

Montaigne's ambition for noble self-representation at the spa went beyond ephemeral activities like balls. He had become acquainted with the custom of displaying the coats of arms of noble spa guests at or in the hostels of Plombières and Baden.[14] Subsequently, he wanted to start the same custom, "prevalent in all the famous baths of Europe,"[15] in Bagni di Lucca. To this end, he had his coat of arms made in Pisa and then "carefully nailed to the wall of the chamber I had occupied, with the understanding that the device should be held to be given to the room itself, and not to Captain Paulino the proprietor, and that it should not be taken down whatever might befall the house in the future. This the captain promised, and confirmed his promise with an oath."[16]

Many spa publications of the early eighteenth century describe noble amusements and the spaces reserved for these activities on the one hand as well as the role of spa guests from the middle class as spectators on the other. Spa customs thus aligned with early modern customs at courts and in residence towns.[17] Sigismund Beermann, for example, wrote about Pyrmont in 1706, "that in good weather, under these green trees, the nobility almost daily hold assemblies and ballets, while the others usually come together as spectators."[18] Similarly, Johann Friedrich Henkel in his *Bethesda Portuosa* of 1746 pointed out that the prince of Saxe-Merseburg "built beautiful pleasure-houses [*Lust-Häuser*] in Lauchstädt for the delectation of the spa guests, especially nobles."[19]

Spa publications about Karlsbad also describe entertainments that were tailored to the nobility, reporting on the "assemblies" of the "noble estates" in the "pleasure-houses" and on "prize-shooting" by noblemen.[20] In his 1754 travelogue about Karlsbad, Christoph Gottlob Grundig, a Protestant pastor and theologian, made a point of describing his role as that of a spectator to the practices of aristocratic pleasure and noble representation at the spa. Looking out from his lodging house, Grundig saw "the noblest social groups" going on "pilgrimages of pleasure."[21] The author describes the so-called Bohemian hall or Bohemian house

(*Böhmischer Saal* or *Böhmisches Haus*) in Karlsbad as a "magnificently decorated . . . building, where especially spa guests from the noble estate . . . entertain themselves with dancing and other amusements."[22] Grundig thus draws attention to the separation of spaces and practices at the spa. Furthermore, he underlines his own social status as a member of the (educated) middle class: he asserts that he did not participate in any of these activities but that he had come to Karlsbad for other reasons. This implies that he, like Paumgartner, had come to the spa primarily to care for his health.[23]

Before the middle of the eighteenth century, there was evidently little social integration between the nobility and the bourgeoisie at the spa. In addition, members of the middle class primarily traveled to the spa to find a cure for illnesses or to maintain their health. But the spa already functioned as a space where members of the educated bourgeoisie socialized among themselves and formed friendships based on their shared appreciation for humanist and later enlightened learning. The educated bourgeoisie saw the spa as a space for intellectual exchange and for meetings with other educated members of the middle class. Since the late Middle Ages humanist scholars met and interacted at the spas or exchanged letters and gifts between spas. These interactions formed the basis for the perception of the spa as a social heterotopia during the Enlightenment.

As Birgit Studt has shown, humanists exchanged spa gifts that suited their intellectual interests. In contrast to Montaigne's spa gifts that consisted of items of clothing like leather belts and taffeta aprons,[24] humanists exchanged literary gifts that were meant to contribute to entertainment and diversion at the spa.[25] While staying in Wildbad and Baden-Baden in 1481, the Strasbourg humanist Peter Schott and Johannes Geiler von Kaysersberg sent each other spa gifts that included "jokes, riddles, poems, and burlesques" for mutual amusement.[26] In a letter to Geiler, Schott expressed his gratitude "for the burlesques that his friend and his bathing companions had sent to him in Wildbad and that he had found very entertaining."[27]

In the eighteenth century, the published discourse often explicitly commented on scholarly interactions between members of the educated bourgeoisie at the spa. Beermann wrote about Pyrmont in 1706, "Furthermore, in the bookstores one [a learned man] has not only the pleasure to see and acquire the latest books there, but one generally meets a pleasant company of scholars and polished people, with whom one can enjoy discourses and other pleasures."[28] The Breslau physician Balthasar Ludwig Tralles dedicated his *Ode* to Karlsbad of 1756 to his colleague and "dearest beloved friend," the court physician Johann Caspar Sulzer from Saxe-Gotha.[29] The two physicians had met during a visit to Karlsbad and "in the company of a few additional dear friends" had spent their days with "useful conversations and . . . innocent pleasures."[30] Tralles emphasized his great appreciation for "the casual way of our interaction . . . in the company of old and new friends" who belonged to the educated bour-geoisie.[31] The author celebrated virtue, wisdom, and "like-mindedness" as the basis for the formation of an enlightened bourgeois friendship circle at the spa.[32]

Contemporary fiction for educated bourgeois readers also presented bourgeois circles of friends and acquaintances as their main protagonists. For example, *Innocent Pastimes in Karlsbad* (*Unschuldiger Zeitvertreib im Carlsbad*), a gallant novel published in 1751, uses the spa as a setting and recommends itself as light reading material for a stay at the spa. The narrative revolves around a bourgeois circle of spa visitors who, strik-ingly, also interact with the owner of their lodging house, a member of the urban middle class.[33] Similarly, the protagonists of the frame narrative in *Amusements at the Waters of Kleve* (*Amusemens des eaux de Cleve*) of 1748 are Protestant German and Dutch burghers. The author of this spa publication, Johann Heinrich Schütte, thus depicts middle-class interac-tion at the spa as crossing boundaries between countries, but not religious and class boundaries.[34]

The early modern spa was characterized by the separation of social classes, thus reflecting the hierarchical society of which it was a part. The experiences of Lucas Rem in the sixteenth century and Christoph Gottlob Grundig in the eighteenth century showed that a spa visitor's access to spaces and activities was directly related to his or her social status. The early modern "society of estates" (*Ständegesellschaft*) at the spa allowed all groups to enter the space of the spa, but gave precedence to the highest estate, the nobility. Nobles dominated the spa's interior spaces, and the spa's leisure facilities catered to aristocratic practices of self-representation. Or, as Balthasar Ludwig Tralles put it, at the spa "the lower estate [*Stand*] was crowded out by the higher estate."[35] This resulted in the separation of noble and bourgeois elites, who socialized mostly within their own circles. Even in the spaces that were also open to the upper middle class – the avenues, the gardens, and (with restrictions) the "pleasure houses" – the social orders did not mingle because group boundaries were easily recognized (and enforced) through habitus and clothing. Again, Tralles put this in a nutshell: although the "small space" of the spa reflected "the game of the world," he pointed out that "different measures of clothes and steps" defined and demarcated social groups.[36]

At the same time, Tralles' description of Karlsbad provides us with a first glimpse of the role the published spa discourse was soon to play in the formation of bourgeois identity. The author does not only describe early modern spa society but also criticizes the nobility, if only mildly. "Is a rigid gaze an expression of your ancestors' grandeur?," Tralles asks, and then he asserts, "Virtue is much more important than honor and estate."[37] He offers the educated bourgeoisie a sense of self-worth, the core of an identity contrary to the hereditary nobility: "Wisdom creates a nobility that one was not born into," and "my [social] estate [*Stand*] is content and therefore enviable."[38] Tralles thus represents the change in the perception of the spa that began in the middle of the eighteenth century and led to increasing demands for bourgeois equality.

A New Demand for Bourgeois Equality

In the mid-eighteenth century, statements emerged in the published discourse that hint at a new perception of the spa. Publications increasingly demanded that spas function as meeting places of the nobility and the middle class. The spa was described as a social heterotopia where certain forms of interaction figured as "test cases" for the relationship between these groups. Typical spa practices like dancing and seating arrangements during meals became flashpoints for noble-bourgeois encounters at the spa. As we shall see later, it was only during the narrower period of the late eighteenth and early nineteenth centuries that the published discourse became embroiled in such questions and entered a full-fledged debate about the spa as a social heterotopia. Nevertheless, the middle decades of the eighteenth century up to the 1770s marked an important period of change with calls for bourgeois equality at the spa growing louder. Personal narratives of the 1760s reveal the possibilities and limits of noble-bourgeois interaction during this period.

One of the earliest *Amusemens* works, *Amusements at the Waters of Schwalbach* (*Amusemens des eaux de Schwalbach*) of 1739, explicitly discusses noble and bourgeois access to spaces at the spa and the extent of social interaction between the two groups. In this instance, balls are described as a test case: "It has to be noted that only the nobility dances at a ball in Schwalbach, but some privy councillors of W** are allowed to enjoy this honor as well. For whoever is not noble may not mingle with the nobility. Nevertheless, everyone can attend the ball and the concert, but he must stay behind the chairs. This is a custom on which the German nobility is not willing to budge in the slightest bit."[39] This statement criticizes noble attitudes and demands access to spaces and activities for the members of the upper middle class. At the same time, it indicates a gradual change in expectations about social interactions at the spa. Considering that the presence of bourgeois court officials at balls and other courtly entertainments in residence towns remained highly problematic even in the late eighteenth century,[40] admitting non-nobles to balls as spectators and permitting individual bourgeois privy councillors to dance indicates a new perception of the spa as a space where different social rules should apply. The same text, however, draws attention to the persistent boundaries that the bourgeoisie was not supposed to cross at the spa. The narrator warns that in the Schwalbach theater a member of the bourgeoisie might find him-or herself removed without ceremony if he or she occupied what was considered spaces of the nobility: "It is certainly true that nobles always sit right in front of the stage, and if a bourgeois

[*Bürgerlicher*] were also in that place, one [the nobility] would not first ask him nicely to make way for a lady of the nobility."[41]

In the ballad *The Beauties of Pyrmont* (*Die Schönheiten Pyrmonts*) of 1750, Charlotte Wilhelmine Amalie von Donop creates another scene in a ballroom. Donop makes a typical Enlightenment argument in favor of the equal status of the educated bourgeoisie and the nobility on account of the bourgeoisie's achievements:

A well-decorated hero asks, content with himself,
While his handsome foot taps along with the music,
A charmingly beautiful child [a young woman] to grace the dance
 floor [with him],
. . .
She bows. Says not a word, and pulls with a prim glance,
While he is still pleading assiduously, her comely arm away,
Leaves him, sits down, he goes with quiet lamentations,
And asks others: he is rejected again.
Why? He dared too much! Thus speaks a beautiful mouth,
The insolent man! Is he not acquainted with noble manners?
A bourgeois approaches, a bourgeois dares,
A bourgeois is so proud to ask us to dance?
If one day we lack noble dancers at the ball,
It will be honor enough for him to be chosen then.
But now he may go, and find there among the lower linden trees
Enough of bourgeois extraction, of his own kind.
She is silent. What folly! Oh laugh who can laugh.
Lament the dancer [*Tänzerin*]! She has a fever.
Consider, foolish child! I admonish you.
He is made noble by his great mind, you only by coincidence [of
 birth].[42]

While Donop's enlightened criticism focuses specifically on noble conduct toward the bourgeoisie at the spa, Koromandel-Wedekind in his poem *The Spa Guest* (*Der Brunnengast*) of 1744 constructs the entire spa of Pyrmont as a social heterotopia. In this heterotopia, the early modern social order is abolished and "spa freedom" – a concept that became ubiquitous during the following decades – replaces courtly etiquette:

Here birth and status and title are not considered,
While sitting, just motley rows are made.
Soon a nobleman, a count, a mayor,
A merchant, a student, a narrow-minded person,
Soon a clergyman, a doctor, and a privy councillor,
Tartuffe and Don Quixote,[43] whoever has money in his pouch,
Soon above, below, to the right and left sides,

A mish-mash of learned, noble, and bad people.
For everyone here is considered a spa guest,
Freedom is loved, courtly manners hated.[44]

Koromandel-Wedekind combines a description of Pyrmont as a social
heterotopia with a reference to a spa practice that over time acquired
considerable significance as an expression of equality between spa guests:
sitting at a table in random fashion without regard to social status. This
practice derived from two separate traditions and was transferred to the
spa to avoid problems at the so-called public tables, the communal meals
open to all members of spa society. As we saw in the bathing ordinance
of Wildbad, seating according to rank was an important feature of early
modern society – from the bathing pool at a spa to the imperial diet.
Rank-based seating served as an immediate visual indicator of each person's place in the social hierarchy. Conflicts over the order of precedence
were therefore common in early modern society.[45]

On the one hand, the practice of seating at random had its origins in
court society, where seats at banquet tables were allocated by lot in order
to avoid conflicts over precedence when numerous monarchs and princes
of similar rank were gathered.[46] Random seating had also been used during the so-called Pyrmont Summer of Princes of 1681, when the elector of
Brandenburg, the queen of Denmark, as well as numerous other electors
and imperial princes met to discuss the Reunion policy of Louis XIV.[47] By
the early eighteenth century, this had become a more common practice
among the nobility at the spa, as described in *Amusements at the Waters
of Schwalbach* (*Amusements des eaux de Schwalbach*): "The princess
[of Nassau-Weilburg] usually takes the seat of precedence at one table,
and the prince [of Nassau-Weilburg] at the other. One sits down without
consideration of rank at either the prince's or the princess' table. However, only noble persons or privy councillors from W** are present."[48]
On the other hand, the practice of random seating became a feature of
Enlightenment societies – from reading societies to Masonic lodges. At
these societies' meetings, members adhered to a nonhierarchical seating
arrangement based on the length of their membership.[49]

These traditions were incorporated into spa practices, and seating at
random became one of the defining features of the spa as a social heterotopia by the late eighteenth century. Seating arrangements were regarded
as an effective way to allow the bourgeoisie and the nobility to mingle
and overcome the constraints of social rank. Various modes of seating
arrangements emerged. In some spas, guests simply took a seat. In others, lots were drawn, and yet in other cases, visitors were seated at the
table in the order of their arrival at the spa, so that newcomers sat at the
foot of the table and then moved up during their stay at the spa. Accordingly, Göckingk reported from Brückenau in 1782, "The table forms a
square and during the actual spa season seats one hundred and twenty,

thirty, and more guests. People sit down without distinction, and every-one chooses seatmates according to his or her liking."⁵⁰ And the *Journal of Luxury and Fashions (Journal des Luxus und der Moden)* explained the seating custom in Nenndorf in 1796: "At table one sits according to length of stay, so that the person who arrives first gets the lowest seat and moves further and further up as others arrive after him."⁵¹

During the mid-eighteenth century and up to the 1770s, however, seat-ing at random was still an emerging custom. As we have seen earlier, the published discourse strongly advocated for the abolishment of ranked seating, but actual practices show the complexity of lived experiences at the spa. Duke Karl (or Carl) Eugen of Württemberg's visit to his spa of Teinach in 1770 can serve as an example. During Karl's stay, "every spa guest was invited to one of his tables according to his rank and free operas were played."⁵² Like Montaigne's ball in Bagni di Lucca, banquets attended by all spa guests and free operas served to enhance the duke's princely representation at the spa. Ranked seating at Duke Karl's tables further underlined the prince's status and the order of precedence among his guests.⁵³ The duke's spa entertainments thus reinforced early mod-ern social customs rather than the emerging ideal of the spa as a social heterotopia.

Personal narratives written by princes, nobles, and members of the educated bourgeoisie in the 1760s illustrate the limits to noble-bourgeois interactions at the spa. However, these social boundaries varied according to the people involved and the specific circumstances of their encounter. In 1766, Count Ernst Ahasverus Heinrich von Lehndorff, chamberlain of Queen Elisabeth Christine of Prussia, the wife of Frederick the Great, kept a spa diary during his stay in Ems.⁵⁴ Count von Lehndorff, who had a negative view of life at court, provides us with a brief insight into the self-perception and practices of a nobleman at a spa in the 1760s while also displaying the tensions between his self-image and his actual conduct. He asserts, "The nobility in this area is very high-minded and shuns the company of these good bourgeois people [a group of merchant fami-lies from the imperial city of Frankfurt am Main]. But I defy them [the other nobles], and my example causes the others to also desist somewhat from their stiff conduct."⁵⁵ At the same time, however, he reports that "the [spa] society here is not exactly distinguished" and that "Countess Dönhoff" is "the only lady of rank who is here and also the only one who dines at our table."⁵⁶ Count von Lehndorff thus clarifies that a strict spatial separation between the nobility and the "society of Frank-furt merchant families," who lived "on the second floor," prevailed.⁵⁷ It remains an open question whether he even spoke to the Frankfurt burghers because he only remarks that the women were "quite pretty" and that a Mrs. Sarasin was "very gracious."⁵⁸ It seems likely that Count von Lehndorff's concept of aristocratic "condescension" was limited to greeting the bourgeois women.

A similar picture emerges from the diary of Imperial Count Heinrich XXVI of Reuß Younger Line who visited Karlsbad in 1768 together with his wife and his brother and provided a detailed description of his daily activities at the spa. The three noble spa guests were always in the company of other nobility.[59] They socialized in the avenue, at balls, and playing billiards. They met with "cavaliers and ladies" in the two assembly halls in Karlsbad, the Bohemian and the Saxon halls (*Böhmischer* and *Sächsischer Saal*).[60] The only members of the urban middle class Count Heinrich interacted with were the spa physician Dr. David Becher and the mayor of Karlsbad, Poltz, who owned the lodging house where Count Heinrich's brother stayed. Count Heinrich and his family invited Poltz to dine with them one evening, an honor they afforded Poltz because of his status as mayor, not as the proprietor of a lodging house. Thus, Count Heinrich's interactions with Becher and Poltz were either determined by economic relationships or, on one occasion, by a general recognition of the office of mayor as the highest representative of the royal town of Karlsbad.[61]

Two personal narratives from 1765 provide us with insights into the limits and possibilities of noble-bourgeois interaction at the mid-eighteenth-century spa from the perspective of the educated bourgeoisie: the Rehburg spa diary of Johann Christian Kestner, written for his sisters, and the "daily registry" (*Tageregister*) from Wiesbaden by Ludwig Christoph Schmid, a bailiff and councillor in the town of Uffenheim in Ansbach.[62] Kestner and Schmid were members of the educated upper middle class of princely officials. Kestner's father belonged to the Hanoverian "state patricians,"[63] and Schmid was later promoted to the position of privy councillor in the Margraviate of Brandenburg-Ansbach.[64] They were close in age, as Kestner was 24 and Schmid was 29 years old. However, they differed in one significant aspect. Schmid was already married and visited Wiesbaden with his wife, whereas Kestner was still a law student and a bachelor who traveled in the company of his mother to Rehburg, where they met up with his aunt.[65]

Kestner and Schmid visited mid-sized spas that attracted mostly middle-class visitors and guests from the lower nobility who in their majority came from the surrounding region. This shaped their respective spa experiences. The number of spa guests was manageable at these spas. According to the published discourse, this generally resulted in less friction and more integration between the upper middle class and the nobility. Kestner's and Schmid's personal narratives confirm this, but at the same time, their spa diaries also exemplify the social boundaries that members of the educated bourgeoisie were not able to cross at these mid-sized spas. On the one hand, the two men interacted with other members of the upper middle class as well as members of the lower nobility. The majority of both these groups were princely officials and thus belonged to the same professional class. On the other hand, Kestner and Schmid were keenly aware of the social boundary between themselves and members of the nobility, including the lower nobility.

Schmid interacted with a broad range of people in Wiesbaden: bourgeois, ennobled, and noble princely officials, mostly councillors, merchants from the nearby imperial city of Frankfurt am Main, and the auxiliary bishop of Mainz, von Schebel, among many others.[66] When Schmid encountered ruling princes, social boundaries inevitably emerged. Schmid reports that he made the "acquaintance" of the count and countess of the small territory of Solms-Rödelheim and that the countess was "accostable and friendly."[67] In contrast, Schmid was not introduced to the duchess of Weimar, who arrived in Wiesbaden from Aachen. He only met one member of the duchess' entourage, the lord chamberlain von Witzleben, with whom Schmid had common acquaintances in Brandenburg-Ansbach. Significantly, the duchess' presence in the same lodging house resulted in restrictions for the other spa visitors. When she dined with her retinue in the main hall, the other guests were confined to their rooms.[68]

Schmid's spa experience reflected the contradictions and tensions of the spa as a social heterotopia as discussed in the published discourse. On the one hand, he perceived the spa as a space of noble-bourgeois interaction similar to Masonic lodges. He summarized this succinctly, coining a phrase that could have been an advertising slogan for eighteenth-century spas: "Spa guests are like Freemasons, immediately acquainted and familiar."[69] On the other hand, the early modern social hierarchy was fundamental to Schmid's perception of spa society. For example, shortly after arriving in Wiesbaden, he carefully assessed the other spa guests in his lodging house and noted their social status in his daily registry: "Ten spa guests stay in the [lodging] house, of whom the privy councillor von Beist from Eisenach with his wife and three daughters [*Fräuleins*] have the highest social rank."[70]

For Rehburg, too, Johann Christian Kestner records communal meals, dances, walks, and small outings of a group of spa guests from the upper middle class and the lower nobility, most likely including ennobled bourgeoisie. As was the case in Wiesbaden, the majority of these guests were princely officials and their families.[71] Kestner describes the interactions of these spa guests as largely unrestricted by the boundaries of social rank, but he notes that this was due to conscious decisions: "Fräulein [von] Berger had the idea that in future we always call ourselves people: Hugo's people, Berger's people, Ebeling's people, Kestner's people etc. Such little things often have the best effect on entertainments. . . . You can . . . tell by this the informal atmosphere we live in."[72]

Kestner also addresses the clear limits of this "informal atmosphere." He points out to his sisters that he was very much aware of social boundaries when interacting with *Fräuleins*, that is, young noblewomen. Kestner turns to this question right at the beginning of his diary, reporting that he is not "quite satisfied" with his stay in Rehburg. The reason he gives is "that I do not have my own kind here. Women, young women, I think, could well make up for that, and there are young women here, but most of them are noble. It is not really my cup of tea to interact with them. Do you know why? The others, and even the young noblewomen [*Fräuleins*] themselves, might think one is a bit crazy if one seeks their company too often. People who try to elevate themselves above their social estate [*Stand*] always seem a bit dubious to me, so I think others judge the same way."[73]

Due to the many activities shared by the bourgeois and noble spa guests in Rehburg, Kestner was more or less in constant contact with the *Fräuleins*, and he obviously liked Fräulein von Reden. When he came to sit next to her because of random seating arrangements at the spa, he relates this experience with a mixture of pleasure and uneasiness: "I very much liked the place I occupied at the table, which is otherwise something that rarely turns out as one desires on such occasions, because it depends not on choice but on *etiquette*. In a word, Fräulein von Reden sat on my right side and at my left was our aunt [Kestner's and his sisters' aunt]. As a motley row was the guiding principle of seating, I had this pleasure. Otherwise, according to the rules of rank, I could and would not have desired it."[74] Kestner concludes his positive observations about the character and appearance of Fräulein von Reden with a resolute remark: "She does indeed deserve the highest respect, and I dedicate it to her. You know that I won't get involved with anything more."[75]

Kestner also reflects on the cousin of Fräulein von Reden, Mademoiselle Sobelet [Zobelet], who was the child of a *mésalliance* between a nobleman and an "unnoble" (*unadeliche*) woman: "Fräulein [Zobelet] seems to be very well-behaved and has been brought up well. I pity her because her unnoble mother will do her harm."[76] Kestner, of course, did not mean to say that the young woman's mother would actually harm her child, but rather that Mademoiselle Zobelet's social status was compromised because her mother was not a noblewoman. In sum, Kestner was very aware of not only his own social status in relation to the young noblewomen but also the difference in rank between the two *Fräuleins*. Interaction with the (lower) nobility at the spa became a problem for him when the question of *connubium* appeared on the horizon.

To conclude, in the mid-eighteenth century, both in the published discourse and in personal narratives, a major change in the perception of the spa gradually took hold: the spa was increasingly conceptualized as a social heterotopia. As we have seen earlier, Koromandel-Wedekind captured this new ideal in two sentences: "Here birth and status and title are not considered, . . . Freedom is loved, courtly manners hated."[77] These discursive statements set the standard that every spa was measured against in the late eighteenth and early nineteenth centuries. As a social heterotopia the spa had to aspire to be a "different place" where the early modern social order and the concomitant considerations of rank would be suspended and the usual social rules would not apply. This was a remarkable development. A space created by the prince, where the nobility held sway, was now metaphorically "occupied" by the "bourgeois media society."[78] The ideal of the spa as a social heterotopia established a new discursive regime that started to prevail in the 1770s and successfully took over the published discourse in the late eighteenth and early nineteenth centuries. We shall see in Chapter 6 that even authors who addressed the continued existence of social boundaries at spas and the difficulty of avoiding them were forced to argue defensively or apologetically in view of this prevailing discourse.

In both the published discourse and the personal narratives, certain interactions, spaces, and practices were regarded as test cases for the success of the spa as a social heterotopia. However, the published discourse and the personal narratives differed in one important respect. As Donop's description of noble-bourgeois interaction at the spa indicated, the published discourse usually constructed a binary differentiation between the two social groups. This included using the blanket terms "nobility" (*Adel*) and "bourgeoisie" (*Bürgertum, Bürgerliche*), not taking into account that these were ill-defined social groups during the eighteenth century. In fact, as discussed earlier, bourgeois society was dynamic and in flux, ennoblement was a common occurrence, and even the "old" nobility formed a highly differentiated group.[79] Employing a dichotomy made it possible for the published spa discourse to depict noble-bourgeois encounters as clear-cut and unambiguous, usually assigning blame to the nobility. In contrast, the personal narratives, especially those written by the educated bourgeoisie, reveal the complexity of noble-bourgeois interactions, and the ways in which these interactions also depended on context. On the one hand, the personal narratives show the perceptions and practices of eighteenth-century contemporaries to be situational and individualized, at least to a certain degree. On the other hand, these texts reveal that the social boundary between nobility and bourgeoisie, however situational it may have been, was constantly present in contemporaries' minds, even at the spa.

The Spa as a Social Heterotopia: Spa Freedom and Social Tone

By the late 1770s, a new discursive regime was taking hold in the published discourse: the spa was conceived as a meeting place for the nobility and the bourgeoisie where members of the middle class were supposed to be accepted as equals by members of the nobility. The spa of the late eighteenth and early nineteenth centuries was described as a social heterotopia in two respects. In a narrower sense, the spa was seen as separate from society and therefore practices intended to further social equality were considered to be confined to the spa. This conceptualization of the spa can be summarized as "what happens at the spa, stays at the spa."

In a broader sense, the spa as a social heterotopia was supposed to be a kind of "new society in miniature," and the practices of equality that people became familiar with at the spa were expected to affect society at large in the future. This view conceived of the spa as a "social laboratory" with "real-world" applications. Some authors conceptualized the spa in the narrower sense, but other authors, clearly inspired by a more radical enlightened vision of society as free and equal, wanted the spa to have a broader impact.

Some authors regarded the heterotopia of the spa as clearly separate from the other spaces of society and thus maintained the difference between "being at court and at the spa."[80] These texts argued that, as one author in the *Journal of Luxury and Fashions* (*Journal des Luxus und der Moden*) put it in 1797, "the social hierarchy" was "very well-founded" in "civil society [*bürgerliche Verfassung*]," but "not allowed at the spa."[81] And an article of 1798 in the same journal proclaimed effusively that it was "the dear tolerant spa spirit that in the midst of the most diverse nations in an aristocratic or monarchical country brings together and unites people, whose status, purses, and characteristics are often in the greatest contrast, back into a kind of natural state, that is, as common [human] beings."[82] We can infer from this description that the "tolerant spirit" was confined to the spa and that other, less tolerant "spirits" dominated the "aristocratic and monarchical countries" surrounding it.

In his famous work *Practical Philosophy of Social Life* (*Ueber den Umgang mit Menschen*), first published in 1788, Knigge wrote, "In watering places everyone ought to contribute toward banishing all troublesome restraint from social circles . . . In such places . . . many of those considerations and rules of prudence we submit to in civil life must be waived, tolerance and unanimity must prevail, . . . and on returning to our family [we] resume again the post which the state has intrusted [*sic*] to us."[83] Knigge evidently tried to make his argument as widely acceptable as possible by emphasizing that the spa constituted a space outside of the normal social system. The author of an article entitled "On the [Social] Distinction in Pyrmont" ("Ueber die Distinktion in Pyrmont") in the *Pyrmont Spa Archive* (*Pyrmonter Brunnen-Archiv*) of 1782 addressed precisely this topic. The article, while acknowledging that the spa should serve as a meeting place, is rather critical of the bourgeoisie – a rare occurrence in the published discourse. The anonymous author defends the formation of noble circles in Pyrmont, arguing "that . . . the government there does everything in its power to make the separation of the estates [*Stände*] that is necessary because of our constitution [society] as unnoticeable and as undetrimental to the bourgeoisie as can be done in this world."[84] This position ultimately stabilized the eighteenth-century social order by describing the spa as a separate space in society with its own rules.

However, some authors advocated for the spa as a model for the future of society. Pushing what might be called a more radical enlightened-bourgeois agenda, these spa publications argued that the new, more equal forms of social interaction practiced by the nobility and the upper middle class at the spa should inform changes in society. The heterotopia of the spa was seen as a social experiment that would be directly applicable to society as a whole in the future. These discursive statements directly linked the spa to assessments of the perceived state of development and hoped-for future of society. The most creative way to describe the spa's connection to developments in society as a whole can be found in the *Journal of Luxury and Fashions* (*Journal des Luxus und der Moden*) in 1797. In a report about the season at the small spa of Ronneburg, the author linked toleration in religious matters, a hard-earned and socially transformative accomplishment of the sixteenth and seventeenth centuries, with the spa as a social heterotopia: "What one might perhaps miss here especially is the pleasant and informal blending of the various estates [*Stände*]. Apparently, there was too much separatism here, which should not be tolerated in a cheerful spa circle any more than in well-functioning church governance [*Kirchenpolizey*]."[85]

And in a play about Lauchstädt one of the protagonists declared, "Our best minds [enlightened writers and philosophers] have been uniting for more than thirty years to slay the monster of noble pride, and it is said that it is already convulsing here and there."[86] Marcard discussed the topic in his Pyrmont spa guide: "Enlightened reason finally shows without a doubt that hereditary nobility (for personal nobility has always existed and will always exist) is not a necessary thing in the world, but a prejudice that comes from the darkest times."[87] In this instance, the published spa discourse of the late eighteenth century affirmed enlightened-bourgeois criticism of the nobility. The discourse condemns "noble pride" and advocates for nobility attained through merit over hereditary nobility.[88] Some authors of spa publications, then, saw the spa as a space where society had already embarked on the rocky road toward a "noble-bourgeois elite symbiosis."[89]

No matter which role individual authors ascribed to the spa in society, the published discourse homed in on specific terms to describe the social atmosphere at the spa. In this context, practices and spaces were defined as indicators of how well the spa functioned as a social heterotopia. The terms "spa freedom" (*Brunnenfreiheit*) and "tone" (*Ton*) came to signify the success of a spa in furthering noble-bourgeois interaction. Access to certain spaces like assembly rooms and practices like dancing and greetings then served as test cases to gauge the exact level of interaction between and integration of the nobility and the bourgeoisie. During the late eighteenth and early nineteenth centuries, no spa publication could afford to ignore these questions. Visitors wanted to know whether a spa was able to fulfill its promise as a social heterotopia or not. Moreover, spa guests were interested in learning about specific spaces and about incidences that (supposedly) happened at a spa in order to obtain a better sense of its social atmosphere.

"Spa freedom" (*Brunnenfreiheit, Badefreiheit*) was originally a legal term, meant to ensure that spa visitors sitting defenseless in a bathing pool would be protected from harm to their bodies and belongings: "Then whoever sits in it [the bath] shall be assured of his life and limb as well as his possessions."[90] This concept of the spa as a space that was (or at least should be) exempt from violence and war continued into the nineteenth century. In 1807, Karl Wilhelm Friedrich Grattenauer argued that spas should be recognized under international law as neutral spaces accessible to people from all territories, even in times of war.[91]

In the published discourse of the eighteenth century, however, the term "spa freedom" gradually acquired a more general and vague meaning, hinting at the difference between spa life and everyday life, the freedom to do as one pleased, and the many possibilities for enjoyment. Some of the pleasures the term often referred to were the meetings and conversations between educated members of the bourgeoisie at the spa. Grundig explicitly noted in his travelogue of 1754 that he watched, rather than participated in, noble leisure activities, and he then defines freedom at the spa in terms of a quiet bourgeois life that is attained by not drawing attention to oneself: "But otherwise one lives here, if one is only quiet and calm, as a stranger in the most undisturbed freedom. Yes, almost in the most natural state, as a person who, apart from God, has no overlord and commander to recognize."[92] Johann Christian Kestner, with a dash of irony, associated the term "spa freedom" with varied activities and a certain freedom of choice within the highly regulated daily routine at the spa: "At the *grand café* we again experienced spa freedom. One walked hither and thither without being tied to one place."[93] And Justus Möser wrote to Thomas Abbt from Pyrmont in 1766, referring to his conversations with Gotthold Ephraim Lessing: "Spa-Freedom. Mr. Lessing is here, and I am well."[94]

From the middle of the eighteenth century the definition of "spa freedom" gradually took a further turn. Now it was redefined as a term that referred to overcoming the social boundaries between the nobility and the bourgeoisie. After 1789, when the term was often combined with the word "equality," this inevitably had to evoke the French triad of *liberté, egalité, fraternité* in contemporaries' minds. By the 1790s, this more focused use of the term "spa freedom" became established in the published discourse. For example, in his 1795 *Journey of a Livonian* (*Reise eines Liefländers*) Joachim Christoph Friedrich Schulz remarked about Karlsbad, "The freedom and equality of spa life is less to be found here than elsewhere. One inquires about birth, status, and title; one makes exceptions; one listens to petty gossip and does similar things; one gives balls, picnics, and concerts from which people are excluded [i.e., implying that the bourgeoisie was excluded]."[95] And in 1796, the *Journal of Luxury and Fashions* (*Journal des Luxus und der Moden*) wrote about Nenndorf, "There is a lot of informality here. One tries to uphold freedom and equality as much as possible and to keep down those who come to Nenndorf with arrogance."[96]

The *Journal of Luxury and Fashions* evoked "spa freedom" again in 1798 in an even more striking fashion. In an article about Pyrmont, the author repudiates the "freedom" propagated by revolutionaries, and especially by the French Revolution, but praises social integration at the spa as a means to further "general Enlightenment" and even hints at women's rights:

> Through different circumstances, through the French and other revo-
> lutions that followed upon it, the spirit of freedom became the spirit
> of the times. With the new mass migration resulting from the gen-
> eral desire to travel and visit spas its [freedom's] power spread over
> the customs, fashions, amusements, and tastes of the world in every
> respect. It goes without saying that we are not talking here about
> the reckless spirit that seeks only to whirl about in the revolution
> of states. The spirit of freedom I speak of is that which embellishes
> the scenes of sociability with mild colors, which ousts stiff etiquette,
> which assures the female sex that it possesses its own intellect and
> physical strength, which shows its traces in the wide, dangling over-
> coats of the men and in the light garments of the ladies,[97] and which
> advances toward general Enlightenment by . . . bringing humans
> closer to nature again.[98]

Although the term "spa freedom" figures in prominent places in the published discourse, it is used less often than the term "tone" (*Ton*) or "prevailing tone" (*herrschender Ton*).[99] In the spa discourse of the late eighteenth and early nineteenth centuries, "tone" became the term that expressed in one word the complex relationship between the bourgeoisie and the nobility at the spa. When contemporaries described the tone of a spa, they gauged the spa as a social heterotopia and especially the limits of the spa as a meeting place. The tone at a spa was regarded as "good" when members of the bourgeoisie were treated as equals by the nobility and the social atmosphere was perceived as open and without barriers. The tone at a spa was considered "bad" when the nobility separated itself from the bourgeoisie and insisted on maintaining social boundaries and displaying "noble pride." Spas were judged and categorized according to their "prevailing tone." By the late eighteenth century, the primary criterion for a "good" or a "bad" spa was its social tone – not the healing effects of the spa's water, the services and amusements it provided, or the surrounding landscape. This reveals the outsize significance that the ideal of the spa as a social heterotopia had gained in the published discourse. As Göckingk put it in his report about Brückenau in 1782, "The area, as beautiful as it is, the company, as numerous as it may be, would both give little pleasure if people interacted in the same way as in most spas I know. But fortunately this is different here."[100]

Spa publications again and again use the term "tone" when discussing the spa as a social heterotopia. In his aforementioned article Göckingk remarked about Brückenau, "In this spa the spa guests have not yet changed the tone so as to overemphasize etiquette. I have found that the canons of Fulda, the most distinguished court servants, and the Fulda nobility in general were extremely accommodating to every stranger, regardless of his birth or rank in civil society [*bürgerliche Welt*]."[101] The *Journal of Luxury and Fashions* (*Journal des Luxus und der Moden*) alleged in 1800, "The tone that prevails here [in Hofgeismar] among people from all estates is so warm, so moral, honest, and friendly that it is difficult to part from them."[102] In Franzensbad, the author of a travelogue argued, the tone is "just the right one, whereby morality, sociability, pleasure, and health can prevail."[103] Often the metaphor is extended by referring to the act of "tuning" (*stimmen*) a musical instrument. Scherf, for instance, wrote about Meinberg in 1794, "What is the tone in Meinberg? I am happy to tell you that it is tuned [*gestimmt*] according to the maxim that a spa is a rural sojourn and not life at court."[104] Käppel, who defended Pyrmont against Frankenau's attacks, dedicated an entire section of his spa guide to "Social Entertainment [and] the Dominant Tone":[105] "Now people link themselves to each other without being fearful of differences in birth and rank, diligently tuning [*stimmen*] themselves lower, facilitating the path to [making] close acquaintances, and in so far animating the soul of social entertainment. Here the noble pedant is compelled to yield and to join in the general gentle, friendly tone."[106]

In contrast, in the 1798 travelogue *Journey to the Spas of Karlsbad, Eger [Franzensbad], and Teplitz* (*Reise nach den Badeörtern Karlsbad, Eger und Töplitz*), Karlsbad's social tone is described in a negative light: "In general, the tone in Karlsbad is nothing less than corporative. It is a cold, stiff, heartless, and soulless complimentary tone: . . . Still they [the nobles] separate themselves from the bourgeoisie [*den Bürgerlichen*] with a visible and striking aloofness. They are actually the creators and maintainers of this tone that has such a magical effect on the inhabitant of Karlsbad that he [*sic*] believes he is paying no small tribute to the bourgeois guest when he puts the blessed little word 'von' in front of his name and calls him 'Your Lordship.'"[107]

Contemporaries often considered small and mid-sized spas to have a better social tone because, they argued, there was either no tradition of keeping up social boundaries, or the smaller interior space and lower number of guests made it impossible to form separate circles. In contrast to Karlsbad,[108] Franzensbad is presented in the published discourse as a spa where a manageable number of guests met regularly throughout the day, for example at the communal lunch table. Hoser argues,

> Perhaps nowhere do numerous spa guests make up . . . a family almost in the true sense of the word as here in Franzensbrunn. One

only needs to be present for one or two days to get to know the whole society at once, . . . Obviously the nature of the place, the close circle of daily doing and weaving, which is more limited than elsewhere, but not oppressive, the necessary gathering of all parts of the [spa] society at the well and in the dining hall, is responsible for the fact that people are brought closer together and become acquainted with each other in the shortest possible time.[109]

Hoser transfers the idea of the intimacy of the bourgeois family to the spa. He argues that Franzensbad's spatial construction almost inevitably guaranteed interpersonal encounters through the shared use of spaces. This leads to the assertion that Franzensbad possessed a certain *genius loci* that rubbed off on spa guests: "It is strange enough that even those who in Karlsbad live either in an offish and constrained or in a glamorous and luxurious fashion often within half a day, during which they travel from there [Karlsbad] to here [Franzensbad], change their tone and adopt the kind of amiable informality that is the basis for all the comforts of life at any other place, but especially at a spa. Nowhere does one here become aware of the sharply marked boundary that separates the two estates [*Stände*], the noble [*den Adelichen*] and the bourgeois [*Bürgerlichen*]."[110] Hoser's claim about Franzensbad evokes two characteristics of Enlightenment optimism about human nature: he assumes that people can change and that society at large can therefore change for the better.

In his 1796 article about Rehburg in the *German Monthly* (*Deutsche Monatsschrift*), Deneken provides a more pragmatic reasoning than Hoser for the relative success of social integration at most small and mid-sized spas:

The spa of Rehburg is mostly only visited by people from the neighboring areas who have already known each other as countrymen or who will soon and easily get to know each other. Therefore, a like-minded, sociable tone prevails here, which is not disturbed by any striking differences in the way of life, by any cold politeness or mistrustful distance from each other, as is the case at spas where people from far-flung countries meet. Here one lives as in a family, into which every person who arrives [at the spa] and does not want to be an eccentric is introduced without ado.[111]

Deneken also describes the spa as a (bourgeois) family, but the similarities with Hoser's argument end there. For Deneken, it is not the *genius loci*, but rather the limited catchment area and the socially more homogeneous spa society that differentiates Rehburg from larger spas. His analysis matches Schmid's and Kestner's experiences in Wiesbaden and Rehburg in 1766.[112] Deneken does not, however, identify the social boundaries that also existed at smaller and mid-sized spas, which became obvious in the personal narratives.

As I will show in detail in the following chapter, both the published discourse and personal narratives focused on spaces and practices that were seen as test cases for a spa's social tone and as indicators of whether the spa could be considered a success as a social heterotopia. These spaces and practices either furthered noble-bourgeois interaction or created social boundaries between the two groups. First, contemporaries were concerned about access to spaces. Access signified social integration, even if this was, of course, not an automatic consequence. While access to certain spaces like the prince's summer residence always remained restricted, the published discourse postulated that all interior spaces at the spa should be accessible to the upper middle class. Examples of contested spaces were the Bohemian and Saxon halls in Karlsbad and the ballroom in Lauchstädt. Second, practices that were regarded as test cases occurred in the context of seating arrangements, usually during meals, but also in the theater and at concerts – that is, at events that were described as "public" in the eighteenth-century sense of "not excluding the bourgeoisie."[113] In Pyrmont, for example, the breakfast on the main avenue became one such test case for the social tone of the spa (Figure 2.2). Other contentious practices included dancing and clothing, especially female clothing.[114] All these elements were discussed in the published discourse and in personal narratives as flashpoints of noble-bourgeois interaction.

During the late eighteenth and early nineteenth centuries, discursive statements about spas increasingly employed terms and concepts like "freedom," "equality," "reason," "merit," and "enlightened." These were used in opposition to "birth," "rank," "etiquette," and "noble pride" – early modern concepts that would be overcome at the social heterotopia of the spa. This reveals how deeply the published spa discourse was rooted in the general Enlightenment discourse. The climax of this discursive regime in spa publications occurred in the decades between the late 1770s and about 1820. This period is generally described as encompassing the Late Enlightenment, the Counter-Enlightenment, and early conservatism in Germany. Similar to the periodization historians have proposed for the popular Enlightenment,[115] however, it is more appropriate to characterize this period in the spa discourse as a prolonged late Enlightenment period.[116]

The published spa discourse thus served as a powerful multiplier of Enlightenment ideas about social equality. It supported the creation and dissemination of a new bourgeois identity, combining self-assertion based on Enlightenment principles with vocal demands to be accepted as equals by the nobility. When social boundaries between the bourgeoisie and the nobility remained firm, the published discourse usually constructed the nobility as the guilty party. In the following chapter, I will explore the different ways in which noble-bourgeois interactions were constructed and experienced both in the published discourse and in personal narratives. I will also describe the limits of these interactions at the spa.

Notes

1. See, e.g., [Grundig], *Beschreibung seiner, im Jahr 1751 in das Käyser Carls-Bad gethanen Reise*, 1754, 80–81.
2. [Jormann], *Das Schwalbacher Sommer-wehrende Perpetuum Mobile*, 1690, 5: "Die Fürsten/ Grafen/ Herrn/ die Edelleuth und Pfaffen/ | Domm-Herren/ Nonnen/ Münch/ und viel unedle Affen/ | Juristen, Medicos, Doctores ohne Zahl | . . . | Die Dames und die Mägd/ ins Ohr dem Artzte beichten/ | . . . | Viel Männer/ Weiber/ Knecht/ viel Jungfern . . . | Seugammen/ Huren auch/ und kleine Kinderlein/ | Laqueyen/ Kutschers/ und viel Bürger auch viel Bauren/ | Viel Beutelschneider und viel lose böse Lauren/ | Auch Hoch- und Nidrige/ der Officirer da/ | Fuß-Knecht und Reuters er [Merkur] mit samt Kauffleuten sah. | Gelehrt und Ungelehrt/ Gastgeber/ Wirth und Kramers/ | . . . | die gantze Bettler Zunfft/ viel lahme/ krumme Leut." See also [Wasserbach], *Perpetuum mobile Pyrmontanum aestivum*, 1719, 109–132.
3. Tralles, *Das Kaiser-Carls-Bad in Böhmen in einer Ode entworfen*, 1756, 20: "In kleinem Raum seh' ich das Spiel der Welt."
4. See Föhl, "Wildbad," 475; Miller, Taddey, *Handbuch der historischen Stätten: Baden-Württemberg*, article "Wildbad," 888.
5. "Badeordnung von Wildbad 1549," 165: "Zum fünften soll keiner dem Andern an sein geordnete Statt sitzen, ob aber einer eins hohers Stands dann der ander were, soll der, so des niders Stands, wie billig ime statt geben und wychen." See also "Badeordnung von Liebenzell, c. 1530."
6. Rem, *Tagebuch*, 23: "um daz [es] wermer und mer geselschaft."
7. See Montaigne, *Tagebuch*, 19.
8. Montaigne, *Journal*, vol. 1, 77.
9. See Paumgartner, *Briefwechsel*, 245–246, 264–265.
10. Paumgartner, *Briefwechsel*, 44–45: "gnueg und mein hend vol zu thon hett" – "paradeyß" – "aus der nohtt ein tugennd machen" – "also schier wider meinen willen guett leben habenn."
11. See Montaigne, *Tagebuch*, 18, 35–36, 228–229, 233–234, 263.
12. See Montaigne, *Tagebuch*, 219–224.
13. See Montaigne, *Tagebuch*, 34, 233, 261, 264.
14. See Montaigne, *Tagebuch*, 22, 33.
15. Montaigne, *Journal*, vol. 3, 75.
16. Montaigne, *Journal*, vol. 3, 144.
17. See Chapters 1 and 3.
18. Beermann, *Einige Historische Nachrichten*, 1706, 54–55: "daß bey gutem Wetter unter denen grünen Bäumen fast täglich Assembléen und Balletten von der Noblesse pflegen angestellet zu werden/ da dann die übrigen sich insgemein attrouppiren und Zuschauer abgeben."
19. Henkel, *Bethesda Portuosa*, 1746, 8: "schöne Lust-Häuser zu deren Bade-Gäste Ergetzlichkeit, insonderheit vor Standespersonen."
20. *Neu-verbessert- und vermehrtes denckwürdiges Kayser Carls-Baad*, 1736, 31–33: "Assembleen" – "hohen Ständen" – "Lust-Häuser" – "Frey-Schiessen."
21. [Grundig], *Beschreibung seiner, im Jahr 1751 in das Käyser Carls-Bad gethanen Reise*, 1754, 54: "die vornehmsten Gesellschaften" – "zur Lust wallfahrten."

22. [Grundig], *Beschreibung seiner, im Jahr 1751 in das Käyser Carls-Bad gethanen Reise*, 1754, 49: "prächtig ausgeziertes . . . Gebäude, allwo sich sonderlich hohe Badegäste . . . mit Tanzen und anderen Lustbarkeiten zu unterhalten pflegen."

23. See [Grundig], *Beschreibung seiner, im Jahr 1751 in das Käyser Carls-Bad gethanen Reise*, 1754, 49.

24. See Montaigne, *Tagebuch*, 219.

25. See Studt, "Badenfahrt," 45–48.

26. Studt, "Badenfahrt," 47: "Witze, Rätsel, Gedichte und Schwänke."

27. Studt, "Badenfahrt," 46: "für die Schwänke, die sein Freund und dessen Badegenossen ihm ins Wildbad geschickt hätten und über die er sich köstlich amüsiert habe."

28. Beermann, *Einige Historische Nachrichten*, 1706, 53: "Ferner hat man in den Buchläden nicht nur das Vergnügen/ daß man daselbst die neuesten Bücher sehen und haben kan/ sondern man trifft insgemein in selbingen eine angenehme Compagnie Gelehrter und Politer Leute an/ mit welchen man sich durch Discours ergötzen und sonst vergnügen kan."

29. Tralles, *Das Kaiser-Carls-Bad in Böhmen in einer Ode entworfen*, 1756, dedication sheet: "herzinnigst-geliebten Freunde." Tralles was a member of the German Academy of Natural Scientists Leopoldina (*Deutsche Akademie der Naturforscher Leopoldina*) since 1755. Sulzer became a member in 1763.

30. Tralles, *Das Kaiser-Carls-Bad in Böhmen in einer Ode entworfen*, 1756, 4v: "in der Gesellschaft noch einiger geliebten Freunde" – "nützlichen Unterhaltungen und . . . unschuldigen Ergötzlichkeiten."

31. Tralles, *Das Kaiser-Carls-Bad in Böhmen in einer Ode entworfen*, 1756, Vorrede: "die ungebundene Art unseres Umganges . . . in der Gesellschaft alter und neuer Freunde."

32. Tralles, *Das Kaiser-Carls-Bad in Böhmen in einer Ode entworfen*, 1756, 23: "Gleichheit am Gemüthe."

33. See *Unschuldiger Zeitvertreib im Carlsbad*, 1751.

34. See [Schütte], *Amusemens des eaux de Cleve*, 1748.

35. Tralles, *Das Kaiser-Carls-Bad in Böhmen in einer Ode entworfen*, 1756, 21: "Den niedern Stand durch höhern Stand verdrängt."

36. Tralles, *Das Kaiser-Carls-Bad in Böhmen in einer Ode entworfen*, 1756, 20–21: "kleinem Raum" – "das Spiel der Welt" – "Verschiednes Maaß an Kleidern und an Schritten."

37. Tralles, *Das Kaiser-Carls-Bad in Böhmen in einer Ode entworfen*, 1756, 22: "Drückt steifer Blick den Glanz der Ahnen aus?" – "Die Tugend geht weit über Ehr und Gut."

38. Tralles, *Das Kaiser-Carls-Bad in Böhmen in einer Ode entworfen*, 1756, 22–23: "Beneidens werth ist mein zufriedner Stand" – "Die Weisheit schafft den ungebohrnen Adel."

39. [Merveilleux], *Amusemens des eaux de Schwalbach*, 1739, 7: "Dabey ist noch zu merken, daß nur blos der Adel auf einem Ball zu Schwalbach tanzet, doch läßt man auch wohl einigen Herrn Cammer-Räthen von W** diese Ehre mit genießen; denn was nicht Adelich ist, darf sich auch nicht unter den Adel machen. Gleichwohl kan idermann dem Ball und dem Concert beywohnen, er muß aber hinter den Stülen sich aufhalten. Dieses ist ein Gebrauch, wovon der Deutsche Adel nicht das geringste nachläßt." It is not entirely clear from the context which residence town "W**" stands for. See note 48.

40. See Berger, *Anna Amalia*, 469–470, on an inquiry from the Weimar court to the Brunswick court in 1760 regarding the extent of integration of bourgeois

court, government, privy, or consistory councillors: whether they were to be allowed to *watch* court balls, participate in card games at court, and attend courtly meals. The privy council in Brunswick responded negatively. See also Kreutzmann, *Zwischen ständischer und bürgerlicher Lebenswelt*, 244, 246.

41. [Merveilleux], *Amusemens des eaux de Schwalbach*, 1739, 19: "Das ist zwar wohl wahr, daß sich Standes-Personen allemal gerade vor die Schaubühne setzen; und wenn sich auch ein Bürgerlicher an dem Orte befänd, so würde man ihm nicht erst viel gute Worte geben, einer Dame von hohem Stande Platz zu machen."

42. Donop, *Die Schönheiten Pyrmonts*, 1750, C4 r-v: "Ein wohlgeschmückter Held ersucht, mit sich vergnügt, | Indem sein stolzer Fus sich nett nach Noten biegt, | Ein reizend schönes Kind, den Tanzplatz auszuschmücken, | . . . | Sie neigt sich. Sagt kein Wort, und zieht mit sprödem Blick, | Noch weil er emsig fleht den holden Arm zurück, | Verlässt ihn, sezt sich hin; er geht mit stillen Klagen, | Und fordert andre auf: auch dis wird abgeschlagen. | Warum? zu viel gewagt! So spricht ein schöner Mund, | Der Freche! ist ihm nichts von edlen Sitten kund? | Ein Bürger nähert sich, ein Bürger wil es wagen, | Ein Bürger ist so stolz uns Tänze anzutragen? | Wens etwan einst beim Ball an edlen Tänzern fehlt, | Ists ihm noch Ehre gnug, wenn man ihn dan erwählt: | Nun aber kan er gehn, und dort in nidren Linden | Genug von Bürgerart, von seines Gleichen finden. | Sie schweigt. Der Tolheit Wort! o lacht, wer lachen kan. | Beklagt die Tänzerin! ihr stöst ein Fieber an. | Bedenk dich blödes Kind! ich steh dir für den Tadel. | Ihm gibt ein grosser Geist, dir nur das Glück den Adel."

43. "Tartuffe" is a reference to the protagonist in the comedy *Tartuffe, or The Impostor, or The Hypocrite* by Molière. "Don Quixote" is a reference to the novel *The Ingenious Gentleman Don Quixote of La Mancha* by Miguel de Cervantes.

44. Koromandel-Wedekind, *Der Brunnengast*, 1744, 13: "Hier wird Geburt und Stand und Würde nicht betracht, | Im Sitzen blosserdings nur bunte Reih gemacht. | Bald sitzt ein Edelmann, ein Graf, ein Bürgermeister, | Ein Kaufmann, ein Student, ein Held der kleinen Geister, | Bald sitzt ein Geistlicher, ein Doctor und ein Rath, | Tartuf und Donqvirot; wer Geld im Beutel hat, | Bald oben, unten an, zur rechten und linken Seiten, | Ein Mischmach von gelehrt-vornehm und schlechten Leuten. | Denn jeder gilt allhier so viel als Brunnengast, | Die Freyheit wird geliebt, die Hofmanier gehasst."

45. See Stollberg-Rilinger, "Zeremoniell als politisches Verfahren."

46. See the report by Margravine Wilhelmine of Bayreuth, the Prussian king's daughter, about her wedding celebration in Berlin in 1731: "whereupon one went to the [banquet] table. The king had the places drawn by lot to avoid disputes over order of precedence of the foreign princes." ("worauf man sich zur Tafel begab. Der König hatte die Plätze auslosen lassen, um die Rangstreitigkeiten der fremden Fürsten zu vermeiden.") Wilhelmine von Bayreuth, *Eine preußische Königstochter*, 280.

47. See in detail Engel, "Pyrmonter Fürstensommer," esp. 142–143, 161.

48. [Merveilleux], *Amusemens des eaux de Schwalbach*, 1739, 3: "Die Fürstin nimmt gemeiniglich an der einen Tafel, und der Fürst an der andern den ersten Platz ein. Man läßt sich ohne Unterschied des Ranges bald an des Fürsten Tafel, bald an der Fürstin ihrer nieder. Gleichwie auch sonst niemand als Standes-Personen, oder Kammer-Räthe von W** zugegen sind." This quote again emphasizes that privy councillors from a residence town that cannot be clearly identified, but was probably Weilburg, were the only members of the bourgeoisie admitted to noble activities in Schwalbach, echoing the description of the balls above. See note 39.

49. See, e.g., Schlögl, "Die patriotisch-gemeinnützigen Gesellschaften," 75.
50. Göckingk, "Von dem Kurbrunnen bei Brückenau," 1782, 338: "Die Tafel läuft ins Viereck und besteht in der eigentlichen Kurzeit aus hundert und zwanzig, dreissig und mehreren Personen. Man sezt sich ohne Unterschied, und jeder wählt sich Nachbarn nach seinem Gefallen."
51. See "Teutsche Badechronik," *JLM* (October 1796), 524: "Bey Tische sitzt man nach der Anciennität, so daß der, welcher erst ankommt, den untersten Platz erhält und immer weiter hinan rückt, so wie mehrere nach ihm ankommen." See also "Badechronik," *JLM* (December 1798), 679–680; Wilhelm I. von Hessen, *Wir Wilhelm*, 164.
52. Böckmann, *Journal*, 16: "wurde jeder Brunnengast zu einer seiner Tafeln seinem Range nach eingeladen und man spielte freie Opern."
53. See about the question of seating orders at courtly tables in general Stollberg-Rilinger, "Ordnungsleistung."
54. See Lehndorff, *Aus den Tagebüchern.*
55. Lehndorff, *Aus den Tagebüchern*, 191–192: "Der Adel ist hierzulande sehr hochfahrend und meidet die Gesellschaft dieser guten Bürgersleute. Ich setze mich indes darüber hinweg, und mein Beispiel bewirkt, daß auch die anderen etwas von ihrem steifen Wesen ablassen."
56. Lehndorff, *Aus den Tagebüchern*, 191: "die hiesige Gesellschaft nicht gerade hervorragend" – "die Gräfin Dönhoff" – "die einzige Dame von Stande, die hier ist, und auch die einzige, die mit an unserer Tafel speist."
57. Lehndorff, *Aus den Tagebüchern*, 191: "Gesellschaft Frankfurter Kaufmannsfamilien" – "in der zweiten Etage."
58. Lehndorff, *Aus den Tagebüchern*, 191: "recht hübsch" – "sehr liebenswürdig."
59. Reuß, "Tagebuch einer Reise nach Karlsbad, 1768."
60. Reuß, "Tagebuch einer Reise nach Karlsbad, 1768," 220: "Cavaliers und Damen."
61. Further economic contacts existed with "dawdlers and Jews" as well as with the "Messerschmied Damm." See Reuß, "Tagebuch einer Reise nach Karlsbad, 1768," 221.
62. See Kestner, *Die wahre Brunnenfreiheit*; Schmid, *"Wer an seinem Schöpfer sündiget . . .".*
63. Kestner, *Die wahre Brunnenfreiheit*, 48: "Staatspatriziat." See Lampe, *Aristokratie.*
64. See Schmid, *"Wer an seinem Schöpfer sündiget . . ."*, 10–11.
65. Kestner mentions his aunt only in passing in his spa diary. It is therefore not possible to identify her.
66. See the list of spa guests in Schmid, *"Wer an seinem Schöpfer sündiget . . ."*, 75–96.
67. Schmid, *"Wer an seinem Schöpfer sündiget . . ."*, 58: "Bekanntschaft" – "leutselig und freundlich."
68. See Schmid, *"Wer an seinem Schöpfer sündiget . . ."*, 63–64.
69. Schmid, *"Wer an seinem Schöpfer sündiget . . ."*, entry of 30 June 1765, 31: "Badgäste sind wie Freymäurer gleich bekannt und vertraut."
70. Schmid, *"Wer an seinem Schöpfer sündiget . . ."*, 29: "Im Hause logieren 10 Badgäste, worunter der Geheime Rath von Beist aus Eisenach mit seiner Gemahlin und 3 Fräuleins der vornehmste ist."
71. See the list of spa guests in: Kestner, *Die wahre Brunnenfreiheit*, 100–103.
72. Kestner, *Die wahre Brunnenfreiheit*, 37: "Das Fräulein [von] Berger hatte den Einfall, dass wir uns künftig immer Leute nennen wollten: Hugos Leute, Bergers Leute, Ebelings Leute, Kestners Leute p. Solche Kleinigkeiten haben

oft zum Vergnügen die beste Wirkung. . . . Sie können . . . daraus erkennen, auf was für einem ungezwungenen Fuße wir leben."

73. Kestner, *Die wahre Brunnenfreiheit*, 17: "dass ich Meinesgleichen hier nicht habe. Frauenzimmer, junge Frauenzimmer, meine ich, könnten dieses wohl ersetzen; und es sind auch deren hier, aber die meisten sind adlich. Mit diesen mich sehr abzugeben ist nicht recht meine Sache. Wissen Sie warum? Die übrigen und selbst auch wohl die Fräuleins möchten denken, wenn man ihre Gesellschaft viel sucht, man wäre ein bisschen angeschossen. Solche Leute aber, die sich auf diese Weise über ihren Stand versteigen, kommen mir immer zweideutig vor, darum denke ich, andere urteilen ebenso."

74. Kestner, *Die wahre Brunnenfreiheit*, 32: "Die Stelle am Tische, welche ich hatte, gefiel mir am besten, welches sonst eine Sache ist, welche selten bei solchen Gelegenheiten nach Wunsch ausfällt, weil sie nicht von der Wahl, sondern von der *Etiquette* abhängt. Mit einem Worte, ich saß der Fräulein von Reden zur Rechten und unserer Tanten zur Linken. Weil eine bunte Reihe die Richtschnur des Sitzens war, so hatte ich dies Vergnügen, sonst hätte ich es nach der Regel des Ranges nicht begehrt und begehren können." (Italics in the original.)

75. Kestner, *Die wahre Brunnenfreiheit*, 32: "Sie verdient in der Tat Hochachtung und ich weihe ihr diese. Sie wissen schon, dass ich mich auf mehrers nicht einlasse."

76. Kestner, *Die wahre Brunnenfreiheit*, 16: "Die Fräulein scheint wirklich sehr artig und wohl angeführt zu sein. Ich bedaure sie, dass ihre unadliche Mutter ihr Schaden tun wird."

77. Koromandel-Wedekind, *Der Brunnengast*, 1744, 13: "Hier wird Geburt und Stand und Würde nicht betracht, . . . Die Freyheit wird geliebt, die Hofmanier gehasst."

78. See Faulstich, *Die bürgerliche Mediengesellschaft*.

79. See, e.g., Fehrenbach, *Adel und Bürgertum im deutschen Vormärz*.

80. Göcking, "Von dem Kurbrunnen bei Brückenau," 1782, 337: "am Hofe und im Bade sein." See also [Hassencamp], *Briefe eines Reisenden von Pyrmont*, 1783, 24.

81. See "Badechronik," *JLM* (November 1797), 555: "diese in der bürgerlichen Verfassung sehr wohlgegründeten, aber nur in dem Badeorte unstatthaften Rangordnungen."

82. "Badechronik," *JLM* (March 1798), 190: "der liebe tolerante Badegeist, der mitten unter den verschiedensten Nationen in einem aristokratischen oder monarchischen Lande Menschen, deren Stände, Geldbeutel und Eigenschaften oft im größten Contrast stehen, wieder in eine Art von Naturzustand, das heißt als gemeine Wesen, zusammenbringt und vereinigt."

83. Knigge, *Practical Philosophy of Social Life*, 226; Knigge, *Ueber den Umgang mit Menschen*, part 2, 249: "In Bädern soll Jeder dazu mitwürken, allen lästigen Zwang, nicht aber Sittsamkeit und Gefälligkeit, aus den gesellschaftlichen Cirkeln zu verbannen. Hier, besonders wenn der Kreis der Gäste klein ist, muß eine Menge Rücksichten und Vorsichtigkeits-Regeln, denen man sich im bürgerlichen Leben unterwirft, wegfallen, Duldung und Einigkeit herrschen . . . Nach Ablauf dieser Zeit rückt Jeder wieder in die Rolle ein, die der Staat ihm anvertraut hat."

84. *Das Pyrmonter Brunnenarchiv*, 1782, 65: "daß . . . die dasige Regierung alles anwendet, um die durch unsre Verfassung nothwendig gewordene Absonderung der Stände so wenig auffallend, und für den Bürgerlichen so unnachtheilig zu machen, als sich in dieser Welt thun läßt."

85. "Badechronik," *JLM* (October 1797), 516: "Was man vielleicht vorzüglich hier noch vermissen dürfte, ist die angenehme und zwanglose Mischung der verschiedenen Stände. Offenbar herrschte hier dießmal zu viel Separatismus, der in einem fröhlichen Badezirkel ebensowenig geduldet werden sollte, als in einer gut eingerichteten Kirchenpolizey."

86. [Möller], *Der Adelsstolz im Bade zu Lauchstädt*, 1791, 18: "Unsre besten Köpfe vereinigen sich seit mehr als dreißig Jahren, das Ungeheuer Ahnenstolz zu erlegen, und es soll schon hier und da Zuckungen haben."

87. Marcard, *Beschreibung von Pyrmont*, vol. 1, 1784, 87–88: "Die erleuchtete Vernunft zeigt endlich unwidersprechlich, daß der Erbadel (denn persönlichen Adel gab es immer und wird es immer geben) kein nothwendiges Ding in der Welt, sondern ein Vorurtheil sei, welches aus den allerfinstersten Zeiten herstammt."

88. See Maurer, *Biographie des Bürgers*, 589–590; Möller, "Aufklärung und Adel"; Langewiesche, "Bürgerliche Adelskritik."

89. Langewiesche, "Bürgerliche Adelskritik," 16: "adelig-bürgerliche Elitensymbiose."

90. City description of Baden in Switzerland by Heinrich Pantaleon, 1578, quoted in Martin, *Deutsches Badewesen*, 322: "Dann welcher in dem sitzet, ist seines leibs und lebens auch haab und gut versichert."

91. See Grattenauer, *Über Neutralität, Erhaltung und Sicherheit der Bäder*.

92. [Grundig], *Beschreibung seiner, im Jahr 1751 in das Käyser Carls-Bad gethanen Reise*, 1754, 82: "Sonst aber lebt man hier, wenn man nur still und ruhig ist, als ein Fremder in der ungestörtesten Freyheit: Ja fast im nätürlichsten Zustand, als ein Mensch haben kann, der, ausser Gott, keinen Oberherrn und Gebiether zu erkennen hat."

93. Kestner, *Die wahre Brunnenfreiheit*, 16: "Bei dem *grand Caffée* äußerte sich wiederum die Brunnenfreiheit. Man ging ab und zu, ohne sich an den Ort zu binden." (Italics in the original.) Schröcker's argument that Kestner's use of the term *Brunnenfreiheit* reflects the desire of the middle class to be treated as the nobility's equals is not borne out by Kestner's diary. Kestner never uses the term in such an explicit way. Rather, he always employs it in a mildly ironic fashion to describe typical spa activities in which the bourgeois and noble guests at Rehburg participate together. See Kestner, *Die wahre Brunnenfreiheit*, 69–71; for another example of Kestner's use of the term, see 20.

94. Möser, *Briefwechsel*, letter from Möser to Thomas Abbt, 5 July 1766, 409: "Brunnen-Freyheit. Herr Lessing ist hier; und ich befinde mich wohl."

95. [Schulz], *Reise eines Liefländers*, 1795, 97: "die Freyheit und Gleichheit des Badelebens ist hier weniger zu finden, als anders wo. Man erkundigt sich nach Geburt, Stand und Würde; man macht Ausnahmen, man hört kleine Klätscheryen an und macht dergleichen; man giebt ausschließend Bälle, Pickenicke, Koncerte."

96. "Teutsche Badechronik," *JLM* (October 1796), 523: "Es herrscht im Ganzen hier viel Zwanglosigkeit. Man sucht Freyheit und Gleichheit möglichst aufrecht zu halten und diejenigen nieder zu halten, die mit Anmaßungen nach Nenndorf kommen."

97. On the role of clothing at the spa, see Chapter 6.

98. "Badechronik," *JLM* (September 1798), 500: "Durch mancherley Umstände war der Geist der Zeit Geist der Freyheit geworden, durch die französische und andere darauf folgende Revolutionen. Durch die neue Völker-Wanderung der allgemeinen Reise- und Bade-Lust hatte sich seine Macht über die Sitten, die Moden, die Belustigungen und über den Geschmack

der Welt in jeder Hinsicht verbreitet; versteht sich, daß hier nicht die Rede von dem Schwindelgeiste seyn kann, der nur in Umwälzung der Staaten sich herumwirbeln möchte. Der Geist der Freyheit, von dem ich rede, ist jener, der mit mildern Farben die Scenen der Geselligkeit verschönert, der die steife Etikette verdrängt, der dem weiblichen Geschlecht gehöriges Eigenthum über Geist und Körperkräfte zusichert, der in den weiten schlotternden Ueberröcken der Männer, in den leichten Gewändern der Damen seine Spur zeigt, und der der allgemeinen Aufklärung entgegen kommt, indem er das . . . Menschengeschlecht wieder der Natur näher bringt."

99. See the definition of "tone" (*Ton*) in the Adelung dictionary (*Grammatisch-kritisches Wörterbuch*): "the entirety of outward manners in human society" ("das ganze äußere Betragen in der menschlichen Gesellschaft").

100. See Göckingk, "Von dem Kurbrunnen bei Brückenau," 1782, 333: "Die Gegend, so schön sie auch ist, die Gesellschaft, so zahlreich sie auch sein mögte, würden beide wenig Vergnügen gewähren, wenn die Art des Umgangs auf dem Fuß der mehrersten Bäder, die ich kenne, eingeführt wäre. Aber zum Glück ist das hier anders." See also Krieger, *Alexisbad*, 1812, 36.

101. Göckingk, "Von dem Kurbrunnen bei Brückenau," 1782, 336–337: "In diesem Kurort haben die Brunnengäste den Ton noch nicht etiketmässig überspannt. Ich habe gefunden, daß die Domherren aus Fulda, die vornehmsten Hofbedienten, und überhaupt der fuldische Adel gegen jeden Fremden, ohne Rücksicht auf seine Geburt und seinen Rang in der bürgerlichen Welt, überaus gefällig war."

102. "Badechronik," *JLM* (November 1800), 587: "Der Ton, welcher hier unter den Menschen aus allen Ständen herrscht, ist so herzlich, so sittlich, bieder und freundschaftlich, daß man sich nur mit schwerem Herzen von ihnen trennen kann."

103. *Reise nach den Badeörtern*, 1798, 233: "gerade der rechte, wobei Sittlichkeit, Geselligkeit, Vergnügen und Gesundheit bestehen kann."

104. Scherf, *Briefe für das Publikum*, 1794, 219: "Wie der Ton in Mainberg ist? Ich freue mich Ihnen sagen zu können, er ist nach der Maxime gestimmt, ein Kurort sey ein ländlicher Aufenthalt und kein Hofleben."

105. Käppel, *Pyrmonts Merkwürdigkeiten*, 1810, 43: "Gesellschaftliche Unterhaltung. Herrschender Ton."

106. Käppel, *Pyrmonts Merkwürdigkeiten*, 1810, 45: "Man kettet sich nun ohne ängstlichen Unterschied der Geburt und des Ranges näher an einander an, stimmt sich geflissentlich herab, erleichtert den Weg zu vertraulichen Bekanntschaften, und belebt in sofern die Seele der gesellschaftlichen Unterhaltung. Der Adelspedant sieht sich hier gezwungen, nachgiebig zu werden, und in den allgemeinen sanften, freundlichen Ton mit einzustimmen."

107. *Reise nach den Badeörtern*, 1798, 171–172: "Im Allgemeinen genommen, ist also der Ton in Karlsbad nichts weniger als gesellschaftlich; es ist kalter, steifer, herz- und geistloser Komplimentier-Ton: . . . Noch immer sondern sie sich von den Bürgerlichen mit einer sichtlichen und auffallenden Zurückhaltung ab. Sie eigentlich sind die Schöpfer und Unterhalter jenes Tons, der so zauberisch auf den Karlsbader Einwohner wirkt, daß er dem bürgerlichen Gaste keine geringe Ehren zu erweisen glaubt, wenn er das gebenedeite Wörtlein von seinem Namen vorsetzt, und ihn Ihr Gnaden nennt."

108. We find isolated voices in the published discourse that contradict the general wisdom that social boundaries were inflexible at large spas like Karlsbad. For example, the author of a 1789 article in the *Journal des Luxus und der Moden* argues about the "prevailing tone during the morning walks at the spring" at Karlsbad: "the nobility mingles with every other estate in a very

informal way. . . . in short, I have always seen human beings interact with human beings there." ("herrschenden Ton bey den Morgenspaziergängen des Brunnens" – "der Adel vermischt sich da ganz ungezwungen mit jedem anderen Stande. . . . kurz ich habe dort immer Menschen mit Menschen umgehen sehen.") "Badechronik," *JLM* (November 1798), 626–627.

109. Hoser, *Beschreibung von Franzensbrunn*, 1799, 104: "Nirgend macht vielleicht eine zahlreiche Brunnengesellschaft . . . beinahe im eigentlichsten Verstande so eine Familie aus, als hier in Franzensbrunn. Es bedarf der Anwesenheit von ein oder zween Tagen, um sogleich die ganze Gesellschaft zu kennen, . . . Offenbar ist hieran die Beschaffenheit des Lokals – der mehr als anderwärts beschränkte, aber doch nicht drückend enge Kreis des täglichen Thun und Webens, das nothwendige Zusammenfinden aller Theile der Gesellschaft beym Brunnen und im Speisesaale, Schuld, daß die Menschen einander näher gebracht und in kürzester Zeit mit einander bekannt werden."

110. Hoser, *Beschreibung von Franzensbrunn*, 1799, 107: "es ist sonderbar genug, dass selbst diejenigen die in Karlsbad entweder auf einem steifen gezwungenen, oder glänzenden luxuriösen Fusse leben, oft innerhalb eines halben Tages, während welchen sie von dort hierher reisen, diesen Ton verändern, und jene liebenswürdige Ungezwungenheit annehmen, die die Grundlage aller Annehmlichkeiten des Lebens an jeden anderen, vorzüglich aber in einem Brunnenorte ausmacht. Nirgend wird man hier jene scharf bezeichnete Gränzlinie gewahr, die die beiden Stände, den Adelichen und Bürgerlichen unterschieden und von einander entfernen." See also *Reise nach den Badeörtern*, 1798, 234–235.

111. Deneken, "Bemerkungen bey dem Rehburger Gesundbrunnen," 1796, 197: "Der Rehburger Brunnen wird größtenteils nur von Personen aus den benachbarten Gegenden besucht, die vorher sich schon als Landsleute kennen oder sich doch bald und leicht kennen lernen. Es herrscht daher hier ein gleichgestimmter-geselliger Ton, der durch keine auffallende Verschiedenheit in der Lebensweise – durch keine kalte Höflichkeit oder mistrauische Entfernung von einander, wie an Brunnen-Oertern, wo Leute aus weitentlegenen Ländern zusammentreffen, gestöhrt wird. Hier lebt man, wie in einer Familie, in welche jeder Ankommende, der kein Sonderling seyn will, ohne Umstände eingeführt wird."

112. See Chapter 5.

113. See Hölscher, "Die Öffentlichkeit begegnet sich selbst," 30.

114. See Chapter 6.

115. See Müller, *Aufklärung*, 94–100; Borgstedt, *Zeitalter der Aufklärung*, 60, 90–98.

116. On the problem of the periodization of the German Enlightenment in general, see Whaley, "Transformation."

6 Nobility and Bourgeoisie at the Spa

Creating Unity and Maintaining Differences

As we have seen in Chapter 5, the spa discourse of the late eighteenth and early nineteenth centuries was increasingly influenced by Enlightenment ideas and by bourgeois demands for social equality. A new discursive regime came into being that described the spa as a social heterotopia, a space where the nobility and the bourgeoisie were expected to practice new and more equal forms of social interaction. Contemporaries thus constructed spas as spaces similar to Masonic lodges, reading societies, salons, and other institutions of Enlightenment sociability. This chapter explores the aspirations, tensions, and limits that characterized the spa as a social heterotopia. In the first section of this chapter, I will analyze the expectations and demands laid out in the spa discourse, and I will examine how the nobility and the bourgeoisie were represented both in the published discourse and in personal narratives. In the second section, I will focus on the limitations of noble-bourgeois integration at the spa. In this context, enlightened social circles played an important role in maintaining the ideal of the spa as a meeting place, even when many contemporaries were well aware of the spa's shortcomings as a social heterotopia.

Noble-Bourgeois Interactions: Representations and Experiences

A close reading of the representations of noble-bourgeois interactions at spas in the published discourse and in personal narratives reveals deeply ingrained argumentative patterns. As we will see in this section, the published discourse and the way people reported their personal experiences at spas often converged in surprising ways. The sometimes striking overlaps and parallels between the published discourse and the personal reflections about spa visits by members of the educated elite leave no doubt that personal narratives were embedded in the contemporary discourse and that spas and spa-goers were part of a circle of communication. The range of statements about noble-bourgeois interactions in the published discourse and in personal narratives was, in fact, limited – or, considering the infinite possibilities of language, even "scarce."[1] They can be categorized into three basic types of discursive statement based on the following characteristics: first, forcefully pro-bourgeoisie and critical of the nobility; second, seeking middle ground; and third, critical of the bourgeoisie. These descriptions are, of course, only shorthand. It is important to note that all three types of discursive statement accepted – and operated within – the prevailing discourse that stipulated social integration at the spa. The three types of discursive statement were often, but not always, mutually exclusive. Some spa publications fall neatly into one of these categories, while others employed combinations of the three types of statement. Clearly, some authors did not strive for internal textual coherence but tried to broaden the appeal of their publications as much as possible.

In the *first* type of discursive statement, demands for bourgeois equality are made forcefully, at times even aggressively. These authors presented noble-bourgeois equality at the spa as a natural outcome of enlightened thinking. Moreover, they actively engaged in creating and defining a new, self-confident bourgeois identity. They also defined the spa as a space for social interactions that was to serve as a model for the future of society as a whole. As a result, these authors placed the blame for noble-bourgeois conflicts at the spa solely on the nobility. This type of discursive statement revolves around one main argument, namely a criticism of the nobility for being "proud" and "unenlightened." It is, in short, the most "radical" form of discursive statement about the spa as an Enlightenment social heterotopia. This type of statement is often found in travelogues (including fictional travelogues), in journal articles, and in some of the middlebrow literature that used the spa as a setting, such as the play *Noble Pride at the Spa of Lauchstädt* (*Der Adelsstolz im Bade zu Lauchstädt*).[2] Here the thesis is presented directly in the title.

The *second* type of discursive statement, which seeks compromise, encompasses a more diverse range of arguments. These arguments still have one common goal, namely to maintain a sense of bourgeois identity, while at the same time not criticizing the nobility in an overly forceful or aggressive fashion. These statements can be characterized as searching for a middle ground yet insisting on the validity of enlightened ideals of social equality. On the one hand, some spa publications present an enlightened aristocrat as a proponent of noble-bourgeois equality at the spa. In this case, the published spa discourse, which otherwise takes a bourgeois viewpoint, is transformed into an enlightened discourse that consciously seeks to broaden its appeal and address members of the nobility who regarded themselves as enlightened. We find this type of argument in travelogues, journal articles, advertising pamphlets, and spa guides. On the other hand, some authors directly address members of the middle class as customers, making the case for their equal role in society without the kind of biting criticism of the nobility that was common in the first type of discursive statement. Still, these authors affirmed a self-assured bourgeois identity. This kind of argument appears above all in advertising pamphlets and spa guides.

The *third* type of discursive statement holds the bourgeoisie partially responsible for a breakdown in the heterotopian ideal and thus seeks to spread the blame for failed noble-bourgeois integration at the spa. This type of statement usually appears in spa guides and advertising pamphlets that tried to address a wide audience and attract as many people as possible to the spa. Tellingly, it is most prevalent in texts about spas like Pyrmont that had come under attack in other spa publications for their "prevailing tone" and the nobility's alleged tendency to shun the bourgeoisie. As a result, spa guides employing the third type of discursive statement sometimes take on a defensive attitude. These authors either reject or try to minimize the criticism that the majority of spa publications leveled at the spa's social tone. These texts often refer to social barriers not mentioned in other spa publications, especially the role that "bourgeois pride" played in hindering noble-bourgeois interaction at the spa. Nevertheless, the authors' carefully chosen wording and defensive posture reveal their keen awareness of the existing discursive regime. Their attempts to extend the boundaries of the prevailing discourse were rather limited, and they always sought to convince their readers that the social heterotopia at their particular spa was fundamentally intact, even if occasionally disrupted.

A detailed analysis of these three types of discursive statement reveals both their general rootedness in Enlightenment ideas and specific argumentative patterns.

In the *first* type of statement, a spa's social tone is described either as "free" and sociable or as formal and "court-like." In the published discourse, the two most popular spas of Karlsbad and Pyrmont are regularly criticized for the alleged "separation" (*Absonderung*) of the nobility from the bourgeoisie. The Saxon spa town of Lauchstädt was also regarded as a spa where "noble pride" (*Adelsstolz*) prevailed. Authors expressed these sentiments through a (late) Enlightenment criticism of the nobility that was sometimes biting and often mixed with a good dose of sarcasm and ridicule. Göckingk, for instance, stated, "In Pyrmont and Lauchstädt (says Professor Schlözer)[3] there are sometimes said to be spa guests who make such a big difference between the nobility [*Adelichen*] and the bourgeoisie [*Bürgerlichen*] as if the former had a completely different Adam [the Adam in Genesis, the first man] than the latter."[4]

In the 1793 issue of the *German Magazine* (*Deutsches Magazin*), Ludwig Giseke reported, "The . . . nobility show their love of splendor, and no impartial person can say truthfully that the prevailing tone in Karlsbad is as free and pleasant as it should be at a spa. Etiquette rules here as at one of the most formal courts, and measures every difference in rank precisely."[5] Giseke then effectively declares hereditary nobility invalid and demands that the nobility accept bourgeois values: "Such old lineage is no longer valid in itself, and she [a noblewoman] will be well-advised to only refer to the fact that her father was an honest man and that she is a good mother and housewife. This gives the greatest value today, and therefore we say that we live in a philosophical [enlightened] time. Others want to call it a bad time. I don't know anything about that."[6]

In the play *Noble Pride at the Spa of Lauchstädt* (*Der Adelsstolz im Bade zu Lauchstädt*), a chamberlain named von Strehwalde appears as a stock character, personifying a proud, unenlightened nobleman. He has this to say about the educated "bourgeoisie" (*Bourgeoisie*): "Everyone must remain in his own estate [*Stande*]. How should the world persist if persons of our birth [*naissance*] compromised themselves with people who only exist to serve us. . . . The learned gentlemen [*Herren Gelehrten*] should . . . remain only with their estate and not mingle with cavaliers and noble persons, who want to have nothing to do with these fighters with blunt feathers [*stumpfen Federfechter*, i.e. learned men]."[7] Here a nobleman, who defines the boundaries between the early modern social estates as immovable, is constructed as a stereotype so that the play can satirize the nobility and their behavior at the spa.

In a 1798 fictional travelogue we find a similarly harsh criticism of the nobility:

Tell us, you gentlemen brothers [*Herren Brüder*],
What do you think?
Has nature only given
To you, again and again?
Are you more and are we less
Adam's or Noah's children?
Did He who created mankind
Give you power and profession to be idolized?
Is it mind, reason, and courage?
Is it in the flesh? Is it in the blood?
No! It is but three letters [the word "von" designating nobility in
    German]
And a feathered hat.
By this division between two of the first classes of men, a great rift in
the general sociability must necessarily arise, which [general sociability] only spreads pleasure and happiness everywhere in general, and
especially at spas.[8]

It is highly significant that the address *Herren* (translated imperfectly as "gentlemen" here) is used in the two texts; the authors skillfully exploited the increasingly vague nature of this term in late eighteenth-century Germany.[9] On the one hand, in the play about Lauchstädt, the author engages in a kind of ironic doublespeak. The unenlightened nobleman derisively calling educated members of the bourgeoisie *Herren Gelehrten* adds to the ridicule directed at this stock character because the audience knows better. The implication is that, by using the term at all, the nobleman inadvertently admits that the learned men of the middle class deserve respect and status. On the other hand, the address *Herren Brüder* used by the fictional bourgeois narrator of the travelogue reinforces that he is not willing to accept the nobility's claim to an elevated status. Combining "brothers," the form of address used among Freemasons and sympathizers with the French Revolution to signify social equality, with the term *Herren* ("lords," "sirs") effectively negates the early modern status boundary, renders *Herren* meaningless, and even gives it an ironic twist. As a result, the narrator simultaneously criticizes the nobility and expresses bourgeois self-confidence.

Even though criticism of noble pride and social separation mostly focused on the large fashionable spas, smaller spas were not spared the condemnation of the published discourse. For instance, in 1798 the *Journal of Luxury and Fashions* (*Journal des Luxus und der Moden*) published a scathing article about Freienwalde in Brandenburg: "Guests have been as numerous during this year's spa season as during one of the previous ones. But never before has the partition between the nobility – nobles from Brandenburg, Mecklenburg, and Pomerania dominate here – and the bourgeoisie [*den Bürgerlichen*] been so ironclad and impenetrable as this time. And while other spas are becoming more and more humanized and popularized, [here] noble separatism holds its scepter as stiffly as King Solomon on the lion throne in the Nuremberg illustrated bibles [*Bilderbibeln*]."[10] In this article, criticism of the nobility's conduct is wrapped up in a reference to one of the most important cultural accomplishments of early modern burghers, the impressive Lutheran *Bilderbibeln* produced in the imperial city of Nuremberg and other German cities. By using the well-known illustrations of King Solomon as shorthand for eighteenth-century noble pride, the author of the article about Freienwalde does not stop at a critique of the nobility. He also appeals to bourgeois self-confidence: the *Bilderbibeln* and the illustrations of King Solomon were, after all, creations of educated burghers and therefore proof of urban civic achievements.[11]

Spa publications that employ the first type of discursive statement accuse the nobility of actively preventing the bourgeoisie from crossing the social boundary between the two estates. As we have already seen in Chapter 5, access to spaces became a point of contention in this context. The nobility was blamed for insisting on preferential access to spaces or even for seeking the exclusive right to use certain spaces at the spa. Such behavior was then seen as an indicator of noble pride and thus of the nobility's unwillingness to accommodate bourgeois demands for social equality.

In the discourse about Karlsbad, access to one of the assembly halls, the Saxon hall, is often seen as a crucial test case. Ludwig Giseke stated in 1793, "The nobility effectively regards this [Saxon] hall as their own, . . . They hold their evening assemblies only here, and people of the other estate [*Gens de l'autre monde*, literally 'people of the other world'] can then appropriate the Bohemian hall."[12] The anonymous author of *Journey to the Spas of Karlsbad, Eger [Franzensbad], and Teplitz (Reise nach den Badeörtern Karlsbad, Eger und Töplitz)*, published in 1798, confirmed this observation: "The nobles claim this place [the Saxon hall] for their exclusive use, so that a bourgeois [*ein Bürgerlicher*] rarely goes there nor does he dare to go there."[13] In his 1795 travelogue *Journey of a Livonian (Reise eines Liefländers)*, Joachim Christoph Friedrich Schulz argued that this kind of strict spatial separation also extended to the accommodations in Karlsbad: "But one has even seen sick nobles leave Karlsbad again because they could not find accommodation in the fashionable areas of town. All this to avoid having to set up their lodgings between priests, merchants, bourgeois councillors [*bürgerlichen Räten*], and the like, with whom they have the misfortune, by the way, to have to drink from the same well."[14]

In *Lauchstädt, a Small Painting (Lauchstädt, ein kleines Gemählde)*, the author constructs a vivid episode about the occupation of space. He describes the alleged experience of an "artist," a violin player, who wanted to smoke tobacco and make acquaintances in Lauchstädt. The violinist entered the spa pavilions (Figures 3.14 and 3.15) for this purpose: "This artist believed that he did not need any further privilege than that of being a human being [*Mensch*] in order to exercise his freedom to act according to his inclination and habit."[15] The author comments that, to the misfortune of the violinist, the nobility in Lauchstädt had successfully claimed the spa pavilions for their exclusive use. The nobles thus regarded the artist's attempt to participate in their entertainments as bourgeois "impertinence."[16] As an act of revenge the nobility then used their social privilege to not only deny the artist access to other spaces but also threaten his livelihood: they held a dance in an assembly hall that the violinist had already booked for a performance.[17] The author concludes with a comment that clearly places this episode in the first category of discursive statement:[18] "And now tell me, after incidents like this, can we still make claims to Enlightenment? May we believe that we are more advanced in the art of being human? Hardly would one [a member of the nobility] have allowed oneself to do something similar at the beginning of this century, when mankind was still suffering enormously and when [bourgeois] merit had not yet broken the bonds of slavery."[19]

Personal narratives only occasionally mention the question of access to spaces, and rarely do the published discourse and personal recollections overlap in such a striking way as in an incident Adele Schopenhauer recorded in her diary in 1816. During a visit to Schwalbach, Schopenhauer witnessed noble conduct toward bourgeois musicians: "In the evening there was a concert. For the first time I thought that the writers who scold the elegant world [the nobility] are right. Nearly all the [noble] ladies, the princes, etc. were furious that they had to play [cards] in the next room. [They said that] it was terribly rude and impertinent to disturb the society with a concert, the tootling was unbearable. We attended and were very satisfied."[20] Although the musicians in Schwalbach, unlike the violin player in Lauchstädt, were able to perform, Schopenhauer's recollections and the fictional incident in Lauchstädt exhibit striking parallels. It is not surprising that Schopenhauer relates the event she witnessed back to the published spa discourse and asserts that authors who criticized the nobility had gained credibility with her as a result. This is a powerful reminder of the circle of communication encompassing spa-goers and spa publications.

Other test cases for noble-bourgeois integration and thus for the social tone at a spa were practices like dancing and seating arrangements during meals. From an early modern noble standpoint, it was regarded as permissible for a nobleman to lead a bourgeois woman to dance – this was a part of noble "condescension" and many early modern noblemen had, after all, mistresses of middle-class origin.[21] The reverse, however, a bourgeois man asking a noblewoman to dance, was not acceptable in early modern society. Therefore, the published spa discourse focused on one question in particular: did noblewomen accept or reject offers to dance from bourgeois men? If bourgeois men met with rejection, this was seen as a sign that the spa's social heterotopia was disrupted. If noblemen even refused to ask bourgeois women to dance, the social tone at the spa was regarded as beyond repair.

One of the recurring themes in the published spa discourse was thus the role of noblewomen, especially young noblewomen, at balls. As we saw in Charlotte Wilhelmine Amalie von Donop's 1750 ballad *The Beauties of Pyrmont* (*Die Schönheiten Pyrmonts*),[22] this was one of the earliest flashpoints identified in the published discourse. By the late eighteenth century, authors vigorously complained about noblewomen who refused to be led to the dance floor by a bourgeois man. For example, in his 1799 book about Pyrmont, Rasmus Frankenau warned bourgeois men,

> However, I absolutely do not want to recommend to anybody to ask to dance the *marchionesses*, countesses, baronesses, and whatever they are all called, who teem around here like a swarm of bees, unless one can lay one's family tree at the lady's feet, or a title, even if it were

only the title "councillor." In this case, one may just barely participate;[23] . . . Everyone who is below these ranks can be sure that their
[the ladies'] backs will be turned at them and they will be looked at
over their [the ladies'] shoulders.[24]

Similarly, in the 1782 novella *The Hollandaise Sauce: A Lauchstädt
Spa Story* (*Die holländische Sauce: Eine lauchstädtsche Badgeschichte*),
Sophie, a young noblewoman, is admonished by her guardian, who wants
to marry her off to a rich aristocrat: "Look, here in Lauchstädt the young
noblewomen [*Fräuleins*] are less generous with their favors than you
are. Do you see one of the *Fräuleins* von B.-- dancing with a bourgeois
[*einem Bürgerlichen*]?"[25] The narrator's comment provides the broader
conclusion that readers were to draw from this episode: "Noble pride and
avarice are powerful motivators in this world, and love and humility are
too insignificant to defeat these enemies."[26]

In the aforementioned article about Freienwalde in the 1798 *Journal of
Luxury and Fashions* (*Journal des Luxus und der Moden*), which sharply
criticizes the nobility, dances and meals became the ultimate proof of
"noble separation" because noblemen did not ask bourgeois women to
dance: "The addiction to separation [*Absonderungssucht*] indeed went
so far this time that there was an actual agreement among the nobles
according to which no nobleman was allowed to ask a bourgeois woman
to dance without being severely reprimanded by his peers [*Standesgenossen*]. Nobody but nobles organized the communal breakfasts, and the
bourgeoisie [*die Bürgerlichen*] did of course not intrude."[27]

In contrast, in his 1782 article about Brückenau, Göckingk argues that
the "good" social tone at this spa resulted from the nobility's conduct
toward the bourgeoisie by explaining

that the noble lords [*Herren*] who were chiefly positioned to set the
tone here danced with a bourgeois mademoiselle [*mamsell*, i.e. an
unmarried woman] as well as with a noble lady of the highest rank,
without making the slightest difference even in the manner of dancing; that at the table an honest tenant sat down next to an excellency
[*eine Exzellenz*] without this seeming strange to the latter. In short,
that one was sensible enough to not only recognize the difference
between "being at court and at the spa," but also to behave accordingly. A few years ago, a lady of old nobility found it insulting that
a bourgeois [*ein Bürgerlicher*] was so bold as to ask her to dance.
People did not rest until she left the spa.[28]

And finally, clothing, especially women's clothing, became a major indicator of the spa as a social heterotopia. Göckingk's reports on Lauchstädt
and Brückenau offer an instructive comparison. As we have already seen
previously, Lauchstädt was generally regarded as a spa characterized by

social separation, whereas Brückenau was praised for social integration. Accordingly, Göckingk criticizes Lauchstädt's social tone that prevents "equality and informal general pleasure from being the dominant tone."[29] He directly connects this shortcoming with the "splendor of dress" that allegedly prevailed in Lauchstädt: "A lady must present herself in the avenue, differently in the morning, differently in the afternoon, and differently in the evening, . . . This vanity, which is in fact most ridiculous here [at the spa], has also spread to the men."[30] Göckingk presents Brückenau as the exact opposite of Lauchstädt. Here, the simplicity of dress is described as being directly responsible for the "good" social tone prevailing at the spa: "Of the dozen spas I have visited, I do not know one that can be compared in the least with this one [Brückenau] in terms of the informal way of life. I have not noticed any rivalry to distinguish oneself by the splendor of one's clothes here, but rather I have seen ladies of rank who came to the table several days in a row dressed in plain travel clothes."[31]

The call for the abolishment of the "splendor" of dress culminated in suggestions for a "spa uniform" (*Badeuniform*) in the published discourse. Early modern clothing ordinances that stipulated a certain dress and level of luxury for each social estate were no longer enforceable and therefore were often not renewed in the eighteenth century.[32] In addition, late eighteenth-century consumer society provided larger swaths of the population with opportunities to consume fashion.[33] These changes meant that expressing status, including noble status, through dress became more difficult, leading to an increased display of fashion[34] and, as a result, an increase in calls for various forms of a national dress code.[35] Consequently, contemporaries regarded women's clothes as one of the most important manifestations of the "addiction" to fashion and luxury. Therefore, they argued, if spas were to successfully facilitate the crossing of social boundaries, the clothes of female spa guests in particular needed to be standardized. Women's clothes, in short, became the ultimate symbol of social equality at the spa.

In a 1778 article in the *German Museum* (*Deutsches Museum*), Göckingk proposed a female spa uniform made of "white nettle cloth." The text is full of irony – Göckingk was keenly aware that his ideas would not be implemented. He suggests that women who refuse to wear the spa uniform should be denied "access to the general entertainments of the spa." These measures, Göckingk maintains, would result in "a better understanding among people of such different ranks" at the spa.[36] In the 1788 *Journal of Luxury and Fashions* (*Journal des Luxus und der Moden*), the Brückenau spa physician Conrad Anton Zwierlein again made a "suggestion for a general spa uniform for women," which was repeated and discussed in 1789, 1792, 1797, and 1803.[37] In 1789 and 1792, the *Journal* even included engravings of suggested spa uniforms.[38] The 1792 uniform is a simple dress in an olive color, worn with a hat, a

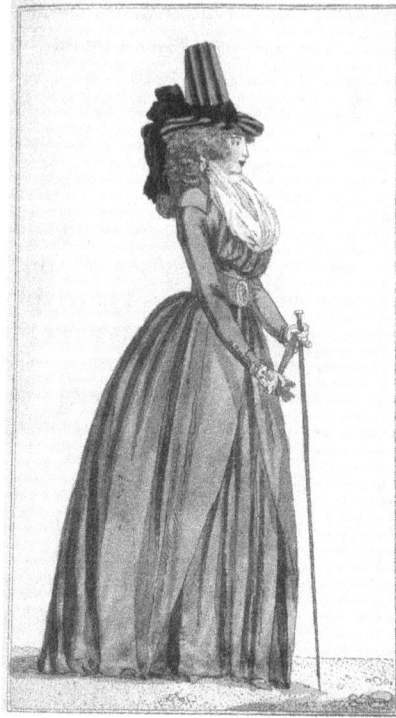

Figure 6.1 General spa uniform for ladies, colored engraving, 1792. ("Junge teutsche Dame in der neuen allgemeine Bad-Uniforme [*sic*]." *Journal des Luxus und der Moden* 7 [April 1792]: figure 11. Klassik Stiftung Weimar/Herzogin Anna Amalia Bibliothek/shelf mark ZA 2011.)

belt, a handkerchief, and shoes – all in red – as the only adornments. In addition, the "young German lady" depicted in the engraving was supposed to wear her spa uniform with a white scarf covering her bosom (Figure 6.1). According to its creators, the spa uniform enabled women to engage "without any effort" in activities like "walking, dancing, driving [in a carriage], and riding [on horseback]."[39] The article also argued that an "equivalent uniform" should be worn by male spa guests.[40] Civilian and military male uniforms were a common demand and, in the case of the military, also an increasing reality in the eighteenth century.[41] In contrast, spa uniforms remained an aspiration, but their close association with the spa as a social heterotopia draws our attention once again to the specific ways in which general ideas of the Enlightenment period were applied to and multiplied by the spa.[42]

As dress became a less reliable indicator of social status in late eighteenth-century society, it also became increasingly difficult to distinguish between a nobleman and a bourgeois at the spa, at least at first sight. The spa discourse often addresses this, for example by pointing out that noblewomen were not able to recognize bourgeois men by their clothing. This raised the question of whether a noblewoman could accept an offer to dance from a man she was not acquainted with.[43] And in Joachim Heinrich Campe's *Travels from Braunschweig to Karlsbad* (*Reise von Braunschweig nach Karlsbad*), a grandfather explains the conduct of the inhabitants of Karlsbad toward spa guests to his grandchildren. With plenty of sarcasm directed at the nobility, the narrator asserts:

> Here in Karlsbad, . . . so many nobles flock together that often the second or third man one encounters is a [noble] lord [*gnädiger Herr*] or an excellency [*Exzellenz*]. But since one cannot tell by people's noses, and often not even by their speech when they are talking, whether they are lordly [*gnädige*], excellent [*exzellente*, a play on the word "excellency"], or just common [middle-class], if not sub-common [lower-class] human beings, people [the inhabitants of Karlsbad] would rather call them "Your Lordship" [*begnädigen*] and "Excellency" [*beexzellenzen*] lock, stock, and barrel, especially if they are foreigners and unknown to them, rather than run the risk of treating a born lord [*gebornen Gnädigen*] or an excellency stamped by letter and seal like a simple bourgeois [*Bürgersmann*].[44]

In the first type of discursive statement, which mainly criticized the nobility, some authors also constructed a new social identity for the bourgeoisie. These authors wanted to convince their bourgeois readers that the middle class could stand tall and that it should define its social identity independently of the nobility. However, this strong sense of bourgeois self-worth was combined with a defiant attitude toward the nobility, indicating that middle-class identity could not be constructed without reference to the highest social estate. For example, at the end of the aforementioned 1798 fictional travelogue *Journey to the Spas of Karlsbad, Eger [Franzensbad], and Teplitz* (*Reise nach den Badeörtern Karlsbad, Eger und Töplitz*), the (bourgeois) narrator moves from his criticism of the nobility to a statement about the accomplishments of the bourgeoisie. He emphasizes the contributions of the middle class to society and aims at creating or strengthening bourgeois identity in the spirit of the Enlightenment: "Fortunately, the bourgeois [*Bürger*] can do without the noble [*Adlichen*] if he [the noble] wants and can do without him [the bourgeois] (to whom he [the noble] owes so many advantages of literature, Enlightenment, necessities, or taste). In the end, the inhabitant of Karlsbad finds our money just as pretty and round as the nobility's!"[45] And in a fictional travelogue of a Leipzig burgher about his visit to Lauchstädt, the narrator advises the bourgeoisie not to get upset about noble arrogance but to counter such noble conduct with disregard: "If, for example, a noble [*Hochadelicher*[46]] had his nose so high that it loomed over me, I walked underneath it pretending not to notice that a nose was above me."[47]

Other authors, in contrast, occasionally reveal the ambivalence of the bourgeois search for a new social identity vis-à-vis the nobility. For example, a travelogue about Karlsbad that heavily criticizes noble spa visitors for their arrogance toward the bourgeoisie also calls on the nobility to do more for the improvement of the spa and its surroundings. The author wants nobles to pay for walkways or spa pavilions. In true Enlightenment fashion, he makes the case that such improvements would provide lasting benefit to "humanity" and compare favorably with noble "free balls" as an ephemeral activity.[48] By asking the nobility to pay for spa improvements, the author accepts such activities as expressions of aristocratic self-representation. Thus, the author also conveys an implicit recognition of Karlsbad as a space where the nobility could claim precedence.

This kind of bourgeois ambivalence was also reflected in Johann Stephan Pütter's autobiography. Pütter's account of his experiences in Pyrmont fluctuates between bourgeois uncertainties about how to interact with the nobility on the one hand and bourgeois self-confidence on the other. Here again we can see that the published discourse mirrored the perceptions of contemporaries. The large communal breakfast in Pyrmont, held at a long table in the avenue (Figure 2.2), was a flashpoint for noble-bourgeois interaction at that spa. It was customary for nobles among the spa guests to take turns as hosts of this communal meal. As a result, they determined who was invited.[49] Pütter describes how he, after making subtle inquiries, decided to sign up as a host of the breakfast, thereby effectively breaching one of the privileges of the nobility in Pyrmont:

> Thus, only gentlemen of the nobility or members of the high estates [*höhere Standespersonen*, i.e. the high nobility] signed up for this table [the large communal breakfast]. But at times others [members of the bourgeoisie] were invited to it, for example when the prince of Waldeck, or one of his entourage, hosted the [morning] coffee, or if it was the turn of someone who perhaps had a special friend among the rest of the [spa] society. This honor was bestowed on me several times in a row, . . . When I finally had reason to believe that no one would take it amiss if I signed up as well, so that is what I did, and thus it was my turn, . . . Then [Justus] Möser, who was famous and popular among all people, followed my example. In general, this helped somewhat to gradually, but noticeably soften the separation of the nobility from the non-nobility, which had hitherto in part been too pronounced.[50]

Pütter starts out by describing his insecurity in the face of a practice that was reserved for the nobility and his awareness of his (inferior) social status. At the end, however, he ascribes to himself a decisive role in overcoming social boundaries in Pyrmont and initiating a permanent change in the interactions of spa visitors.

The *second* type of discursive statement either constructs the enlightened nobility as being in accord with the bourgeoisie or addresses only the middle class without reference to the nobility. In either case, these statements can be described as a form of compromise. They provide their readers with a strong sense of bourgeois identity and still express the bourgeoisie's demand for equality. On the one hand, some authors directly addressed enlightened nobles and either praised them for already interacting with the bourgeoisie at the spa or invited them to do so. These authors carefully differentiated between enlightened and unenlightened nobles and did not use the nobility in its entirety as a negative foil.[51] The discourse formed by these texts can be described as "enlightened" rather than "bourgeois" because it created the enlightened nobility as an ideal type and subscribed to the broader idea of an emerging new social formation, an enlightened educated elite. As a result, the British social group of the "gentry" sometimes appears in these texts as an example to be followed. On the other hand, some spa guides and advertising pamphlets construct the spa as an exclusive heterotopia for the middle class. These texts only address the bourgeoisie and do not mention or criticize the nobility. The emerging discourse formed by these texts created an ideal of "ourselves alone" because it offered the bourgeois reader a vision of the spa as a space reserved for the middle class and its needs.

In order to address both the enlightened nobility and the bourgeoisie, some authors constructed a (fictional) enlightened noble friend of the bourgeois narrator and/or included anecdotes illustrating the division of the nobility into "enlightened" and "unenlightened" groups. Johann Matthaeus Hassencamp, in his 1783 *Letters of a Traveler* (*Briefe eines Reisenden*), skillfully combines a fundamental critique of the early modern social system with "philosophical stoicism"[52] toward the continued existence of hereditary nobility in German society. The author criticizes the (allegedly few) remaining unenlightened nobles, and he invites the enlightened nobility to overcome social boundaries by befriending members of the bourgeoisie at the spa. Hassencamp thus highlights the formation of a new, enlightened social elite as part of the bourgeois spa experience. He adds a compliment directed at the enlightened nobility represented by a fictional friend: "However, I have met many wonderful people in this estate [the nobility], who completely compensate one [the bourgeois] for their [the proud nobles'] presence, and who actually bring more honor to their noble status than their noble status brings honor to them. Among this group you yourself, my dear friend, do not occupy the least significant place."[53]

Just as we have seen previously with regard to the role of dress at spas, Hassencamp then introduces a gendered element. He distinguishes between bourgeois men and women in terms of their level of Enlightenment (and, by implication, education) as well as their resulting social self-confidence. Allegedly, enlightened bourgeois men had already advanced to a state where they no longer wished to interact with proud, unenlightened nobles. Bourgeois women, in contrast, had not yet fully internalized enlightened principles so as to render them immune to noble slights, and therefore they could still be offended by noble conduct. In this context, Hassencamp uses many of the catchphrases that served as signposts in the published discourse, such as "children of Adam" (*Adamskinder*), noble "pride" (*Stolz*), noble "separation" (*Absonderung*), "at court and at the spa" (*am Hof und im Bade*):

> In this way, even there [in Pyrmont], I have not yet missed an hour of good company from all estates [*Stände*] when I so desired. In any case, I have never mingled with weak, uneducated minds, of whom in our enlightened and philosophical age there are, fortunately, only a few [left] who come from one or another remote village and who, regardless of personal merit, simply because of birth, look down upon other of Adam's children who are not of such [noble] birth with pride and contempt. I have therefore not had any cause to complain about their affectatious separation, which I am not only indifferent to, but even find desirable. However, I have heard the bitterest complaints from many others, especially [bourgeois] ladies, who do not yet have enough philosophy to rise above such meanness. It cannot be denied that some people there maintain an extravagant tone and a certain stiff, proud attitude, which is completely unknown in most other spas, where one does not seem to forget that there is still a great difference between being at court and at the spa, even in terms of our conventional manners.[54]

In his *Travels from Braunschweig to Karlsbad* (*Reise von Braunschweig nach Karlsbad*), Campe refers to the social division between the noble Saxon hall and the socially more mixed Bohemian hall in Karlsbad in order to praise enlightened nobles for their attitude toward the bourgeoisie:

> Unfortunately! [*sic*] here, as in many other spas, people are still not sufficiently educated, so that they draw a rather sharp boundary between the two estates [*Stände*] in a place where civil circumstances [*die bürgerlichen Verhältnisse*] should not be taken into consideration at all. But I must add, to the honor of many nobles, that one usually finds the society in and around the Bohemian coffeehouse very mixed, because a large, perhaps the largest part of the nobility has so much

good sense that they prefer to linger and enjoy themselves in mixed company rather than to be bored in the limited circles of their peers [in the Saxon hall].[55]

In 1800, the *Journal of Luxury and Fashions* (*Journal des Luxus und der Moden*) reported an alleged incident in Karlsbad. As in Campe's description, the story features a group of enlightened noblemen. It starts out by praising the circle of the duchess of Courland for its socially inclusive atmosphere and continues to relate the following episode: "Here [in the circle of the duchess], then, there was no rigid separation of the estates [*Stände*], who, after all, come together here at one healing spring, and no insulting exclusion was considered, of the kind that later on in the Saxon hall caused a very offensive incident through the insult of a brave merchant from Annaberg [in Saxony] that could only be alleviated by the emphatic mediation of a few gentlemen [*Herren*] of the nobility who loudly disapproved of this impropriety."[56]

In both these stories about Karlsbad, readers were expected to draw on a considerable amount of background knowledge, based on either spa visits or familiarity with the published discourse. Through the mention of an insult directed at a merchant from Annaberg in the Saxon hall, readers had to infer that this man – bravely or daringly, depending on one's perspective – entered an exclusive noble space and probably was verbally attacked. The cryptic reference in the *Journal of Luxury and Fashions* in effect counted on its readership having heard or read such stories before. And most importantly, readers implicitly understood that the nobles who were praised in the first story for mingling with the bourgeoisie in the Bohemian hall and in the second story for defending the Annaberg merchant against their peers were enlightened members of their estate. The authors clearly assumed that readers were already aware of this differentiation among the nobility.

In her diary, Elisa von der Recke, who saw herself as an enlightened aristocrat and cultivated friendships with members of the bourgeoisie, recounted events in Karlsbad that led her to reflect on the distinction between "enlightened" and "proud, unenlightened" nobles. Her account also throws another spotlight on the question of dress as a distinguishing feature at the late eighteenth-century spa. In 1795, she recorded in her diary that Count Nieuport had willingly filled in one day for her maid and had carried the coats of all her friends, among them bourgeois women, to the well. Recke contrasts this episode with another experience:

Here I remembered another count who, when I used the Karlsbad water here five years ago and a sick man fell unconscious on Dorothea's meadow[57] and I asked the count to help the sick man, whom I could not help up alone, he asked, "Forgive me, what estate [*Standes*] does the man belong to?" I replied, "I don't know, he is a human being and needs our help." Afterward it turned out that the sick man was the servant of a merchant from Prague, and the lofty count could not forget for a long time that he had been used to serve such a common man [*gemeinen Mann*]. In Nieuport, I did not notice even a trace of noble pride.[58]

Strikingly, the unnamed count was no longer able to tell the unconscious man's social status by his clothes. Clearly, the count suspected that he was not helping a nobleman or at least a member of the bourgeois elite, but his question indicates that he simply could not be sure.[59] For Elisa von der Recke, the two noblemen's actions revealed their true nature as individuals. At the same time, however, she employs terms and concepts that were common in the published spa discourse. Recke attributes the actions of individuals to general characteristics such as being a "lofty count" or being free of "noble pride" and thereby constructs a contrast between an unenlightened and an enlightened nobleman. One can therefore easily imagine Recke's stories appearing as anonymous episodes in the published discourse – the two aristocrats and the servant seem almost like stock characters. This, in turn, confirms that nobles who regarded themselves as enlightened would have had no problems with the published spa discourse, specifically with texts that emphasized the formation of an enlightened educated elite and the role enlightened nobles played in this context.[60]

Occasionally, the authors of spa publications used the British social formation of the "gentry" as an example to talk about the type of social change they hoped to see in Germany. Without going into the details of the actual nature of the gentry and what it meant to be considered a gentleman in the early modern and eighteenth-century British Isles,[61] these authors defined the gentry as an enlightened educated elite, that is a social group encompassing the enlightened nobility and the bourgeoisie. As Wilhelm Ferdinand Chaßot von Florencourt explains in his travelogue, the goal was to distinguish between "people of education and good manners (gentlemen) and their opposites (not gentlemen)" in order to ensure the "comfort of society." He points out that Germany still had a long way to go to reach that goal: "But what giant steps must the Enlightenment take before we reach that point!"[62] In his spa guide for Pyrmont, Marcard also explains the concept of the "gentleman" in the spirit of the Enlightenment as "not . . . a nobleman . . . , but a man of good breeding, of refined manners and noble mind [*edler Denkungsart*]. In England, such a man has all the rights to participate in the life of society that the nobility in Germany claims exclusively for itself. He [the English gentleman] belongs in the first and best society."[63]

In spa guides and advertising pamphlets we also find another variation of the second type of statement that affirms bourgeois identity without explicitly criticizing the nobility. These texts often combine an argument about the bourgeoisie as a social group with statements about the new landscape perception. By the early nineteenth century, some spas sought to compete with the larger and more fashionable spas by appealing only to bourgeois spa guests. These spas advertised themselves as rural idylls in a mountainous landscape where "simple pleasures" prevailed. Spa guides and advertising pamphlets created the image of a bourgeois social heterotopia, where the middle class could find rest and recreation after hard work.

In the *Driburg Pocketbook* (*Driburger Taschenbuch*) of 1811, the author tried to convince his readers to visit the spa by appealing to their perceived needs and interests:

> The businessman [*Geschäftsmann*] and scholar [*Gelehrte*] who, glued to his desk all year round, strained his mind at the expense of his body . . . , all such sick people often gladly escape the noise of large cities and long to enjoy for a few undisturbed weeks all that makes a stay in the country so attractive to every soul that is not yet completely corrupted. If one wishes to find the life of big cities with all its splendor . . . everywhere, if one prefers noisy pleasures . . . to quiet social interaction with educated people and innocent pastimes in a charming rural area, then one may find, especially if one is or wants to be grand, the stay in Driburg sad and boring, however beneficial for one's health it may be. One can hurry to Pyrmont, Spa, and other glamorous spas and avoid above all the . . . trip to Driburg, where sick people from big cities, released for a while from the hustle and bustle and the worries of an exhausting life, can learn again to enjoy the pleasures of nature.[64]

The author of this spa guide gives the bourgeois man a distinct sense of his own situation and identity. He is "sick" because he is exhausted from hard mental labor at his desk. Here, the author clearly appeals to work and diligence as bourgeois values. The dietetics of the soul call for a stay at the spa in the countryside and the enjoyment of unspoiled nature. At the spa, the bourgeois man (and, presumably, his family) can not only escape the city and attend to his health; at the same time, he can remain true to his values of thrift and "innocent pastimes" and meet other "educated people" who share his values. In part, these statements refer back to the spa as a meeting place for humanists and enlightened scholars in the early modern period and the first half of the eighteenth century.[65] But the new conception of the spa as a bourgeois heterotopia goes further than that. It appeals to a broad bourgeois identity that embraces the "scholar" as well as the "businessman," and it converts the spa into a space that (allegedly) caters solely to the bourgeoisie. Thus, this new conception implicitly affirmed the independent worth of the middle class vis-à-vis the nobility.

The *third* type of discursive statement usually appears in spa guides and advertising pamphlets. These publications attempted to appeal to the broadest possible audience. Therefore, they sought to deflect the heavy criticism leveled at the nobility in the first type of discursive statement. The most common argument employed by these authors held the bourgeoisie partly responsible for the tensions between the nobility and the bourgeoisie and thus for the shortcomings of the spa as a social heterotopia. Authors argued that both the nobility and the bourgeoisie had to move out of their comfort zones to make the spa function as a social heterotopia, or that the bourgeoisie was too timid in their interactions with the nobility or even displayed their own type of social "pride."

Nevertheless, it is striking that none of these publications denied the ideal of noble-bourgeois integration at the spa. In fact, authors usually began by acknowledging this ideal and often explicitly formulated demands directed at the nobility and then moved on to arguments that were clearly more controversial in their readers' eyes. Criticizing the middle class often appears to be an addendum or an afterthought. The authors are careful to argue these points in a balanced and cautious way so as not to antagonize the bourgeoisie in a prolonged fashion. The prevailing discourse clearly imposed limits on what was sayable in spa publications.

Gottfried Käppel's spa guide titled *Pyrmont's Noteworthy Features* (*Pyrmonts Merkwürdigkeiten*) of 1800 exemplifies this type of discursive statement. He confirms the prevailing discourse and at the same time criticizes the middle class. Käppel writes, "Before, the German noble pride is said to have shown itself here in all its preposterous bareness, to have drawn a thick partition between itself [the nobility] and the bourgeoisie [*den Bürgerlichen*], and to have done extraordinary damage to the spirit of general social entertainment. The torch of the Enlightenment, and even more so, the greater reputation of this spa . . . have finally triumphed over this German prejudice."[66] At this point, Käppel inserts a footnote that voices his criticism of the bourgeoisie: "Many have written about noble pride, and very few seem to have considered that the seed of arrogance lies in every human heart, . . . How ridiculous is the pride of scholars and merchants!"[67]

In her memoirs, Johanna Schopenhauer reflects on just this question of "merchant pride." Schopenhauer, who later in her life founded a salon in Weimar, wrote about her 1787 visit to Pyrmont when she was the young wife of a merchant from Danzig (today Gdańsk in Poland). At the time of her spa visit, Schopenhauer was 21 years old and, as she herself admitted, not well versed in the ways of the world and rather naive. When she wrote her memoirs in the 1830s, she looked at her younger self with detached amusement, and she criticized some of her own behaviors in Pyrmont at the time as foolish "burgher pride."

Schopenhauer describes how her husband, after arriving at the spa, gathered a circle of urban upper-middle-class acquaintances from Hamburg,

Bremen, and Lübeck: "Hanseatic people just like us, with whom I soon felt completely at home."[68] The Schopenhauers' circle established a break-fast table in the main avenue before the duchess of Brunswick arrived with her entourage and also occupied "a long table in the avenue" for breakfast.[69] This juxtaposition of a burgher and an aristocratic table in the same space led to a memorable encounter. Schopenhauer gives a detailed account of the incident in her memoirs, diligently describing the function-ing of the spa as a social heterotopia.

The women of the burgher circle had "gotten into a kind of superficial acquaintance with a lady-in-waiting of the duchess, as it happens so eas-ily in such places."[70] This resulted in an offer from "Frau von V . . . " to present Schopenhauer and another burgher woman from Hamburg to the duchess: "Very kindly she remarked that we would thereby be given the advantage of being allowed to join the large breakfasts. In vain I reminded our protectress of our social estate as burghers who were not presentable at court [*nicht hoffähigen Bürgerstand*]. She replied that in places like this court etiquette was not followed so strictly."[71] But the noble lady also reminded Schopenhauer and her friend that during the presentation they would at least have to indicate their intention of kissing the duchess' hand or the hem of her skirt, "in which case the very gracious duchess would never let things go further than a mere demonstration."[72]

This proved too much for the burgher women, though, and they rejected the invitation: "We, not subject to any prince, freeborn women, we should kiss the hand of another woman who was not our mother or grandmother, or bow down to the ground to grasp the hem of her garment? . . . The thought that we might be required to do so made my republican blood boil over."[73] As Schopenhauer observed in hindsight, she felt that she and her fellow burgher woman had acted with "imperial-city [*reichsstädtischen*] stubbornness."[74] In retrospect, Schopenhauer realized that she had made herself the object of aristocratic ridicule: "Praised by our men, . . . [and] receiving profuse compliments from our other Hanse-atic friends, we did not even think about how much material for humor-ous remarks our burgher pride [*Bürgerhochmut*] might have provided to the table on the opposite side of the avenue."[75]

Here Schopenhauer and her spa circle personify the "merchant pride" criticized in the published discourse. In contrast, the lady-in-waiting and the duchess appear as (sufficiently) enlightened members of the nobility since they recognize the difference between "being at court and at the spa" and extend an offer to the burghers to cross the social boundary. When Schopenhauer and her friend rejected the opportunity for social integra-tion, they exhibited a strong burgher identity rooted in the early modern tradition of imperial cities and the Hanseatic League. Affirming this tra-ditional burgher identity as "republican" and "freeborn" vis-à-vis the nobility in general and the members of ruling princely houses in particular clearly came naturally to Schopenhauer at the time. She insisted that they "remained apart from that [noble] sphere, to which we never wished to be close."[76] Later in life, Schopenhauer came to think that, as Käppel wrote, the "pride of merchants" was just as "ridiculous" as noble pride and described her own conduct with ironic distance. She thus confirmed the criticism some authors in the published spa discourse directed at the behavior of different groups among the middle class at the spa.

In his 1812 spa guide for Alexisbad, Johann Friedrich Krieger expressed a similar critique of middle-class conduct at the spa but hinted at the emergence of a new social boundary. A section titled "Sociability" ("Das Gesellschaftswesen") at first seems to echo the usual criticism of the nobility. A close reading of this passage, however, reveals that Krieger saw the upper classes, comprised of the nobility, princely officials who were members of the educated bourgeoisie (*gebildetes Bürgertum*), and wealthy bourgeois, presumably members of the economic bourgeoisie (*Wirtschaftsbürgertum*),[77] as a group that was potentially walling itself off from the less educated or less prosperous members of the middle class:

> If of course the higher rank, the wealth [wealthy people], . . . even at the spa, wants to only be an object of homage, and does not want to sacrifice even one of the customary servilities, only demand, and not grant anything, only command, and not give an inch; . . . if he [*sic*, i.e. the higher rank] regards only those who are his equals as worthy of rapprochement or integration, and if he allows no access to people who cannot show the certificates of lineage, of civil honors, or of wealth; . . . if in confidential whispers he regards it as one of the evils of visiting a spa that the [spa] society is corrupted and divided by so many unlearned, i.e. less grand and wealthy, fellow guests; . . . where things are like this, there is certainly no consideration of nourishing and refreshing sociability. Yet so often at the spas it [sociability] is shattered into pieces against this cliff, or so the general complaint goes.[78]

However, immediately afterward Krieger reproaches the less privileged members of the middle class for their failure to promote social integration at the spa: "But the reverse expresses with equal truth the complaints of the other party [the upper classes]. The pride, stubbornness, and jealousy of the less fortunate directed at the apparent favorites of destiny, or baseless mistrust and fearfulness have no small share in the disruption of the social tone."[79]

Finally, it is instructive to take a closer look at authors who combined all three types of discursive statement in a single spa publication. As mentioned earlier, while many authors did maintain consistency in their arguments about noble-bourgeois interaction at the spa, others did not strive for internal consistency but sought to make their texts as broadly appealing as possible. This may have been a successful strategy because readers bought these publications for entertainment and in preparation for spa visits and therefore did not read them as closely as one might read a philosophical treatise. It is also likely that readers recognized the fundamental nature of these texts as advertising tools and thus took everything the authors said with a grain of salt. Or, finally, it is conceivable that confirmation bias worked in these authors' favor and that from the arguments offered, readers picked those that already fit their own worldview. However, as we will see, none of this was successful with more perceptive readers.

In the 1780 travelogue *News from a Spa Visit to Karlsbad* (*Nachrichten von einer Carlsbader Brunnenreise*) by Johann Peter Willebrand, the first part of the book, titled "News" ("Nachrichten"), contains a statement in line with the first discursive type. The author argues about "institutions of pleasure" (*Lustanstalten*) like "dance balls" in Karlsbad that "certain spa guests, who seem to think that they are not begotten from sinful seed, at public gatherings have no qualms to misbehave toward deserving men of dignity, who certainly have no need to fearfully seek their merits in the splendor of their ancestors."[80] However, in the second part of his book, titled "Travel Memories" ("Reiseerinnerungen"), the author rolls the second and the third types of discursive statement into one. He asserts:

> When often spa guests who belong to the first bourgeois estate [*ersten bürgerlichen Stande*] complain that they want for a meeting with this or that noble, of which they consider themselves worthy, this refers first and foremost only to uneducated, uncivilized [*ungesitteten*] country squires. . . . For he who is well-educated and civilized [*gesittet*], and has merits and true dignity, cannot be harsh, grand, and proud. Meanwhile, these complaints are often the consequences of a mere prejudice. For I have often noticed that bourgeois [*Bürgerliche*] of importance are unnecessarily . . . timid in terms of interacting with the nobility. . . . Certainly, wise nobles know well that they cannot do without the bourgeois estate [*bürgerlichen Stand*] for long.[81]

At the beginning of his travelogue Willebrand criticizes the nobility and affirms bourgeois "dignity" and "merit" using many of the catchwords readers expected in the context of the definition of the spa as a social heterotopia. He includes a version of the oft-used biblical reference to Adam ("sinful seed") and the even more common reference to the nobility's preoccupation with lineage. As we saw earlier, Hassencamp argued that the few unenlightened nobles who disrupted social integration at the spa were from "remote villages." Willebrand likewise claims that unenlightened nobles come from the countryside. These authors employed the old town-country cliché that depicts townspeople as educated and refined and countrypeople as uneducated and uncivilized. Finally, Willebrand accuses the bourgeoisie of being prejudiced toward the nobility and therefore not sufficiently outgoing. He has thus effectively turned his initial argument on its head, but his readers may not have even noticed because the arguments appear in different parts of his book.

Heinrich Matthias Marcard's *Description of Pyrmont* (*Beschreibung von Pyrmont*) contains a 65-page chapter on "social life in Pyrmont"[82] that includes all three discursive statements about noble-bourgeois interaction. Marcard's argumentative balancing act, however, is more obvious than Willebrand's because it is more condensed. First, he upholds the ideal of the spa as a social heterotopia and echoes the demand for integration by employing the first type of discursive statement: "It is indisputable that the institution of the nobility, a principle that has a powerful influence on the social life of the Germans, is one of the true reasons why the Enlightenment does not altogether flourish among us. . . . In Germany, noble pride apparently draws a line between itself [the nobility] and the rational and enlightened part of the people, [and] removes from itself those who, through real qualifications, have elevated themselves all alone."[83]

Second, Marcard seeks to present "noble pride" and "noble separation" – major points of criticism that were leveled against Pyrmont in the published discourse – as rare phenomena: "I do not claim in any way that there have never been individual cases in Pyrmont in which such complaints [about the nobility] were based on facts. . . . at some point a proud boorish nobleman [*bauernstolzer Edelmann*] may have found his way to Pyrmont, or a fat lady, bloated by her nobility, may have been . . . rude toward a non-noble [*einen Unadelichen*]."[84]

Third, Marcard introduces the second type of discursive statement by describing the enlightened nobility as antithetical to these "boorish" nobles: "Nevertheless, today there are already . . . many admirable noble persons worthy of respect . . . , who were not only born noble, but also have a noble mind, and think about the nobility in the way one should reasonably think about it [i.e., who know that the nobility should not seek precedence merely on the basis of birth]."[85]

Fourth, Marcard employs the third type of discursive statement by criticizing bourgeois behavior: "Some complain about the aloofness of the nobility, but they must simply complain about themselves. They show such reserve and such deferential fear that they themselves thereby bring about all the [social] separation they complain about, because in doing so they seem to acknowledge that a nobleman or a noblewoman is a being of a nature completely different from themselves."[86]

Fifth and finally, Marcard attempts to dispel the image of Pyrmont as a spa marked by noble separation, an image that dominated the published discourse. He claims that the social heterotopia is intact: "By the way, social interaction is pleasant and informal in Pyrmont, and has a certain ingeniousness, which can otherwise not easily be found in this northern region. Without hesitation, one addresses everyone to whom one has been introduced, or introduces oneself. One approaches every [social] circle as one pleases, in order to take part in the conversation. . . . This altogether leads to a not unpleasant freedom and ease."[87]

Marcard's strikingly convoluted argument, however, turned out to be a hard sell to a sophisticated reader like Justus Möser. In a 1784 letter, Möser thanked Marcard for sending him his recently published *Description of Pyrmont* (*Beschreibung von Pyrmont*). In this letter, the interplay between the published discourse and the perception of a reader who was also a spa visitor is evident. In fact, rarely do primary sources provide us with such insight into the reception of texts. It is significant that Möser focused his attention on the chapter about social life, a topic that clearly preoccupied the published discourse and mirrored the interests of its readers. Both perceived the spa as a meeting place and were interested in the functioning of this social heterotopia.

In his letter, Möser indirectly refuted Marcard's attempts to portray Pyrmont – despite all statements to the contrary in the published discourse – as an intact social heterotopia. Instead of contradicting Marcard outright, Möser made detailed suggestions as to how social integration could be achieved in Pyrmont in the future. He favored the idea of a so-called spa king (*Brunnenkönig*), a kind of master of ceremonies who would organize the social entertainments at the spa. This was not Möser's idea; rather, he was inspired by the practices at English spas, especially Bath, where Beau Nash served as master of ceremonies between 1705 and 1761:[88]

> If the spa king, whom the prince [of Waldeck and Pyrmont] would have to appoint, but without the title,[89] only directed it so that a great man [*ein Grosser*, i.e. a prince] who thinks equitably would always give the first breakfast [of the season], that would make a great difference. And in general, he [the spa king] would have to convince the great men [princes], who are generally accommodating [*herablassend*] and about whom one rarely has to complain in Pyrmont, to preempt the lesser nobles and make it their business to follow the example of the prince [of Waldeck and Pyrmont, who regularly invited members of the bourgeoisie to his table]. The little worms [the lesser nobility] will then crawl after them.[90]

Möser laid out his argument in accordance with the first type of discursive statement. He indirectly criticized Pyrmont for not living up to the ideal of noble-bourgeois integration, emphasizing that the spa should be "without distinction of rank."[91] Strikingly, Möser not only exempted ruling princes from his otherwise harsh criticism of the nobility; he even praised them for their behavior toward the bourgeoisie. His argument points us to the limitations of bourgeois demands in the published discourse and to the limitations of the spa as a social heterotopia in general.

Limitations of the Spa as a Social Heterotopia

In the published spa discourse, demands for social integration were omnipresent. However, there were clear limits on what was sayable in spa publications and on the functioning of the spa as a social heterotopia in practice. *First*, ruling princes were not subjected to the same criticism as the rest of the nobility in the published discourse but rather stylized as enlightened rulers sharing bourgeois values. *Second*, the spa as an actual meeting place was never able to live up to the demands voiced in the published discourse. The lofty ideal of the spa as a social heterotopia faced evident limits, but nevertheless this ideal persisted in people's minds because contemporaries regularly experienced the spa as a space where social boundaries were less stringent than in everyday life. Smaller groups of friends and acquaintances, so-called circles (*Zirkel*), facilitated noble-bourgeois integration at the spa and thus upheld the concept of the spa as a heterotopia. *Third* and finally, social integration encompassed only the nobility and the upper middle class, especially the educated bourgeoisie. The spa as a social heterotopia remained confined to the social elites, as holds true for other institutions of Enlightenment sociability.[92]

These limitations and exclusions, however, contributed to the preservation and even stabilization of the ideal of the spa as a social heterotopia among the participating elites. Spa guests from the upper middle class could perceive the social heterotopia as at least partially intact because spa publications depicted ruling princes as enlightened friends of the bourgeoisie, spa visitors experienced social integration in small circles, and spas created spaces for the exclusive use of the noble and bourgeois elites and actively excluded the rest of society from these spaces.

In this section, I will explore the three major limitations of the spa as a social heterotopia during the transitional period of the late eighteenth and early nineteenth centuries. Then I will describe how this period that had focused larger societal goals on spas as heterotopic spaces came to an end. In the era of the German Confederation (*Restaurationszeit*) and especially in the aftermath of the 1819 Karlsbad Decrees, the vocal demands for noble-bourgeois integration in the published spa discourse largely fell silent. Yet at the same time, a new social elite bridging the upper middle class and the nobility had emerged and continued to play an important role at the nineteenth-century spa.

As to the *first* limitation, the late eighteenth-century published spa discourse, which always found fault with the nobility to varying degrees, did not criticize the highest nobility, the ruling princes. Rulers were depicted as benefactors of mankind, as enlightened sovereigns who served the common good and embodied bourgeois values and virtues. Authors expressed the hope that these enlightened rulers would act as founders and supporters of spas for the benefit of humanity. This is a consistent feature of the published discourse. While praise of a ruling prince who supported a particular spa can certainly be expected in spa guides and advertising pamphlets, journal articles and travelogues were equally flattering toward the ruling nobility and their actions in general beyond their role in spa development.

For example, the 1798 travelogue *Journey to the Spas of Karlsbad, Eger [Franzensbad], and Teplitz (Reise nach den Badeörtern Karlsbad, Eger und Töplitz)* praised the prince of Clary-Aldringen for rebuilding the spa town of Teplitz after a fire. The author points out that the spa was "rebuilt very well" thanks to "the generous provision of its prince, who must be a very excellent man, since everything in this place, public order, cultivation, and plantings, bears witness to wisdom, good taste, and philanthropy. He does everything possible for the comfort and pleasure of the spa guests."[93] Göckingk, in his 1782 article about Brückenau in the *German Museum (Deutsches Museum)*, not only emphasized the improvements the prince-bishop of Fulda, Heinrich von Bibra, had realized at the spa, investing "more than one hundred thousand florins," but also praised the prince for his "tireless" efforts to improve his territory in general "without burdening his subjects."[94] Göckingk concluded, "Life under a bishop's crosier would be good [*Unter Krumstab ist gut wohnen*[95]], if all ecclesiastical princes were like him [Prince-Bishop Heinrich]. Every foreigner who travels through his territory will find traces everywhere of his excellent way of thinking and acting."[96]

Predictably, Marcard in his 1784 spa guide of Pyrmont praised Prince Friedrich Karl August of Waldeck and Pyrmont. He underlined that the prince was enlightened and did not support noble separation at the spa: "Whoever has the fortune to know the ruling prince of Waldeck will gladly believe that such an enlightened, unprejudiced prince, such a trusted friend and connoisseur of scholarship, does not protect the foolish addiction to [noble] distinction in Pyrmont. Regardless of birth, decent people from all walks of life are asked to join the princely table."[97] Hassencamp pursued a similar line of argument about the prince of Waldeck and Pyrmont in his 1783 travelogue, and he added a comparison with the prince-bishop of Fulda and his spa of Brückenau: "The prince of Waldeck ..., a very affable and accommodating [*herablassend*] lord, as well as his entire court, where there are many excellent men, ... do everything that is remotely possible, as matters stand, to eliminate this East Indian caste difference [in Pyrmont], but they are not yet as successful with it as the prince of Fulda was in Brückenau."[98] And Hirschfeld described the prince of Waldeck and Pyrmont in his 1785 *Theory of Garden Art (Theorie der Gartenkunst)* as "the excellent prince, who with noble, open kindness of the heart ... combines so much of his good taste and so much care for the pleasure of all strangers who flock together here [in Pyrmont], who loves to dwell amongst them, and hides his princely status to be a full member of the [spa] society, and [who] spreads freedom, sociability, and cheerfulness all around him."[99]

When writing about Wilhelmsbad, Hirschfeld paints a similar picture of Wilhelm, the ruling count of Hanau and hereditary prince of Hesse-Kassel: "One sees here a prince who, when he builds, plants, and embellishes, is wholly a prince, but who, in order to enjoy nature and sociability, and allow them to be enjoyed, becomes a private individual who has his quiet apartment among the guests at the spa, lingers at their table, and even at their games and dances."[100] In an article about Nenndorf, the *Journal of Luxury and Fashions* (*Journal des Luxus und der Moden*) casts Wilhelm, by then landgrave of Hesse-Kassel, as a benevolent ruler oriented toward the common good rather than economic profit: "People say that some expressed doubts to the landgrave [as to] whether his capital investment [in Nenndorf] would produce any gains, to which he answered that it would be sufficient interest if only a few gained their health there."[101]

Reinforcing the theme of the ruler as a "private individual" and casting his family as the equivalent of a bourgeois nuclear family, Hirschfeld remarks about Wilhelm's wife, Countess Wilhelmina Caroline of Hanau, in 1785 that she was "a princess . . . , who, as much as she is the glory of Denmark[102] among the Germans . . . , does not remember these rare privileges, and . . . the love of all hearts all around her flows to her in the circle of the happy young family [of the count and countess]."[103] This was an entirely fictitious argument and an obvious attempt to project bourgeois values onto a ruling prince's family. We know from other sources, including Wilhelm's own memoirs, that the image of a happy marriage and family created in the published discourse was far from true. The spa of Wilhelmsbad was, in fact, a flashpoint of Wilhelm's marital problems as he utilized the relaxed social atmosphere of the spa to introduce his mistress, Rosa Dorothea Ritter (ennobled as Freifrau von Lindenthal), into noble society.[104]

The stylization of the prince as an enlightened ruler with bourgeois values in the published spa discourse points to the complexity of the historical relationship between the bourgeoisie and the rulers of small and medium-sized German territories at the end of the eighteenth century. As Maiken Umbach has argued, the "minor rulers of the Holy Roman Empire" and the bourgeoisie formed a kind of symbiosis: the princes could use the characteristics of being bourgeois (*Bürgerlichkeit*) as a "powerful trope" to stylize themselves as enlightened and justify their existence, while the bourgeoisie constructed princes as allied partners of the Enlightenment program.[105] And as Michael Maurer has stated, "The bourgeoisie celebrates itself and sanctions its values by ascribing them [its values] . . . to princes."[106] The published spa discourse, in accordance with its statements affirming bourgeois enlightened identity, voiced these expectations for princes. Rulers of small and mid-sized territories were supposed to take a leading role in establishing and stabilizing spas as social heterotopias. Thus, the *Journal of Luxury and Fashions* (*Journal des Luxus und der Moden*) stated about Alexandersbad in 1798, "For social improvements must come from above even more than most others."[107] This statement expresses in a nutshell the prevailing sentiment about political and social change in the territories of the Holy Roman Empire and the German Confederation during the late eighteenth and early nineteenth centuries.[108]

Only a few personal narratives by members of the bourgeoisie explicitly reflect on encounters with ruling princes. Those that do largely echo the image propagated in the published discourse. For example, in her memoirs Johanna Schopenhauer described watching the duke of Mecklenburg-Schwerin as he "waltzed down the avenue" with a "flower girl" in Pyrmont in 1787. She was astonished and delighted by his "humanity":[109] "I had known for a long time that they [the ruling princes] were no longer walking around with crowns on their heads [and] scepters in their hands, but to find the high lord so accommodating [*herablassend*] and humane, so free of any nimbus that I thought would be inseparable from the outward appearance of such a master over the life and freedom of his subjects, I would never have guessed."[110]

In his autobiography, Johann Stephan Pütter also reported about encounters with ruling princes during his visits to Pyrmont. Pütter confirms the published discourse's description of the prince of Waldeck and Pyrmont as a ruler who invited members of the bourgeoisie to his table: "Usually, the ruling prince of Waldeck came with his entire court from Arolsen to Pyrmont every year during the spa season. . . . With the way in which he . . . tried to enliven the whole [spa] society with the engagement of good actors, as well as with concerts, and with illuminations or fireworks organized at his own expense, and how he almost daily invited a number of guests to his table without considering differences in estate [*Standes*], the benefits of staying in Pyrmont were increased even more."[111] Furthermore, Pütter displays a deep respect, even deference, for ruling princes that again mirrors the attitude of the published discourse. Pütter lists the ruling princes and the members of their families present in Pyrmont (among others, the crown prince of Prussia, the duke of Weimar, the duke of Mecklenburg-Schwerin, and the duke of Oldenburg) and states, "To only see persons of such high estate [*erhabenem Stande*], to see them several days in a row in different circumstances, . . . [was] an even greater gain if they waive[d] the privileges of rank [*herablassen*] to talk to one of us [*unser einem*, i.e. a member of the bourgeoisie] – a good fortune that I have had the pleasure of enjoying several times."[112]

In contrast to the Göttingen professor Pütter, the Zurich theologian and philosopher Johann Kaspar Lavater (1741–1801) displayed a striking self-confidence toward Landgrave Wilhelm of Hesse-Kassel[113] during a visit to Hofgeismar in 1793. As a burgher of a Swiss city, Lavater clearly felt that he did not owe any special deference to a German prince unless he received a direct order to be of service. He commented in his travelogue, "Now and then a courtier came . . . , not formally, but only in passing to tell me that the landgrave would like to see me. 'I wait for his orders,' and that's that. I will certainly not approach a prince with even one step that might seem officious."[114] And in small circles, like the one of the duchess of Courland that will be described in more detail later, enlightened nobles admitted the challenges facing rulers in the age of Enlightenment, thus revealing that the praise lavished on ruling princes in the published spa discourse obscured a much more complicated reality. In Pyrmont in 1791, Elisa von der Recke had a long conversation with Prince Friedrich Christian of Augustenburg and Friedrich Nicolai "about the difficult question whether kings and princes could be good [enlightened] people."[115]

Second, "circle" (*Zirkel*) is one of the key terms in contemporary spa descriptions. Similar to the term "tone," "circle" could carry both positive and negative connotations. It referred to a group of friends and acquaintances who participated in, but also separated themselves from, the larger spa society of the nobility and the upper middle class. The "formation of circles" (*Zirkelbildung*) was occasionally seen as positive in the published discourse, but negative views generally prevailed. Authors of spa publications regarded circle formation as detrimental to the spa as a social heterotopia, especially if spa guests formed circles based on social rank. Accordingly, the *Journal of Luxury and Fashions* (*Journal des Luxus und der Moden*) strongly condemned spa guests who "formed small courts" in Karlsbad in 1797.[116] Joachim Christoph Friedrich Schulz was equally critical of the formation of circles in his 1795 *Journey of a Livonian* (*Reise eines Liefländers*): "Small courts are formed that are jealous of each other. One plots little intrigues, criticizes the others, searches for or fabricates absurdities. In one word, one plays the usual pathetic game that appears infinitely important to the people involved."[117] In the aforementioned letter to Heinrich Matthias Marcard, Justus Möser described the dynamics of circle formation in Pyrmont in a more neutral way that reflected lived experience. While he upheld the ideal of the spa as a meeting place for the bourgeoisie and the nobility, he saw the formation of circles as a social process that was unavoidable, even if people did their best to counteract it: "Otherwise it is an old adage: birds of a feather flock together, and acquaintances stick to acquaintances."[118]

As we have seen in the previous section of this chapter, the majority of statements in the published spa discourse created a noble-bourgeois dichotomy without reference to the internal differentiations of these social groups. Some publications, however, addressed the formation of circles *within* the larger social groups of the nobility and the bourgeoisie. Although these discursive statements are comparatively rare, they nevertheless provided readers with brief glimpses of the more complex divisions in German society during the late eighteenth and early nineteenth centuries.[119] For example, the author of *Lauchstädt, a Small*

Painting (Lauchstädt, ein kleines Gemählde) criticized Leipzig merchants for behaving no better than the nobility by "forming their own society" in Lauchstädt: "The scholar is now usually excluded from this society because these gentlemen [the merchants] have their own ideas, too."[120]

In other instances, authors discuss that ennobled members of the bourgeoisie were not accepted by members of established noble families. In the play *Noble Pride at the Spa of Lauchstädt (Der Adelsstolz im Bade zu Lauchstädt)*, a noblewoman from an old noble family denies an ennobled family named "von Radegast" their noble status: "If someone cannot show a [noble] pedigree, so that he can obtain the position of canon in prince-bishoprics and appear at princely courts, and yet, without being a cavalier, allows himself and his wife from the bourgeoisie [*Bürgervolke*] to be called 'Your Lordship' [*gnädig nennen*], we will say that he is not of [noble] family [*von Familie*]."[121] And the author of *Lauchstädt, a Small Painting* summarized the dilemma of the ennobled bourgeois: "Even the man who acquired a noble rank through his qualifications and the services he rendered to his prince has to feel this [noble] separation and has to endure the nobility [*Adel*] looking down upon him from its elevated status."[122]

The published discourse regarded the formation of circles as positive when, as one author said about Karlsbad during the off-season, "small domestic circles" engaged in "the quiet, true pleasures of educated sociability."[123] As we saw in Chapter 5, following a long tradition that began with the humanists, spas became meeting places for circles of enlightened bourgeois scholars during the eighteenth century. By the end of the century, the social composition of these circles of educated sociability had changed. They now encompassed members of the educated bourgeoisie *and* nobles who regarded themselves as enlightened. In short, these circles became meeting places for the enlightened educated elite (*Stand der Gebildeten*). Jens Baggesen, who otherwise had a mostly negative view of Pyrmont, thus praised social circles in general and in particular the circle of the writer Jenny von Voigts (1749–1814), Justus Möser's daughter, at this spa: "Among the special daily pleasures are the small tea parties where a limited circle of acquaintances gathers. Together with [Adam Gottlob Detlef] Moltke, I spent many a pleasant hour in one of them, where the clever, good, very interesting Frau von Voigt [*sic*] from Osnabrück presided."[124]

The circle of Duchess Dorothea of Courland (1761–1821) in Karlsbad and Pyrmont was one of the most prominent. Duchess Dorothea's sister Elisa von der Recke and Recke's bourgeois friend and travel companion Sophie Becker wrote about this circle in their diaries.[125] This circle was one of the very few to be explicitly named in the published discourse. It was depicted as a positive example of circle formation and as a model of noble-bourgeois integration. The *Journal of Luxury and Fashions (Journal des Luxus und der Moden)* reported about Karlsbad in 1800, "The duchess of

Courland together with her beautiful daughters formed a circle in which a very cheerful and informal tone is said to have prevailed."[126] The circle of Duchess Dorothea consisted of nobles, ennobled bourgeois, and members of the educated bourgeoisie.[127] At different times and among others, the circle encompassed Friedrich Christian II, hereditary prince (and later duke) of Schleswig-Holstein-Sonderburg-Augustenburg (1765–1814); Princess Pauline of Lippe (1769–1820), neé Pauline Christine Wilhelmine of Anhalt-Bernburg; Count Nieuport from Brussels, "commander of the Knights of Malta";[128] Count Karl Friedrich von Geßler (1753–1829), Prussian envoy in Dresden; Count Hans Moritz von Brühl (1746–1811), son of the Saxon prime minister and married to Christina, or Tina, von Brühl (neé von Schleyerweber und Friedenau), one of the few female landscape architects of the eighteenth century; the ennobled writer August von Kotzebue (1761–1819); the ennobled writer and Prussian official Leopold Friedrich Günther von Göckingk (1748–1828);[129] the ennobled Johann Wolfgang von Goethe (1749–1832); the aforementioned Sophie Becker (later Schwarz, 1754–1789), daughter of a Lutheran pastor; Ernst Platner (1744–1818), professor of medicine and philosophy and university rector in Leipzig; the writer, publisher, and bookseller Christoph Friedrich Nicolai (1733–1811) from Berlin; the philosopher and general superintendent Johann Gottfried Herder (1744–1803) from Weimar;[130] the writer and publisher Johann Joachim Christoph Bode (1731–1793) from Weimar; and the writer Joachim Christoph Friedrich Schulz (1762–1798),[131] who later became professor at the grammar school in Courland through these spa contacts.

As Recke's and Becker's diaries reveal, noble-bourgeois integration did indeed take place in Duchess Dorothea's circle. However, it is important to note that this circle was composed of individuals who already transcended the social boundary between the nobility and the bourgeoisie in one way or another. The nobles, including the ruling nobility, regarded themselves as enlightened and progressive and sought the company of the educated bourgeoisie. The ennobled bourgeois came from the learned upper middle class (*Bildungsbürgertum*);[132] and, importantly, the bourgeois members of the circle were also part of the educated elite. Members of the traditional *urban* middle and upper middle classes (*Stadtbürgertum*), notably merchants, who appear in the published discourse (e.g., the "merchants from Leipzig"[133] or the "merchant from Annaberg"[134] mentioned earlier), were not part of this circle, a fact that points to the limits of social integration. Ultimately, this and other noble-bourgeois circles did not fulfill the promise of the spa as a comprehensive social heterotopia. Rather, they brought together groups of like-minded people who used the more informal atmosphere of the spa to bring to life their smaller, more restricted version of an Enlightenment social heterotopia. In many ways, these spa circles mirrored eighteenth-century salons.

The personal narratives of the leading noble members of the duchess of Courland's circle reveal their enlightened self-image and confirm their willingness to both criticize their own social estate and socialize with the educated bourgeoisie.[135] In 1791, Princess Pauline of Lippe strikingly wrote the following to the prince of Augustenburg, an educated enlightened aristocrat: "I am of course aware that our class [*Classe*, i.e. the nobility] is not loved by you, that at times I have tried in vain to reconcile you with the same, and that unfortunately more and more experience teaches me that your judgment in general is unfortunately correct."[136] Elisa von der Recke's identity as a member of the enlightened elite made her feel uncomfortable in aristocratic circles: "Unfortunately, my birth places me in the circle of the nobility, the rank of my sister as a duchess, which I find burdensome, draws me to courts and into the circles of the noble [*vornehmen*] world. But in these circles. . . . I seldom find people I can respect. In the enlightened middling estate [*aufgeklärten Mittelstande*] I have always found my dearest and most of my friends."[137] And in 1791, the duchess of Courland wrote playfully to Herder from Pyrmont: "Naturally, I wish that you and your wife could be part of our Pyrmont solitude. Harmony prevails here throughout, the Pyrmont colony [her spa circle] leads a life that surpasses the ideal of the golden age in Karlsbad that [Ernst] Platner described to us. We are pious and happy like good children, enlightened in some respects and religious in the exercise of the commandment: thou shalt love thy neighbor as thyself."[138]

The members of the circle around the duchess of Courland and Elisa von der Recke regularly engaged in joint activities. As we saw in Chapter 4, walks and outings were part of the circle's amusements. In 1785, at the end of their stay in Karlsbad, members of the circle went up the steep Laurentius (or Lorenzo) Hill to the Chapel of St. Laurentius, where an altar of friendship, commissioned by Count von Brühl, had been built. They sang a song to friendship there, laid flowers on the altar, and said goodbye to one another.[139] Several of the activities of this circle became publicized in the spa discourse – among others, Göckingk's *Song to be Sung at the [Karlsbad] Hot Spring* (*Lied am Sprudel zu singen*) for Elisa von der Recke and a gazebo dedicated to the duchess of Courland that was erected in 1791 on Dorothea's meadow (*Dorotheenaue*) in Karlsbad, which was also named after the duchess.[140] The duchess of Courland's circle shared meals, met in the Saxon hall,[141] and in small private settings noblewomen danced with bourgeois men.[142]

However, the descriptions of spa life among Duchess Dorothea's circle also reveal the limitations of and pressures on noble-bourgeois interactions. Noticeably, bourgeois scholars often provided intellectual stimulation in the form of lectures that appeared more to be formal work than informal, spontaneous arrangements. As David Blackbourn has noted, "personal patronage remained the dominant mode of cultural support in late eighteenth-century Germany."[143] For example, Ernst Platner, the

Leipzig university professor, spent the summer of 1791 in Karlsbad and Pyrmont, invited (and reimbursed for the loss of his regular income) by the prince and princess of Augustenburg.[144] He gave several lectures in the rooms of the duchess of Courland.[145]

Moreover, Elisa von der Recke remarked in her diary that even within this small spa circle, noble-bourgeois sociability was not without problems. During her stay in Pyrmont in 1791, Platner approached Recke with a message from the prince of Augustenburg, who wished to participate in a dinner given by Christoph Friedrich Nicolai for the spa circle. The prince wanted to make sure that Nicolai "would not be embarrassed." Recke concludes, "Of course I accepted this gratefully in Nicolai's name and valued the good prince . . . even more. But I fear that our society will now become more formal than it would otherwise have been."[146] She then states that, as expected, the prince's presence changed the "tone" in her circle: "Only the king of Poland [Stanisław II August Poniatowski, 1732–1798] and my Daria [Elisa's sister Dorothea, the duchess of Courland] know how to bring the tone of joyful sociability into any society in such a way that one forgets their estate [*Stand*] and finds their company beneficial. The prince of Augustenburg did not achieve his well-intentioned goal by any stretch of the imagination."[147]

Furthermore, the interior space of this spa circle could not be isolated from the spa society around it. This is revealed by a spiteful "anecdote about [Ernst] Platner" recorded by Karl August Böttiger (1760–1835):

> When he [Platner] embarrassed himself on multiple occasions as court philosopher of the Augustenburg princes in Karlsbad four years ago, he also had the habit of following around the gracious princess of Augustenburg on every walk like a ghost. She did not seem to be dissatisfied with a philosopher wagging beside her instead of a lapdog. But the other chamberlains and nobles among the spa guests were extremely displeased with the school fox [*Schulfuchs*, i.e. learned man, namely Platner], who so often snatched the beautiful princess away from their circles. A Bohemian count had just arrived who had met Platner in Vienna. The others took him [the Bohemian count] aside and instructed him. Suddenly he [the Bohemian count] comes toward him [Platner] in an avenue as he is leading the princess, [tells him that he] is happy to see him [Platner] again, and quite innocently asks, without waiting for an introduction: *and the lady holding your hand, Doctor, surely your patient?* The princess left in a hurry and has since then never again been alone with Platner.[148]

In this instance, lived experience again strikingly resembles the statements about noble-bourgeois interaction in the published discourse. Whether it was true or not, Böttiger certainly thought of Platner as a member of the bourgeoisie who did not behave appropriately by simultaneously being too deferential and too close (both in social and spatial terms) to a female member of the nobility. At the same time, Böttiger described the Bohemian nobleman and his fellow nobles as status-conscious people who did not approve of noble-bourgeois integration, at least not at the level practiced within the duchess of Courland's circle.

Sophie Becker, the daughter of a Lutheran pastor and a member of Duchess Dorothea's spa circle, was a woman from the educated middle class. Her experiences provide an instructive contrast with Elisa von der Recke, who saw herself as enlightened, but as a noblewoman also had access to all aristocratic circles and spaces in society. Becker visited the spas of Karlsbad, Pyrmont, Teplitz, Lauchstädt, Brückenau, Wilhelmsbad, and Wiesbaden as well as numerous princely residence towns as Recke's companion on her trips through Germany in 1784–1786.[149] Her diary reveals that Sophie Becker experienced a noticeable difference between "being at court and at the spa."[150] As a permanent member of the circle around the duchess of Courland in Karlsbad and Pyrmont, she was regularly invited to and fully participated in activities and amusements organized by nobles. For example, in Karlsbad in 1784, she described a ball given by a Polish countess and emphasized that the social atmosphere there was "without any constraint."[151]

In contrast, Sophie Becker's options for interactions with nobles and her access to aristocratic spaces were severely restricted in the princely residence towns she visited with Elisa von der Recke. The circles in these residence towns were still clearly divided into "noble" and "bourgeois." Again and again Becker records in her diary that Recke was at court while she socialized with members of the educated bourgeoisie she had met in the duchess of Courland's spa circle. In 1784, she wrote about her stay in Weimar: "Elise went to court for the first time today, but returned rather dissatisfied with the tone there. I, however, spent my time pleasantly in [Johann Joachim Christoph] Bode's company."[152] In 1785, the same pattern repeated itself in Berlin: "I am often at Herr Nikolai's [Christoph Friedrich Nicolai's] house, and usually spend the evenings there when Elise visits the courts."[153]

For Sophie Becker, sociability at the spa clearly differed from everyday life. At the spa, she was a member of an enlightened circle of nobles and bourgeois, she took part in all forms of activities, and she could enter all spaces. In the princely residence towns, in contrast, she was subject to unambiguously defined restrictions. Joachim Berger has remarked that in the court of Duchess Anna Amalia of Saxe-Weimar-Eisenach, who had been regent for her son Karl August until 1775, "the [Enlightenment] ideals of interaction across the social boundary between the estates could not be transferred to the court as a sphere of action."[154] For Sophie Becker, "being at court and at the spa" therefore constituted two very different experiences. Through her membership in an enlightened circle, Becker experienced the spa as a space outside of everyday life where different social rules applied. In short, the spa circle was a social heterotopia for Becker, where the barrier between the nobility and the bourgeoisie was more permeable.

Goethe's partner and later wife Christiane Vulpius (1765–1816) was another middle-class woman who reported in detail about her spa experiences in the late eighteenth century. While Goethe spent many summers at the two most fashionable spas of the time, Karlsbad and Pyrmont, Vulpius mostly visited Lauchstädt, where she also had an eye on the Weimar court theater that performed there during the summer seasons.[155] Like Sophie Becker's diary, the letters of Christiane Vulpius speak to the limits and possibilities of social interaction at the spa and in spa circles in contrast to the princely residence town of Weimar. Vulpius' social status was, however, of a more complex nature than Becker's. Christiane's father, Johann Friedrich Vulpius, had to quit his law studies for financial reasons and eventually worked as an archivist in the ducal administration. His position was poorly paid and precarious. He died in 1786, leaving behind a destitute family.[156] For many years Christiane Vulpius, who became Goethe's lover and partner in 1788, was despised by Weimar society.[157] She was not well educated, but she could read and write, and her writing style is vivid and engaging. After she had died, Elisa von der Recke described her as having possessed an "undemanding, bright, utterly natural intellect,"[158] perhaps implying a certain naiveté, but also a keen awareness of the world around her. Both qualities become apparent in her reports about her spa trips to Lauchstädt.

Vulpius experienced a sense of social integration in Lauchstädt, even during her visits to the spa before her marriage to Goethe in the fall of 1806.[159] She was a member of a small middle-class circle of educated bourgeois, including the writer Johann Joachim Christoph Bode, actors of the Weimar court theater such as Karoline Jagemann (1777–1848, also mistress of Duke Karl August of Weimar),[160] and Leipzig burghers. Vulpius herself described this circle as a "bourgeois society," and she obviously appreciated the level of acceptance and integration in this circle, which was very different from the treatment she experienced in Weimar.[161] Vulpius also moved in a wider spa circle that included noble spa guests, and she recorded in her letters that noblemen regularly asked her to dance.[162] She was especially delighted to find that some nobles in Lauchstädt were more "well-behaved" towards her "than towards other people."[163] Vulpius took great pleasure in letting Goethe know that, "so many people from Weimar" had to "watch" her interact with nobles and were "surprised."[164] And Vulpius was clearly able to utilize the more relaxed social atmosphere at the spa to her own advantage. As was said in the published discourse, she used "a carriage and four [and] a hat ribbon with diamonds"[165] to elevate herself. In 1803, when she visited Lauchstädt with a servant, a carriage, and beautiful horses, she felt that this immediately lent her a higher social status.[166] Whereas in Weimar before her marriage she sat on a bench on the ground floor of the theater, in Lauchstädt she already sat in a box.[167] The spa signified a degree of social recognition for Goethe's partner that she did not attain in the princely residence town of Weimar.

Vulpius' perception of the spa as a space of freedom and therefore as a social heterotopia was very pronounced. In 1803 she wrote to Goethe, "I feel as if I am only now beginning to live."[168] Nevertheless, Vulpius was not oblivious to the social tensions at Lauchstädt that were front and center in the published discourse. In fact, she mentioned several times that she became aware of what the spa discourse described as "noble distinction" or "noble separation." However, she herself did not feel affected by this: "The nobility [*Adelichen*] are beginning to do all sorts of silly things. All kinds of things are said about what they hold against the bourgeoisie [*die Bürgerlichen*]. I myself know nothing of that, they are all well-behaved toward me."[169] It is difficult to gauge the level of naiveté or even intentional ignorance involved in Vulpius' perceptions, but considering that her experiences in Weimar most likely made her more rather than less aware of social slights, it is plausible that her perceptions reflected her lived reality. And even though Christiane Vulpius can certainly be regarded as a special case because of her unusual social status, her spa visits as well as Sophie Becker's reveal that bourgeois women in the late eighteenth and early nineteenth centuries experienced their spa circles as small social heterotopias set apart from everyday life.

All in all, for the learned bourgeoisie and the enlightened nobility, the German spa of the late eighteenth and early nineteenth centuries functioned as a limited social heterotopia. In smaller social circles at the spa, like-minded friends and acquaintances overcame social boundaries. Nevertheless, even in these circles the new enlightened educated elite (*gebildete Stände*) sometimes struggled to put their convictions into practice. The early modern social hierarchy was always lurking just underneath the surface as these spa visitors negotiated how to interact and how to behave toward one another. The spa viewed in its entirety was never able to fulfill the heightened demands for bourgeois equality voiced in the published discourse. As we saw in the reports about Platner in Karlsbad and from Vulpius in Lauchstädt, social tensions between the nobility and the bourgeoisie and noble resistance to social integration were not merely an invention of the published discourse. Rather, they were lived experiences. But the limited success of the smaller spa circles helped to keep the idea of the spa as a social heterotopia alive and lent a degree of both plausibility and hope to the demands of the published discourse.

Third, noble-bourgeois spa circles obviously encompassed only a small part of society. The published discourse, even though it spoke to a larger portion of the middle class among its readers, ultimately closed its eyes to the broader processes of social demarcation and exclusion that characterized the spa. In fact, the spa could only aspire to function as a social heterotopia because it created clearly delineated times and spaces for the interaction of noble and bourgeois elites and excluded other social groups. This was not unique to the spas; as discussed earlier, other institutions of Enlightenment sociability also excluded groups of lower social status.[170] Besides economic mechanisms like prices for accommodations, meals, and entertainments including theater performances and concerts, other mechanisms of exclusion were also employed to separate the elite spa society from other visitors.

Mechanisms of "opening and closing" marked the spa as a heterotopia on several levels, and the control both of time and of access to spaces was a decisive factor in these processes. As we have already seen, in spite of the ideal that all internal spaces of a spa were supposed to be fully accessible to the nobility and the bourgeoisie, the nobility repeatedly claimed certain spaces for their exclusive use, sometimes only for a certain period of time and sometimes as a general principle. This provoked some of the most vitriolic comments in the published discourse about "noble separation." At the same time, the nobility and the bourgeoisie also sought to separate themselves from the rest of society. This led to very specific questions of spatial access at spas that also throw light on the ambiguous social position of the middle and lower middle classes in the late eighteenth and early nineteenth centuries.

At Pyrmont, for example, the accommodations for the peasants, the lower middle class, and some members of the middle class like small-town officials or petty merchants were located far from the spa district at the edge of town or in the surrounding villages.[171] The "country people" (*Landleute*) were expected to come to the avenue and drink from the healing spring between 3 or 4 and 6 o'clock in the morning, before the upper classes made their appearance at the well at 6 o'clock.[172] The "peasants" (*Bauern*), beggars, and other members of the lower orders were forbidden from entering the main avenue after the upper social classes had appeared there in the morning, and they also did not have access to the spa buildings like the ballroom and the coffeehouse. "Avenue servants" were at hand to remove people who were not supposed to be in the main avenue, but often managed to enter in order to listen to the music, watch the dancers, or just take in the upper classes strolling along the avenue. The authorities fought a continuous uphill battle to enforce these rules of spatial access.[173]

Marcard and Piepenbring strike very different tones when describing the separation of the peasants from the upper classes in Pyrmont. Marcard argued that the peasants were used to getting up early and that they were in the main avenue before the other social groups because the avenue would otherwise be too crowded later on. This is obviously a rather flimsy pretext for what was, in fact, social exclusion. Marcard was clearly trying to maintain the ideal of the spa as an Enlightenment social heterotopia. Piepenbring, in contrast, insulted the peasants as having less "reason"

(*Vernunft*) than some dogs, thus explicitly excluding them from the spa as a space of Enlightenment sociability.[174]

These rules and mechanisms of social exclusion left open the role and options of the large group in the middle of society, that is, the members of the middle and lower middle classes, whose social status ranged from small-town mayors and merchants to valets and personal maids, and included many others.[175] In Pyrmont, these groups were regarded as "proper" spa visitors in terms of their expected inclusion in the guest lists.[176] But in terms of spatial access at the spa, authorities were clearly at a loss. Just like the peasants and lower orders, these groups were not supposed to frequent the more exclusive spaces of the spa like the ballroom, and both their economic and their social status excluded them from the activities shared by the upper classes. At the same time, they did not wish to frequent the taverns of the peasants and lower orders. The problems associated with catering to this large social group "in the middle" became obvious in Pyrmont in the late 1780s when a debate flared up between the spa physician Marcard on one side and the privy councillor Klapp and the treasurer of the public revenues (*Rentmeister*) Scholing on the other. Scholing, supported by Klapp, developed a plan to build a dance hall with a wine tavern at the lower end of the avenue. While Klapp argued that there was a need for such an establishment to serve "honest people of the middle estate," Marcard was adamant that it would ruin Pyrmont because the upper classes would stop visiting the spa.[177]

Jewish spa guests also faced specific mechanisms of inclusion and exclusion. Jews were "the other" in early modern central Europe, which resulted in their spatial separation in towns as well as at spas. Even the newly built spas of the eighteenth century like Wilhelmsbad had bathhouses and lodgings on the peripheries to accommodate Jews.[178] And even during the age of Jewish emancipation starting in the late eighteenth century, the "othering" of Jewish spa guests is palpable in the published discourse and, once again, speaks to the clear limits of the spa as a social heterotopia. Individual educated Jews like the famous philosopher Moses Mendelssohn (1729–1786) were fully accepted by the elites of spa society, but this was clearly an exception.[179] Overall, Jews are rarely mentioned in the spa discourse, and when they are, they generally feature in their roles as merchants, seasonal shopkeepers, and sometimes moneylenders or casino owners at the spas.[180]

In the rare instances when the spa discourse mentions Jews as spa visitors, they are still represented as "the other." In his 1782 report from Brückenau, Göckingk describes a Jewish spa guest as a person who did everything possible to fit in with the majority Christian society, but was, nevertheless, recognized as an outsider by that society: "When I was present [in Brückenau], there was a Jew there, who pretended to be a Christian and also had taken another name, but everyone knew that he was a Jew. However, nobody revealed that he [*sic*] knew it, but encountered him with politeness, even with friendship, because the Jew was a man who knew how to live. From this single detail one can conclude that at this spa of a Catholic ecclesiastical prince there must prevail a great deal of tolerance, and it is indeed so."[181] Even though Göckingk invokes the tolerant spirit of Brückenau, his description expresses considerable social distance toward the Jewish spa guest.

At the turn of the nineteenth century, the ideal of the spa as a social heterotopia that had been a central demand of the published discourse and that had come to life – at least to a certain degree – in the circles of the enlightened nobility and the educated bourgeoisie gradually started to wane. Two important political developments of the age left their mark on the spa and fundamentally changed the concept of the spa as a meeting place: on the one hand, the emergence of national identities and nation states as a result of the Revolutionary and Napoleonic Wars, and on the other hand, the Metternich system and the rise of conservatism and censorship in the era of the German Confederation (*Restaurationszeit*).

The gradual transformation of the early modern Europe of empires, multiple kingdoms, and dynastic territories into the modern Europe of nation states and national identities is reflected in the published spa discourse. These political developments were perceived as having fundamental social and cultural implications as well, including at the spas. During the era of the French Revolutionary Wars, the spa discourse conveyed a strong sense of German identity to its readers that was centered mostly on language. Authors demanded the use of the German language at the spa and rejected the use of French. For example, in his 1793 article about Karlsbad in the *German Magazine (Deutsches Magazin)* Giseke argued, "If the current nations should one day, like the ancient Romans and Greeks, perish and our European languages are preserved as dead languages, then when French inscriptions are found everywhere in the middle of Germany, people will believe that France had a universal monarchy and subjected everything to itself."[182]

The choice of language at the spa was construed as a sign of national identity. Thus, a 1798 article about Karlsbad in the "Spa Chronicle" ("Badechronik") of the *Journal of Luxury and Fashions (Journal des Luxus und der Moden)* declared, "To my great delight I also found the German language to be dominant there. Even though some exchanged the first greetings in French, they later continued their conversation in German. I think that this must please every German, no matter how much he is convinced that the French language is extremely convenient in the field of diplomacy for political deception, or when people . . . want to talk but have nothing to say to each other."[183]

Contemporaries also took note of the formation of social circles at the spas as an expression of the emergence of national identities. In his 1795 *Journey of a Livonian (Reise eines Liefländers)* Schulz observed that a new reason for social separation had been added to the well-known issue of "noble separation" in Karlsbad: "Because it is not simply sick people who come here, but sick people from the Bohemian nation and sick people from the Saxon nation. Now sick people from the Courland nation and from the Polish nation also come. Each of these nations wants to be the first [in rank]."[184] And in an 1806 letter from Karlsbad Goethe remarked to Christiane Vulpius: "Yesterday I met Frau von Brösigke and her daughter, who came over from Egerbrunn [Franzensbad], where things are also not very cheerful because the Austrians and the Poles are making two parties that are working against each other, and neither of them accepts either a Saxon or a Prussian among themselves."[185] During this time of political and military upheaval, social separation into emerging national circles became a common phenomenon at the spas, especially the Bohemian spas that attracted guests from all over Europe. By the late 1830s, national identities and national circles at spas had become the norm. An article about Karlsbad in the 1839 *Newspaper for the Elegant World* (*Zeitung für die elegante Welt*) described spa guests primarily in terms of national origin as "the English," "the Russians," "French," "Poles," and "the German [*sic*]."[186]

The ideal of the spa as a social heterotopia was weakened not only through the formation of national circles. During the 1820s, the discursive backbone of the concept of the spa as a social heterotopia – the demand for noble-bourgeois integration – also faded from the published discourse. This was a gradual process, and it is therefore not possible to determine whether this change in the discourse was due to the effects of intensified censorship after the Karlsbad Decrees of 1819 or the result of authors' self-censorship. As Andreas Würgler has observed, "One of the most effective impacts of censorship was probably the self-censorship that authors preemptively subjected themselves to. The mechanism of self-censorship can only in rare instances be proven in concrete terms."[187] Irrespective of how this transformation came about, the prevailing spa discourse changed fundamentally in the new social and political climate of the era of the German Confederation. In the spa publications of the 1820s, a new discursive formation emerged. Socially homogeneous spa circles were now described as a sensible arrangement that allowed everyone to move in circles that suited them. The aggressive calls for bourgeois equality ended, and the separation of social classes at the spa was no longer called into question.

For example, a Karlsbad spa guide of 1828 explained to its readers, "In Karlsbad, everyone chooses their social circle according to their own tastes, according to the degree of their education, and thus changes [their companions] according to their liking. Some only stick to people of their own [social] rank, others to people who are like-minded."[188] And another spa publication about Karlsbad asserted in 1838:

Of course, one should not take it amiss if one does not get easy access to the circles of the higher estates, and we note that anyone who is not intimately acquainted with the tone of these classes should stay away from them if he does not want to play the role of the Knight of the Sad Countenance.[189] But anyone who masters this tone will certainly find access there, even if he does not come from the *gentry*. By the way, no estate [*Stand*] will have to complain that it is isolated in Karlsbad. Everybody will find enough people here who are of his own kind.[190]

The new prevailing discourse of the 1820s and 1830s differs both from the early modern discursive regime before 1750 and from the prevailing discourse of the transitional period of the late eighteenth and early nineteenth centuries. In the early modern spa discourse, the social estates were clearly divided. The spa discourse of the transitional period, in contrast, had demanded social equality for the bourgeoisie and noble-bourgeois integration. This discourse had also developed and propagated the concepts that started to dominate the published spa discourse in the 1820s, namely the ideas of an educated social elite (a "social circle according to education") as well as of a "gentry" encompassing members of the upper middle class and the nobility. However, these concepts had been of secondary importance in the discourse of the late eighteenth and early nineteenth centuries and had been described as incomplete steps toward a greater goal. In addition, the usage of the term "tone" had also changed. Previously denoting the social atmosphere at the spa as a whole, it was now used in the narrower sense of the manners of the "higher estates."

As David Blackbourn has remarked, while "a true intermingling of wealthy bourgeois . . . with a monarchical and noble élite" took place over the course of the nineteenth century, a process that resulted in "each [taking] on some social coloring from the other as they began to merge into a new upper class, present in the spa towns in their capacity as a new leisure class,"[191] most members of the middle class were excluded from this development. The published spa discourse clearly reflected this changing social and political climate and moved away from overarching demands for social equality and the concept of the spa as a social heterotopia. Rather, social separation and the formation of spa circles according to "education," "rank," "taste," and, in consequence, also wealth were now presented as positive. The transitional period, with its bourgeois demands and aspirations for the spa as a meeting place, had come to an end, but it left a legacy of the spa as a social heterotopia that was to be taken up again later in the nineteenth century.[192]

Notes

1. See the Introduction to this book.
2. [Möller], *Der Adelsstolz im Bade zu Lauchstädt*, 1791.
3. August Ludwig (von) Schlözer (1735–1809), who published the journal *Staats-Anzeigen*, was a vocal critic of the political and social situation in late eighteenth-century Germany.

4. Göckingk, "Von dem Kurbrunnen bei Brückenau," 1782, 336: "In Pyrmont und Lauchstädt (sagt Hr. Prof. Schlözer) sollen manchmal Brunnen- und Badegäste sein, die zwischen Adelichen und Bürgerlichen einen so großen Unterschied machen, als wenn jene einen ganz andern Adam hätten, wie diese."

5. [Giseke], "Fortsetzung der Briefe über Carlsbad," 1793, 805: "Der ... Adel zeigt viele Prachtliebe, und kein Unpartheyischer kann mit Wahrheit sagen, daß der in Carlsbad herrschende Ton so frey und angenehm wäre, als es in Bädern sein soll. Die Etikette regiert hier, wie an einem der steifsten Höfe, und mißt jeden Rangunterschied genau ab." See also [Schulz], *Reise eines Liefländers*, 1795, 97.

6. [Giseke], "Fortsetzung der Briefe über Carlsbad," 1793, 830: "Solche alte Herkunft gilt an und für sich nichts mehr, und sie wird wohle thun, sich nur darauf zu berufen, daß ihr Vater ein ehrlicher Mann war, und sie eine gute Mutter und Hausfrau ist. Dies giebt heutiges Tages den größten Werth, und daher sagen wir, daß wir in einer philosophischen Zeit leben. Andere wollen es eine schlimme Zeit nennen. Ich weiß nichts davon."

7. [Möller], *Der Adelsstolz im Bade zu Lauchstädt*, 1791, 26: "Es muß jeder bey seinem Stande bleiben, wie sollte die Welt bestehen, wenn Personen von unsrer naissance sich mit Leuten, die nur da sind, uns zu dienen, sich compromittieren wollten. . . . Möchten doch . . . die Herren Gelehrten nur bey ihrem Stande bleiben, und sich nicht unter Cavaliers und charakterisirte Personen mengen, die mit keinem stumpfen Federfechter zu thun haben mögen."

8. *Reise nach den Badeörtern*, 1798, 172–173: "Sagt uns doch ihr Herren Brüder, | Was ihr denkt? | Hat nur euch, und immer wieder, | Die Natur beschenkt? – | Seyd ihr mehr, und sind wir minder, | Adams oder Noahs Kinder? – | Gab Er, der die Menschen schuf, | Euch Befugniß und Beruf | Zum Vergöttern? – | Liegts an Geist, Verstand und Muth? | Liegts am Fleische? Liegts im Blut? – | Nein! Es liegt bloß an drei Lettern, | Und am Federhut. Durch diese Spaltung zwischen zweien der ersten Menschenklassen, muß nothwendiger Weise ein großer Bruch der allgemeinen Geselligkeit entstehn, die, so wie überhaupt überall, besonders an dergleichen Brunnenorten, allein nur Vergnügen und Lebensglück verbreitet."

9. See the explanation of the complex meaning of the word "Herr" as both a term reserved for the nobility, but also a general term of address denoting respect in Adelung, *Grammatisch-kritisches Wörterbuch*.

10. "Badechronik," *JLM* (November 1798), 623–624: "Die diesjährige Bade-saison ist so zahlreich gewesen, als eine der vorhergehenden. Aber noch nie war die Scheidewand zwischen dem Adel – der Brandenburgische, Meklenburgische und Pommersche ist hier der vorherrschende – und den Bürgerlichen so eisern und undurchdringlich, als diesmal; und während andere Badeorte sich immer mehr humanisiren und popularisiren, hält der Adelsseparatismus sein Szepter so steif als König Salomo auf dem Löwen-throne in den Nürnberger Bilderbibeln."

11. See Heal, "For Simple Folk and Connoisseurs."

12. [Giseke], "Neue Briefe über Carlsbad, vom Jahre 1792, Zweiter Brief," 1793, 398: "Der Adel sieht gewissermassen diesen [sächsischen] Saal als sein Eigenthum an, . . . Er hält auch nur hier die Abendassembleen, und die Gens de l'autre monde können sich dann den böhmischen Saal zu eignen."

13. *Reise nach den Badeörtern*, 1798, 92: "der Adel maaßt sich dieses Ortes so ausschlüßlich an, daß selten ein Bürgerlicher dahin kömmt, noch hinzukom-men wagen darf." In the 1796 "Teutsche Badechronik" of the *Journal des Luxus und der Moden*, the Saxon hall is described as a "gathering place for

the nobility who eat breakfast, especially the ladies" – "Sammelplatz des frühstückenden Adels, sonderlich der Damen." "Teutsche Badechronik," *JLM* (November 1796), 556.

14. [Schulz], *Reise eines Liefländers*, 1795, 61–62: "Man hat aber schon vornehme Kranke wieder von Karlsbad abreisen sehen, weil sie in den Modege[ge]nden der Stadt keine Unterkunft mehr finden konnten: alles, um nicht zwischen Priestern, Kaufleuten, bürgerlichen Räthen und dergleichen Leuten, ihren Wohnplatz aufzuschlagen, mit denen sie doch übrigens das Unglück haben, aus einerley Brunnen trinken zu müssen."

15. *Lauchstädt, ein kleines Gemählde*, 1787, 35: "Dieser Künstler glaubte also weiter kein Vorrecht nöthig zu haben, als dieses, daß er ein Mensch war, um seine Freiheit gebrauchen und das thun zu dürfen, wozu ihn seine Neigung und die Gewohnheit antriebe."

16. *Lauchstädt, ein kleines Gemählde*, 1787, 36: "Impertinenz."

17. See *Lauchstädt, ein kleines Gemählde*, 1787, 34–36.

18. But see the following section in this chapter for another statement by the same author that points to divisions within the bourgeoisie.

19. *Lauchstädt, ein kleines Gemählde*, 1787, 36: "Und nun sagen Sie mir, können wir nach Vorfällen dieser Art noch Ansprüche an Aufklärung machen? Dürfen wir glauben, daß wir in der Kunst, Menschen zu seyn, weiter fortgeschritten sind? Kaum hätte man sich etwas Aehnliches zu Anfange dieses Jahrhunderts erlaubt, wo die Menschheit noch gewaltig litt, und das Verdienst die Sklavenfessel noch nicht zerbrochen hatte."

20. Schopenhauer, *Tagebücher der Adele Schopenhauer*, vol. 1, 26–27: "Abends war Konzert. Zum ersten Mal fand ich: die Schriftsteller, die auf die schöne Welt schimpfen, haben recht. Fast alle Damen, die Prinzen usw. waren wütend, daß sie im Nebenzimmer spielen mußten; es sei erschrecklich frech und impertinent, die Gesellschaft mit einem Konzert zu belästigen, das Gedudel wäre nicht zu ertragen. – Wir indessen gingen hin und wurden sehr befriedigt."

21. See [Schulz], "Geheime Szenen aus Bädern," 1800, 132–142.

22. See Chapter 5.

23. Frankenau thus confirms the analysis provided in Merveilleux's *Amusemens des eaux de Schwalbach* sixty years earlier: the highest bourgeois court officials could gain acceptance at noble balls. See Chapter 5.

24. Frankenau, *Pyrmont*, 1799, 48–49: "Ich will indessen grade bei Leibe Niemand rathen, die hier, wie ein Bienenschwarm wimmelnden Markisinnen, Comtessen, Baronessen, und wie sie alle heissen, zum Tanze aufzufordern, wofern man nicht seinen Stammbaum der Dame zu Füssen legen kann, oder einen Titel, und wäre es auch nur der Titel, Herr Rath, hat. In diesem Fall kann man schon zur Noth mitlaufen; . . . Alles was unter diesen Graden ist kann gewiss seyn, dass ihnen der Rükken zugekehrt wird, und man sie über die Achsel ansieht." See also [Hesler], *Das Leben eines Farospielers*, 1794, 203.

25. *Die holländische Sauce: Eine lauchstädtsche Badgeschichte*, 1782, 9: "Sieh, hier in Lauchstädt sind die Fräuleins sparsamer mit ihrer Gnade wie du. Siehst Du wohl eine von den Fräuleins von B.-- mit einem Bürgerlichen tanzen?"

26. *Die holländische Sauce: Eine lauchstädtsche Badgeschichte*, 1782, 13: "Adelstolz und Geiz sind mächtige Triebfedern in dieser Welt, und Lieb und Demuth sind zu klein, um diese Feinde zu besiegen."

27. "Badechronik," *JLM* (November 1798), 624: "Es gieng dießmal die Absonderungssucht wirklich so weit, daß eine nahmhafte Verabredung unter den

Adlichen statt fand, nach welcher kein Edelmann eine bürgerliche Tänzerin aufführen durfte, ohne sich von seinen Standesgenossen empfindliche Vorwürfe auf den Hals zu laden. Niemand als Adeliche gaben die Dejeuners, wozu sich natürlich die Bürgerlichen nicht hinzudrängten."

28. Göckingk, "Von dem Kurbrunnen bei Brückenau," 1782, 337: "daß die Herren, welche hier am ersten den Ton angeben könten, mit einer Mamsell so gut wie mit einer adlichen Dame vom höchsten Range, ohne den geringsten Unterschied selbst in der Art des Tanzens zu machen, getanzt haben; daß bei der Tafel sich ein ehrlicher Pachter neben eine Excellenz gesezt hat, ohne daß dieses ihr sonderbar geschienen hätte; kurz, daß man vernünftig genug war, den Unterschied zwischen dem 'am Hofe und im Bade sein' nicht blos einzusehen, sondern sich darnach zu betragen. Eine Dame von altem Adel fand sich vor ein Paar Jahren beleidiget, daß ein Bürgerlicher so kühn war, sie zum Tanz aufzufordern; man ruhte nicht eher, bis sie den Kurbrunnen verließ." See my previous discussion of the definition of *Herr/Herren* in late eighteenth- and early nineteenth-century German.

29. [Göckingk], "Briefe eines Reisenden," 1778, 470: "Gleichheit und zwangloses allgemeines Vergnügen der herrschende Ton."

30. [Göckingk], "Briefe eines Reisenden," 1778, 470: "Kleiderpracht" – "Eine Dame mus sich in der Allee, anders am Morgen, anders am Nachmittag, und anders am Abend zeigen, . . . Diese Eitelkeit, welche hier in der That am lächerlichsten ist, hat sich auch bis auf die Männer ausgebreitet."

31. Göckingk, "Von dem Kurbrunnen bei Brückenau," 1782, 335: "Ich kenne unter den Dutzend Bädern, die ich besucht habe, auch nicht Eins, daß sich mit diesem, was ungezwungene Lebensart betrifft, im geringsten vergleichen liesse. Ich habe hier keinen Wetteifer bemerkt, sich durch Pracht in der Kleidung zu unterscheiden, vielmehr Damen von Range gesehen, die im schlichten Reisekleide mehrere Tage hintereinander zu Tische kamen."

32. See Frey, *Der reinliche Bürger*, 213; Purdy, *Tyranny of Elegance*, 92.

33. See McNeil, "Appearance of Enlightenment," 385–387.

34. See "Badechronik," *JLM* (November 1797), 556.

35. See North, *"Material Delight"*, 55–58; Purdy, *Tyranny of Elegance*, 180–186.

36. [Göckingk], "Briefe eines Reisenden," 1778, 471: "weissem Nesseltuch" – "Zutritt zu den allgemeinen Vergnügungen im Bade haben" – "ein beßres Verständnis unter Leuten von so verschiednem Range."

37. See Dr. Z** in Br** [Conrad Anton Zwierlein in Brückenau], "Vorschlag zu einer allgemeinen Baad-Uniforme für Damen," *JLM* (July 1788); "Ueber den Luxus des Badereisens," *JLM* (July 1789), 324; "Allgemeine Bad-Uniforme für Damen," *JLM* (April 1792); "Anfragen und Anzeigen [Badeuniform für Damen]," *JLM* (October 1797); "Allgemeiner Modenbericht: Neuester geschmackvoller Badeanzug," *JLM* 18 (1803). See also Zwierlein, *Allgemeine Brunnenschrift*, 1793, 30–36.

38. See "Ueber den Luxus des Badereisens," *JLM* (July 1789), 324 with figure 28.

39. "Allgemeine Bad-Uniforme für Damen," *JLM* (April 1792), 206: "ohne alle Mühe" – "spazieren gehen, tanzen, fahren und reiten."

40. "Allgemeine Bad-Uniforme für Damen," *JLM* (April 1792), 207: "nämliche Uniforme."

41. See Purdy, *Tyranny of Elegance*, 197–201.

42. In a similar vein, the question of when to remove one's hat as a sign of deference, which was generally discussed during the late eighteenth and early nineteenth centuries, was also considered as a spa practice by contemporaries.

Spa publications proclaimed that male spa guests should not remove their hats, but indicate a greeting and the associated social deference by only touching their hats, a practice that was taking hold in many German towns at the same time. See "Teutsche Badechronik," *JLM* (October 1796), 523, about Nenndorf. See in general König, *Kulturgeschichte des Spazierganges*, 259–268.

43. See [Möller], *Der Adelsstolz im Bade zu Lauchstädt*, 1791, 6–7, 13.

44. Campe, *Reise von Braunschweig nach Karlsbad*, 1806, 216: "hier in Karlsbad, . . . so viel Adel zusammenströme, daß oft der zweite oder dritte Mann, der Einem aufstoße, ein gnädiger Herr oder eine Exzellenz sei. Da man aber es den Leuten nicht an der Nase ansehen, oft sogar, wenn sie redeten, es ihnen nicht einmahl anhören könne, ob sie gnädige, exzellente, or ganz gemeine, wo nicht gar untergemeine Menschen seien, so wolle man sie, besonders wenn sie Ausländer und unbekannt wären, lieber in Bausch und Bogen begnädigen und beexzellenzen, als Gefahr laufen, einen gebornen Gnädigen, oder eine durch Brief und Siegel gestempelte Exzellenz wie einen schlichten Bürgersmann zu behandeln."

45. *Reise nach den Badeörtern*, 1798, 174: "Zum Glück kann ja wohl der Bürger den Adlichen entbehren, wenn dieser ihn (dem er doch so viele Vortheile der Litteratur, der Aufklärung, des Bedüfnisses, oder des Geschmacks zu verdanken hat,) entbehren will und kann: auch findet am Ende der Karlsbader Einwohner unser Geld eben so hübsch und rund, als das noble!"

46. The term "Hochadelicher," which in modern historiographical language refers to ruling princes, was used as a term denoting respect for nobility of any rank in the late eighteenth and early nineteenth centuries. See Adelung, *Grammatisch-kritisches Wörterbuch*, entry "Hochadelig." In this particular case, using a respectful term to describe what clearly is a defiant attitude toward the nobility adds to the ironic tone of the passage.

47. Flachs, "Ueber Lauchstädt," 1785, 430: "Trug etwa ein Hochadelicher die Nase so hoch, daß sie über mich hinwegragte, so lif ich darunter weg, ohne bemerken zu wollen, daß eine Nase über mir wäre."

48. *Reise nach den Badeörtern*, 1798, 107: "Menschheit" – "Freibälle."

49. See Marcard, *Beschreibung von Pyrmont*, vol. 1, 1784, 59–60.

50. Pütter, *Selbstbiographie*, vol. 2, 753: "So schrieben sich auf diese Tafel immer nur Herren von Adel oder höhere Standespersonen. Doch wurden zu Zeiten auch wohl andere dazu eingeladen, wenn etwa der Fürst von Waldeck, oder einer aus seinem Gefolge, den Caffee gab, oder auch sonst jemand eben aus der Reihe war, der vielleicht einen besondern Freund unter der übrigen Gesellschaft hatte. Diese Ehre widerfuhr mir mehrmal nach einander, . . . Als ich endlich Ursache hatte zu glauben, daß man es nicht übel nehmen würde, wenn ich meinen Namen mit auffschriebe; so that ich es, und kam auf diese Weise mit an die Reihe, . . . Meinem Beyspiele folgte hernach auch der berühmte und überall beliebte Möser. Ueberhaupt half es etwas dazu, daß die bisher zum Theil zu auffallend gewesene Absonderung des Adels von den Nichadelichen seitdem nach und nach merklich gemildert wurde."

51. See, e.g., Piepenbring, *Bemerkungen über die Schrift des Herrn Doctor Frankenau*, 1801, 24–25. On p. 25, he describes enlightened nobles as "rational people" ("vernünftige Menschen").

52. [Hassencamp], *Briefe eines Reisenden von Pyrmont*, 1783, 25–26: "philosophischer Gleichmüthigkeit."

53. [Hassencamp], *Briefe eines Reisenden von Pyrmont*, 1783, 26: "Dagegen aber habe ich in diesem Stande gar viele herrliche Menschen angetroffen,

unter denen Sie selbst, bester Freund, nicht den geringsten Platz einnehmen, die einen wegen jener wieder völlig schadlos halten, und welche eigentlich ihrem Adel mehr, wie der Adel ihnen Ehre macht."

54. [Hassencamp], *Briefe eines Reisenden von Pyrmont*, 1783, 24: "Auf die Art hat es mir auch dort, wenn ich es verlanget habe, noch keine Stunde an guter Gesellschaft aus allen Ständen gefehlt. Mit schwachen unausgebildeten Köpfen hingegen, derem zum Glücke in unserem aufgeklärten und philosophischen Zeitalter doch nur noch wenige aus einem oder dem andern abgelegenen Dorfe hervorkommen, die ohne Rücksicht auf persönliche Verdienste, blos der Geburt wegen, auf andere nicht so vollbürtige Adamskinder mit Stolz und Verachtung herabsehen, habe ich mich ohnedem nie abgegeben, und also auch in Pyrmont keine Ursache gehabt, mich über ihre affectirte, mir wenigstens nicht allein gleichgültige, sondern sogar erwünschte Absonderung zu beschweren. Hingegen habe ich von vielen andern, besonders Damens, welche noch nicht Philosophie genug haben, sich über dergleichen Armseligkeiten hinauszusetzen, die bittersten Klagen gehört. Zu leugnen ist es nicht, daß dort bey manchen ein überspannter Ton, und ein gewisses steifes stolzes Wesen herrschet, das in den meisten andern Brunnen und Bädern ganz unbekannt ist; wo man nicht zu vergessen scheinet, daß zwischen dem am Hofe und im Bade seyn, selbst nach unsern conventionellen Maniren noch immer ein großer Unterschied ist."

55. Campe, *Reise von Braunschweig nach Karlsbad*, 1806, 187–188: "Leider! ist man auch hier, wie in manchem andern Bade, noch unverständig genug, eine ziemlich scharfe Grenzlinie zwischen beiden Ständen an einem Orte zu ziehen, wo die bürgerlichen Verhältnisse gar nicht in Betracht kommen sollten. Doch muß ich zur Ehre vieler Adeligen hinzufügen, daß man die Gesellschaft in und vor dem Böhmischen Kaffeehause gewöhnlich sehr vermischt findet, weil ein großer, vielleicht der größte Theil der Adeligen so viel guten Sinn mit hieher zu bringen pflegt, daß er lieber in vermischter Gesellschaft sich entweilen und vergnügen, als in den beschränkten Kreisen seines Gleichen sich langweilen mag."

56. "Badechronik," *JLM* (November 1800), 590: "Hier war also an keine steife Absonderung der Stände, die ja hier alle zu Einer Quelle des Heils zusammenkommen, und an keine beleidigende Ausschließung zu denken, die später einmal im Sächsischen Saale einen sehr anstößigen Auftritt durch die Beleidigung eines wackern Kaufmanns aus Annaberg veranlaßte, der nur durch die nachdrückliche Vermittlung einiger Herren von Adel, die diese Ungezogenheit selbst sehr laut mißbilligten, ausgeglichen werden konnte." The spa lists show that merchants from Annaberg visited Karlsbad as spa guests. See, e.g., *Liste der angekommenen Kur- und Badegäste in der königl[ichen] Stadt Kaiser-Karlsbad im Jahre 1795*, 63.

57. Dorothea's meadow (*Dorotheens Aue*) was an area with a monument dedicated to her sister, the duchess of Courland.

58. Recke, *Tagebücher und Selbstzeugnisse*, 330: "Hier fiel mir ein anderer Graf ein, der, als ich hier vor fünf Jahren das Karlsbad brauchte und ein Kranker auf Dorotheens Aue ohnmächtig niederstürzte und ich den Grafen bat, dem Kranken beizustehen, dem ich allein nicht aufhelfen konnte – da fragte dieser: 'Um Verzeihung – was Standes ist der Mann?' Ich antwortete: 'Das weiß ich nicht – er ist ein Mensch und bedarf unserer Hilfe.' Nachher zeigte es sich, daß der Kranke ein Prager Kaufmannsdiener war, und der vornehme Graf konnte es lange nicht vergessen, daß er sich zur Dienstleistung für einen so gemeinen Mann hat müssen brauchen lassen. In Nieuport habe ich auch kein Fünkchen aristokratischen Stolz bemerkt."

59. See McNeil, "Appearance of Enlightenment," 387.
60. See also Dewald, *European Nobility*, 185.
61. See Corfield, "The Rivals: Landed and Other Gentlemen."
62. Florencourt, *Sittliche Schilderungen*, 1801, 104: "Leuten von Erziehung und gutem Benehmen (gentlemen) und ihrem Gegentheil (not gentlemen)" – "Annehmlichkeit der Gesellschaft" – "Welche Riesenschritte muß aber die Aufklärung noch machen, ehe wir dahin gelangen!"
63. Marcard, *Beschreibung von Pyrmont*, vol. 1, 1784, 102–103: "Gentleman" – "nicht . . . ein Edelmann . . ., sondern ein Mann von guter Erziehung, von feinen Sitten und edler Denkungsart. Ein solcher Mann hat in England in Absicht auf das gesellschaftliche Leben alle Rechte, die sich in Deutschland der Adel allein anmaßt: er gehört in die erste und beste Gesellschaft."
64. Ficker, *Driburger Taschenbuch*, 1811, 107–108: "Der Geschäftsmann und Gelehrte, der, das ganze Jahr hindurch an den Arbeitstisch geschmiedet, seinen Geist auf Kosten seines Körpers anstrengte . . ., alle solche Kranke entfliehen oft so gerne dem Geräusche grosser Städte und sehnen sich, einige Wochen ungestört alles dessen zu geniessen, was den Aufenthalt auf dem Lande für jede nicht ganz verdorbene Seele so anziehend macht. Wünscht man das Leben grosser Städte mit all seinem Prunk . . . überall wieder zu finden, zieht man geräuschvolle Freuden . . . dem gesellschaftlichen stillen Umgange mit gebildeten Personen und den unschuldigen Zeitvertreiben in einer anmuthigen ländlichen Gegend vor, so mag man vielleicht, besonders, wenn man vornehm ist oder vornehm thun will, den für die Gesundheit auch noch so heilsamen Driburger Aufenthalt traurig und langweilig finden; man eile nach Pyrmont, Spaa und andern glänzenden Brunnenörtern und meide vor allem den . . . Weg nach Driburg, wo Kranke aus grossen Städten, eine Zeit lang dem Gewühle und den Sorgen eines erschöpfenden Lebens entrissen, wieder lernen sollen, Geschmack an den Freuden der Natur zu finden." Hufeland describes Driburg in a similar vein: "The tone is sociable and informal, and more comfortable for those seeking peaceful recreation, especially for members of the middling estate who are used to domestic family life, more comfortable than the noisy spa of Pyrmont." ("Der Ton gesellig und ungezwungen, und für den, der friedliche Erholung sucht, insbesondere für den Mittelstand, der häusliches Familienleben gewohnt ist, behaglicher, als das geräuschvolle Pyrmont.") Hufeland, *Praktische Uebersicht der vorzüglichsten Heilquellen Teutschlands*, 1815, 98.
65. See Chapter 5.
66. [Käppel], *Pyrmonts Merkwürdigkeiten*, 1800, 43–44: "Ehedem soll sich hier der deutsche Adelsstolz in seiner ganzen lächerlichen Blösse gezeigt, zwischen sich und den Bürgerlichen eine dicke Scheidewand gezogen, und dem Geiste der allgemeinen gesellschaftlichen Unterhaltung ausserordentlich geschadet haben. Die Fackel der Aufklärung, und noch mehr, der grössere Ruf dieses Brunnens . . . haben endlich über dieses deutsche Vorurtheil gesiegt."
67. [Käppel], *Pyrmonts Merkwürdigkeiten*, 1800, 44: "Viele haben über den Adelsstolz geschrieben, und die Wenigsten scheinen bedacht zu haben, dass der Saame des Hochmuths in jedem menschlichen Herzen liegt, . . . Wie lächerlich ist nicht der Gelehrten- und Kaufmannsstolz!"
68. Schopenhauer, *Im Wechsel der Zeiten*, 196: "Hanseaten eben wie wir auch, bei denen ich bald ganz heimisch mich fühlte."
69. Schopenhauer, *Im Wechsel der Zeiten*, 198: "in der Allee eine lange Tafel."
70. Schopenhauer, *Im Wechsel der Zeiten*, 198: "in eine Art oberflächliche Bekanntschaft geraten, wie das an solchen Orten so leicht geschieht."

71. Schopenhauer, *Im Wechsel der Zeiten*, 198: "Sehr freundlich bemerkte sie, dass wir dadurch des Vorzugs teilhaftig werden würden, uns den großen Dejeuners anschließen zu dürfen. Vergebens erinnerte ich unsere Beschützerin an unsern durchaus nicht hoffähigen Bürgerstand; sie erwiderte, daß an Orten wie diesem auf Hofetikette nicht so strenge gehalten werde."
72. Schopenhauer, *Im Wechsel der Zeiten*, 199: "bei der es die sehr gnädige Herzogin aber nie weiter als zur bloßen Demonstration kommen lasse."
73. Schopenhauer, *Im Wechsel der Zeiten*, 198–199: "Wir, keinem Fürsten untertan, freigeborne Frauen, wir sollten einer anderen Frau, die nicht unsere Mutter oder Großmutter war, die Hand küssen, oder vollends zur Erde uns beugen, um den Saum ihres Gewands zu ergreifen? . . . Der Gedanke, dass man ein solches uns zumuten könne, brachte mein republikanisches Blut in heftige Wallung."
74. Schopenhauer, *Im Wechsel der Zeiten*, 199: "starren reichsstädtischen Sinn."
75. Schopenhauer, *Im Wechsel der Zeiten*, 199: "Belobt von unsern Männern, . . . von unsern übrigen hanseatischen Freunden bis in die Wolken gehoben, dachten wir gar nicht daran, wieviel Stoff zu witzigen Einfällen unser Bürgerhochmut wahrscheinlich dem Tisch an der entgegengesetzten Seite der Allee geliefert haben mochte."
76. Schopenhauer, *Im Wechsel der Zeiten*, 199: "blieben jener Sphäre fern, in deren Nähe wir uns nie gesehnt hatten."
77. See Introduction to Part III.
78. Krieger, *Alexis-Bad*, 1812, 36–38: "Wenn freilich der größere Rang, der Reichthum, . . . auch an dem Cur-Orte, . . . nur ein Gegenstand der Huldigung seyn, und nicht eine der gewohnten Kriechereien aufopfern, nur fordern, und nichts gewähren, nur gebieten, und nicht nachgeben will; . . . wenn er nur das ihm gleiche seiner Annäherung oder Verschmelzung würdig achtet, und ohne die Certificate der Herkunft, des bürgerlichen Charakters oder Vermögens, nirgends den Zutritt verstattet, . . . wenn er es im traulichen Geflüster sogar zu den Uebelständen des Badebesuchs zählt, durch so viele ungebildete, d.h. minder vornehme und begüterte, Mitgäste die Gesellschaft verdorben und entweiht zu sehen, . . . wo die Sachen so stehen, da ist freilich an kein gehaltvolles und erquickendes Gesellschaftswesen zu denken. Dennoch zerschellt es in den Bädern so oft an dieser Klippe, so lautet die allgemeine Klage."
79. Krieger, *Alexis-Bad*, 1812, 38: "Doch die Kehrseite spricht mit gleicher Wahrheit die Beschwerden der andern Parthei aus. Stolz, Starrsinn und Eifersucht der Minderbegünstigten gegen die scheinbaren Lieblinge des Schicksals, oder grundloser Argwohn und Aengstlichkeit haben keinen geringern Antheil an den Verstimmungen des Gesellschaftstons."
80. Willebrand, *Carlsbader Brunnenreise*, 1780, 75: "Lustanstalten" – "Tanzbälle" – "gewisse Brunnengäste, die dafür zu halten scheinen, daß sie nicht aus sündlichem Samen erzeugt sind, – kein Bedeken haben, gegen verdiente Männer von Würde, die gewiß ihre Vorzüge nicht im Glanz ihrer Vorfahren ängstlich suchen dürfen, sich oft bey öffentlichen Versammlungen nicht sonderlich feyn betragen."
81. Willebrand, *Carlsbader Brunnenreise*, 1780, 197: "Wenn oft Brunnengäste vom ersten bürgerlichen Stande Klage führen, daß sie an diesem oder jenem Adelichen eine Begegnung vermissen, deren sie sich doch würdig halten – so ist zuvörderst nur von unerzogenen, ungesitteten Landjunkern die Rede . . . ; denn wer wohlerzogen und gesittet ist, und Verdienste und wahre Würde hat, kann nicht hart, groß und stolz seyn. – Inzwischen sind oft diese Klagen

Folgen eines bloßen Vorurtheils: – denn ich habe oft bemerkt, daß Bürgerliche von Bedeutung in Betracht des Adels und dessen Umgangs ohne alle
Noth ... scheu sind, ... Gewiß, kluge Edelleute wissen es wohl, daß sie den
bürgerlichen Stand nicht lange entbehren können."

82. Marcard, *Beschreibung von Pyrmont*, vol. 1, 1784, 51–115, quote 51:
"Vom gesellschaftliche Leben in Pyrmont."

83. Marcard, *Beschreibung von Pyrmont*, vol. 1, 1784, 84–85: "So viel ist wol
unstreitig gewiß, daß das Adelswesen, dieses auf das gesellschaftliche Leben
der Deutschen mit mächtigen Einflusse würkende Principium, eine von den
wahren Ursachen sey, warum die Aufklärung unter uns im Ganzen nicht so
gedeiht ... Der Adelsstolz zieht in Deutschland offenbar eine Linie zwischen
sich und dem einsichtsvollen und aufgeklärten Theil der Menschen; entfernt
diejenigen von sich, die durch würckliche Thalente ganz allein sich empor
schwungen."

84. Marcard, *Beschreibung von Pyrmont*, vol. 1, 1784, 100: "Ich behaupte
keinesweges, daß sich schlechterdings niemals einzelne Fälle in Pyrmont
zugetragen hätten, bey welchen dergleichen Klagen sich auf Thatsachen
gründeten. ... so kann gar wol irgend einmal ein baurenstolzer Edelmann
nach Pyrmont verschlagen seyn; oder eine fette, von ihrem Adel aufge-
triebene Dame, sich eine Grobheit gegen einen Unadelichen erlaubt, ...
haben."

85. Marcard, *Beschreibung von Pyrmont*, vol. 1, 1784, 92: "Dennoch giebt
es heut zu Tage schon ... eine Menge vortreflicher hochachtungswürdiger
Personen von Adel, ... die nicht blos edel geboren, sondern auch edel
gesinnt sind, und grade über den Adel so denken, wie man vernünftiger
Weise darüber denken soll."

86. Marcard, *Beschreibung von Pyrmont*, vol. 1, 1784, 111: "Einige beklagen
sich über die Zurückhaltung des Adels, und haben sich schlechterdings über
sich selbst zu beklagen. Sie zeigen einen solchen Scheu und so viel respect-
artige Furchtsamkeit, daß sie selbst hierdurch allein die ganze Distinction
bewürken, über die sie klagen, weil sie damit anzuerkennen scheinen, ein
Edelmann oder eine Edelfrau seyen Wesen von ganz anderer Art als sie."

87. Marcard, *Beschreibung von Pyrmont*, vol. 1, 1784, 74–75: "Uebrigens ist
der Umgang leicht und ungezwungen in Pyrmont, und hat eine gewisse Frey-
müthigkeit, die man sonst unter dieser nordlichen Breite nicht leicht mehr
findet. Man redet ohne Bedenken jedermann an, in dessen Bekanntschaft
man eingeführt ist, oder macht die Bekanntschaft selbst; man nähert sich
jedem Cirkel nach Gefallen, um an der Conversation Theil zu nehmen.
... Alles zusammen führt zu einer nicht unangenehmen Freyheit und
Unbefangenheit."

88. See Schopenhauer, *A Lady Travels*, 115–117. Schopenhauer describes "the
English Master of Ceremonies" as bearing "a slight resemblance to the doctors in some of the German spas, where during the promenade or at public
eating places they flutter around both the healthy and the sick, setting everything in order, knowing everything, being everywhere and nowhere at the
same time" (117). Strikingly, Möser does not suggest that Marcard or any
other spa physician take on the role of "spa king."

89. Obviously, Möser was aware that the prince of Waldeck and Pyrmont would
not be willing to grant someone the title of "king," even if only as a kind of
nickname.

90. Möser, *Briefwechsel*, letter from Möser to Matthias Marcard, 1784, 659:
"Also, wenn der Brunnen-König, welchen der Fürst, jedoch absque titulo,
setzen müßte, es nur dahin leitete, daß immer ein billig denkender Grosser

das erste Frühstück gäbe, so würde das schon vieles würken; und überhaupt müß[t]e dieser die Grossen, die insgemein herablassend sind und worüber man sich in Pyrmont am wenigsten zu beklagen hat, zu bewegen wissen, den Geringeren zuvorzukommen und sich ein Geschäffte daraus zu machen, dem Beyspiel des Fürsten nachzuahmen. Die kleinen Gewürme werden dann von selbst nachkriechen."

91. Möser, *Briefwechsel*, letter from Möser to Matthias Marcard, 1784, 659: "ohne Unterschied des Standes."

92. See Melton, *Rise of the Public*, 12.

93. *Reise nach den Badeörtern*, 1798, 258–259: "sehr gut aufgebaut" – "der großmüthigen Vorsorge ihres Fürsten zu verdancken, der überhaupt ein sehr vortrefflicher Mann seyn muß, da alles an diesem Orte, Polizei, Ordnung, Anbau und Anpflanzung, von Weisheit, Geschmack, Menschenliebe zeugt. Er thut alles mögliche für die Bequemlichkeit und das Vergnügen der Kurgäste."

94. Göckingk, "Von dem Kurbrunnen bei Brückenau," 1782, 329: "über hundert tausend Gulden" – "unermüdet" – "ohne die Untertanen zu drücken."

95. Göckingk here echoes the well-known contemporary proverb "Unterm Krummstab ist gut leben." A few years later, in 1785, the Fulda canon Philipp Anton von Bibra initiated a discussion about this issue with a prize question in the *Journal von und für Deutschland*. The result was a largely uniform condemnation of ecclesiastical territories by Enlightenment authors. See Aretin, *Das Alte Reich*, 266–267.

96. Göckingk, "Von dem Kurbrunnen bei Brückenau," 1782, 329: "Unter Krumstab ist gut wohnen, wenn alle geistlichen Fürsten diesem gleich wären. Jeder Fremde, der durch sein Land reist, wird überall Spuren seiner vortrefflichen Art zu denken und zu Handeln finden."

97. Marcard, *Beschreibung von Pyrmont*, vol. 1, 1784, 107: "Wer das Glück hat, den regierenden Fürsten von Waldeck zu kennen, der wird sehr gern glauben, daß an einem so aufgeklärten, Vorurtheilfreyen Prinzen, an einem so vertrauten Freunde und Kenner der Wissenschaften, die thörichte Distinctionssucht in Pyrmont keinen Beschützer habe. Ohne Rücksicht auf Geburt pflegen anständige Leute aus allerley Ständen zur Fürstlichen Tafel gezogen zu werden."

98. [Hassencamp], *Briefe eines Reisenden von Pyrmont*, 1783, 35–36: "Der Fürst von Waldeck . . . , ein sehr leutseliger und herablassender Herr, wie auch sein ganzer Hof, an dem sich viele vortreffliche Männer, . . . befinden, thun zwar alles was nach der Lage der Sachen nur immer möglich ist, um dieser Ostindische Casten-Differenz aufzuheben, allein sie sind damit noch nicht so glücklich, wie der Fürst von Fulda in Brückenau gewesen."

99. Hirschfeld, *Theorie der Gartenkunst*, vol. 5, 1785, 95: "der vortreffliche Prinz, der mit der edlen, offenen Güte des Herzens . . . so viel seinen Geschmack und so viel Sorgfalt für das Vergnügen aller Fremden vereiniget, die hier zusammen strömen, der so gerne mitten unter ihnen verweilt, und den Fürsten verbirgt, um ganz Mitgesellschafter zu seyn, und rings um sich her Freyheit, Geselligkeit und Heiterkeit zu verbreiten."

100. Hirschfeld, *Theorie der Gartenkunst*, vol. 5, 1785, 102: "Man erblickt hier einen Prinzen, der, wenn er bauet, pflanzt und verschönert, ganz Fürst ist, aber, um Natur und Geselligkeit zu genießen, und genießen zu lassen, sich wieder in dem Privatmann verbirgt, bey den Brunnengästen seine stille Wohnung hat, an ihrer Tafel und selbst bey ihren Spielen und Tänzen verweilt."

101. "Teutsche Badechronik," *JLM* (October 1796), 521: "Es wird wohl erzählt, man habe gegen den Landgrafen Zweifel geäußert, ob die Interessen seines

Capitals herauskommen würden: worauf er geantwortet, es werde sich hin-
länglich verinteressieren, wenn auch nur Einige ihre Gesundheit da fänden."
See also Hufeland, *Praktische Uebersicht der vorzüglichsten Heilquellen
Teutschlands*, 1831, 151–152. See also Chapter 1.

102. Wilhelmina Caroline was the daughter of King Frederick V of Denmark and
Norway.

103. Hirschfeld, *Theorie der Gartenkunst*, vol. 5, 1785, 102: "eine Prinzessin...,
die, so sehr sie Dänemarks Ruhm unter den Deutschen ... ist, sich dieser
seltenen Vorzüge nicht erinnert, und, ... rings um sich her die Liebe aller
Herzen zu sich in den Kreis der jungen glücklichen Familie strömen." Similarly, the *Journal des Luxus und der Moden* reported about King Frederick
William of Prussia and his family during their visit to Pyrmont in 1797:
"The royal family was without doubt the most beautiful pattern of harmony and love here." – "Die königliche Familie war hier ohnstreitig das
schönste Muster von Eintracht und Liebe." "Badechronik," *JLM* (November 1797), 558.

104. See Wilhelm I. von Hessen, *Wir Wilhelm*, 206–207, 229–230.

105. Umbach, "Culture and *Bürgerlichkeit*," 199, see 190–191. See also Outram,
Enlightenment, 124.

106. Maurer, *Biographie des Bürgers*, 591: "Das Bürgertum feiert sich selbst
und sanktioniert seine Werte, indem es sie Fürsten ... zuschreibt." See also
Berger, *Anna Amalia*, 474; Paulmann, *Pomp und Politik*, 209. For the larger
context, see Büschel, *Untertanenliebe*.

107. "Badechronik," *JLM* (December 1798), 680: "Denn gesellschaftliche Verbesserungen müssen noch mehr als die meisten übrigen von oben herab
kommen." Langewiesche agrees that bourgeois criticism of the nobility usually excluded ruling princes. He argues, however, that rulers of small and
mid-sized territories were the targets of bourgeois criticism. See Langewiesche, "Bürgerliche Adelskritik," 19. This is not the case in the published spa
discourse.

108. See Blackbourn, *The Long Nineteenth Century*, 42–43, 102.

109. Schopenhauer, *Im Wechsel der Zeiten*, 197: "die Allee herunterwalzt" –
"Blumenmädchen" – "Humanität."

110. Schopenhauer, *Im Wechsel der Zeiten*, 197: "Daß sie nicht mehr mit der
Krone auf dem Haupte, das Szepter in der Hand herumspazierten, wußte ich
längst, aber so durchaus herablassend und human, so frei von jedem Nimbus, den ich in der äußern Erscheinung eines solchen Gebieters über Leben
und Freiheit seiner Untertanen mir unzertrennlich dachte, den hohen Herrn
zu finden wäre mir nie eingefallen." Of course, as already discussed, it was
not really problematic for a nobleman, even from the high nobility, to dance
with a middle- or even lower-class woman, although the reverse was not
true. Schopenhauer's story about the "flower girl" reads as if it were meant
as an illustration of the general demeanor of the duke of Mecklenburg-
Schwerin in Pyrmont.

111. Pütter, *Selbstbiographie*, vol. 2, 554–555: "Gewöhnlich kam der regierende
Fürst von Waldeck zur Brunnenzeit jährlich mit seinem ganzen Hofstaate
von Arolsen nach Pyrmont ... Mit der Art, wie er ... die ganze Gesellschaft
mit Berufung guter Schauspieler, wie auch mit Concerten, und auf eigne
Kosten veranstalteten Illuminationen, oder Feuerwerken zu beleben suchte,
und wie er meist täglich eine Anzahl Brunnengäste, ohne auf Verschiedenheit
des Standes zu sehen, zur Tafel bitten ließ, wurden die Vortheile des Aufent-
haltes zu Pyrmont noch erhöht."

112. Pütter, *Selbstbiographie*, vol. 2, 847: "Personen von so erhabenem Stande
auch nur zu sehen, – sie mehrere Tage nach einander in verschiedenen

Verhältnissen zu sehen, . . . [war] noch ungleich größerer Gewinn, wenn sie sich bis zu Gesprächen mit unser einem herablassen; – ein Glück, dessen ich mich mehrfach zu erfreuen gehabt habe."

113. Landgrave Wilhelm I of Hesse-Kassel was Count Wilhelm IX of Hanau before succeeding his father to the landgraviate.

114. Lavater, *Reisetagebücher*, 296: "Dann und wann [kam] ein Höfling . . . , nicht förmlich, sondern nur beyläufig zu sagen, der Landgraf würde mich gerne sehen. 'Ich stehe zu seinen Befehlen,' und dabey blieb's. Ich gehe gewiß keinem Fürsten ein Schrittgen, das Zudringlichkeit scheinen könnte, entgegen."

115. Recke, *Tagebücher und Selbstzeugnisse*, 130: "über die Schwierigkeiten, daß Könige und Fürsten gute Menschen sein können."

116. "Badechronik," *JLM* (November 1797), 545: "kleine Höfe bildeten."

117. [Schulz], *Reise eines Liefländers*, 1795, 98: "Es bilden sich Höfchen, die auf einander eifersüchtig sind; man macht kleine Ränke, bekrittelt sich, sucht oder erdichtet Lächerlichkeiten; mit einem Worte: man spielt das gewöhnliche armselige Spiel, das den mitverwickelten Personen unendlich wichtig scheint."

118. Möser, *Briefwechsel*, letter from Möser to Matthias Marcard, 1784, 659: "Sonst ist es ein altes Sprichwort: gleich und gleich gesellt sich gern, und Bekannte halten sich zu Bekannten."

119. See Introduction to Part III.

120. *Lauchstädt, ein kleines Gemählde*, 1787, 34: "formiren eine eigene Gesellschaft" – "Von dieser ist nun gewöhnlich auch der Gelehrte ausgeschlossen, weil diese Herren auch so ihre eigenen Begriffe haben." Note the ironic use of the term "Herren" for merchants, a reference to their alleged arrogance.

121. [Möller], *Der Adelsstolz im Bade zu Lauchstädt*, 1791, 9: "Wenn jemand keinen Stammbaum aufweisen kann, daß er bey hohen Stiftern Domherrenstellen erhalten und an fürstlichen Höfen erscheinen darf, und sich dennoch, ohne Cavalier zu seyn, mit seiner Frau vom Bürgervolke gnädig nennen läßt, so heißt es bey uns, er ist nicht von Familie."

122. *Lauchstädt, ein kleines Gemählde*, 1787, 32: "Selbst derjenige Mann, dem seine Talente und die Dienste, welche er seinem Fürsten leistete, einen adelichen Rang erwarben, muß auch diese Absonderung fühlen, und den Adel von seiner Höhe auf sich herabblicken lassen."

123. "Badechronik," *JLM* (November 1797), 546: "kleine häusliche Zirkel" – "die stillern, eigentlichen Freuden der gebildeten Geselligkeit." See also *Reise nach den Badeörtern*, 1798, 167.

124. Baggesen, *Labyrinth*, 1789, 165–166: "Zu den besonderen täglichen Vergnügen gehören die kleinen Teegesellschaften, bei denen sich ein begrenzter Kreis von Bekannten versammelt. Gemeinsam mit Moltke verbrachte ich manche angenehme Stunde in einer solchen, wo die kluge, gute, sehr interessante Frau von Voigt aus Osnabrück präsidierte."

125. See Becker, *Vor hundert Jahren*; Recke, *Mein Journal*; Recke, *I. Aufzeichnungen und Briefe*; Recke, *II. Tagebücher und Briefe*; Recke, *Tagebücher und Selbstzeugnisse*.

126. "Badechronik," *JLM* (November 1800), 589–590: "Die Herzogin von Curland nebst ihren schönen Töchtern bildete einen Kreis, in welchem ein sehr fröhlicher und zwangloser Ton geherrscht haben soll." The year 1800 is unfortunately not covered by the diaries analyzed here.

127. See Recke, *II. Tagebücher und Briefe*, 426–442. See also [Schwarz], *Briefe einer Curländerin*, 89, for a slightly different list of members. The composition of the circle clearly changed both over time and from year to year.

128. See *Liste der angekommenen Kur- und Badegäste in der königl[ichen] Stadt Kaiser-Karlsbad im Jahre 1795*, 3: "Herr Graf von Nieuport, Kommandeur des Malterserordens, aus Brüßel."

129. Göckingk, who was ennobled in 1789, contributed journal articles to the spa discourse, in which he praised Brückenau for its informal atmosphere and condemned Lauchstädt for "noble separation," but these articles were published several years before his own ennoblement.

130. Herder was ennobled in 1802, one year before his death.

131. Schulz is the author of *Reise eines Liefländers*. On Schulz, see also Recke, *II. Tagebücher und Briefe*, 344.

132. Significantly, the Frankfurt burgher Goethe constructed his status as an ennobled bourgeois as a confirmation of his patrician origins. See Recke, *Tagebücher und Selbstzeugnisse*, 9–33; Maurer, "Goethe als Prototyp."

133. *Lauchstädt, ein kleines Gemählde*, 1787, 34.

134. "Badechronik," *JLM* (November 1800), 590.

135. This, in turn, confirms the potential of the published spa discourse to convince the enlightened nobility of the validity of its arguments.

136. Pauline zur Lippe and Herzog Friedrich Christian von Augustenburg, *Briefe*, 5 July 1791, 165: "Freylich weiß ich, daß unsre Classe von Ihnen nicht geliebt wird, daß ich mich schon bisweilen vergebens bemühte, Sie mit derselben auszusöhnen und daß leider immer mehr Erfahrung mich lehrt, Ihr Urtheil im Allgemeinen sei leider richtig."

137. Recke, *Tagebücher und Selbstzeugnisse*, 15: "Meine Geburt setzt mich leider in den Zirkel der Adeligen, der mich drückende Rang meiner Schwester als Herzogin zieht mich an Höfe und in die Kreise der vornehmen Welt. Aber in diesen Zirkeln . . . finde ich nur selten Charaktere, die ich hochachten kann. Im aufgeklärten Mittelstande fand ich von jeher meine liebsten und meisten Freunde."

138. Quoted in Recke, *II. Tagebücher und Briefe*, 418: "Daß ich sie nebst ihrer Frau in unsrer Pirmonter Einsamkeit wünsche, werden Sie nathürlich finden. Es herrscht hier durchgehends Harmonie, die Pirmonter Colonie führt ein Leben, welches das Ideal übertrift, das Platner uns vom goldnen Zeitalter in Carlsbad machte; wir sind fromm und froh wie gute Kinder, in mancher Rücksicht aufgeklärt und religioese in der Ausübung des Geboths: Du sollst deinen Nächsten lieben als dich selbst." The published spa discourse often uses the term "golden age" as a general reference to a carefree life at the spa. See also Krieger, *Alexis-Bad*, 1812, 48.

139. See Recke, *II. Tagebücher und Briefe*, 164; Becker, *Vor hundert Jahren*, 157. In a letter to Duke Carl August of 15 August 1785, Goethe described the atmosphere in Karlsbad as being very sociable. See Goethe, *Briefe – Tagebücher – Gespräche*, 3401 (i.e. Goethe-WA-IV, vol. 7, 74). On the cult of friendship in the eighteenth century, see, e.g., Adam, "Freundschaft."

140. See Göckingk, "Lied am Sprudel zu singen," 1785; [Giseke], "Fortsetzung der Briefe über Carlsbad," 1793, 807–808.

141. See Recke, *II. Tagebücher und Briefe*, 338. According to the published discourse, the Saxon hall in Karlsbad was usually monopolized by the nobility.

142. See Recke, *Tagebücher und Selbstzeugnisse*, 132.

143. Blackbourn, *The Long Nineteenth Century*, 39.

144. See Nowitzki, "Curriculum Vitae," 365.

145. See Recke, *Tagebücher und Selbstzeugnisse*, 126, 127, 129, 131, 132.

146. Recke, *Tagebücher und Selbstzeugnisse*, 122: "nicht geniert würde" – "Natürlich nahm ich dies in Nicolais Namen dankbar an und schätzte den guten Prinzen . . . noch höher – doch fürchte ich, dass unsre Gesellschaft jetzt steifer wird, als sie sonst gewesen wäre."

147. Recke, *Tagebücher und Selbstzeugnisse*, 122: "Nur der König von Polen und meine Daria wissen in jeder Gesellschaft den Ton froher Geselligkeit so hinein zu bringen, daß man ihren Stand vergißt und ihren Umgang wohltätig findet. Der Prinz von Augustenburg erreichte seine gute Absicht beim besten Willen nicht."

148. Böttiger, *Literarische Zustände*, 338–339: "Anekdote von Platner" – "Als er [Platner] vor 4 Jahren im Carlsbade als Hofphilosoph der Augusten-burger Herrschaften so manche Blöße gab, hatt er unter [anderm] auch die Gewohnheit, die liebenswürdige Prinzessin von Augustenburg bey jedem Spaziergang, wie ein Gespenst, zu verfolgen, u[nd] diese schien auch kein Misbehagen daran zu finden, statt des Schooßhündchens einen Philosophen neben sich her wedeln zu lassen. Allein den übrigen Cammerherrn u[nd] Nobili unter den Badegästen war der Schulfuchs, der ihren Cirkeln die schöne Prinzessin so oft entführte, äussert fatal. Eben war ein Böhmischer Graf angekommen, der Platnern in Wien hatte kennen lernen. Diesen nehmen die andern auf die Seite und instruiren ihn. Plötzlich kommt dieser in einer Allee auf ihn zu, als er eben die Prinzessin führt, freut sich seines Wiedersehns, und fragt ganz unschuldig, ohne eine Präsentation abzuwarten: *und die Dame an ihrer Hand, Herr Doctor, gewiß ihre Patientin?* Die Prinzessin ging eilig davon, u[nd] seitdem nie wieder mit Platnern allein." (Italics in the original.)

149. See Becker, *Vor hundert Jahren.*

150. [Hassencamp], *Briefe eines Reisenden von Pyrmont*, 1783, 24: "am Hofe und im Bade seyn." See also Göckingk, "Von dem Kurbrunnen bei Brü-ckenau," 1782, 337.

151. Becker, *Vor hundert Jahren*, 45: "ganz ohne Zwang."

152. Becker, *Vor hundert Jahren*, 82: "Elise ist heute zum erstenmal bei Hofe gewesen, aber ziemlich unzufrieden mit dem Tone an selbigem zurückgekehrt. Ich habe meine Zeit indessen recht angenehm in Bodes Gesellschaft ver-bracht." After leaving Weimar, Bode, Becker, and Recke had a conversation in the carriage that once again contrasted the enlightened convictions of their (spa) circle with the social atmosphere in the residence town of Weimar under Duke Karl August: "Bode frightened Elise [Elisa von der Recke] with his usual whim, [arguing] that she had made many enemies in Weimar by expressing her view about the value of the word 'von' so freely, . . . I then asked Bode how one could still have such limited notions about the nobility of human beings in such an enlightened town, squeezed my Elise's hand with the assurance that her correct view of the nobility was only the least of her merits in my eyes, and I expressed my surprise once again that the people in Weimar were still sitting in such darkness [were unenlightened]." ("Bode machte Elisen mit seiner gewöhnlichen Laune bange, daß sie sich durch ihr freies Bekenntnis über den Wert des Wörtchens von viel Feinde in Weimar gemacht hätte, . . . Ich fragte Bode hierauf, wie man denn in seinem so aufgeklärten Orte noch so eingeschränkte Begriffe über den Adel des Men-schen haben könnte, drückte meiner Elise mit der Versicherung die Hand, daß dieser ihr richtiger Blick über den Adel bei mir nur ihr allergeringstes Verdienst wäre, und wunderte mich nochmals, daß die Leute in Weimar noch in solcher Dunkelheit säßen.") Becker, *Vor hundert Jahren*, 82–83.

153. Becker, *Vor hundert Jahren*, 187: "In dem Hause des Herrn Nikolai bin ich oft, und bringe meistens die Abende da zu, wenn Elise die Höfe besucht."

154. Berger, *Anna Amalia*, 474: "Die überständischen Beziehungsideale ließen sich nicht in den Handlungsraum Hof übertragen." See also note 152.

155. See Goethe, Vulpius, *Goethes Briefwechsel mit seiner Frau*, vols. 1 and 2 (passim).

156. See Damm, *Christiane und Goethe*, 20–101 (passim).

157. On Christiane's isolated life and the hostilities she experienced in Weimar, see Goethe, Vulpius, *Goethes Briefwechsel mit seiner Frau*, vol. 1, XL–XLI.
158. Quoted in article "Goethe, Christiane von," in: Jeßing, Lutz, Wilds, *Metzler Goethe Lexikon*, 184: "anspruchsloser, heller, ganz natürlicher Verstand."
159. See, e.g., Goethe, Vulpius, *Goethes Briefwechsel mit seiner Frau*, vol. 1, letter-diary from Lauchstädt, 27 June–4 July 1803, 399; letter-diary from Lauchstädt, 4–10 July 1803, 410.
160. Karl August was duke of Saxe-Weimar and Saxe-Eisenach. In 1809 he became duke, and in 1815 grand duke of Saxe-Weimar-Eisenach. He ennobled Karoline Jagemann in 1809 as Baroness von Heygendorff.
161. Goethe, Vulpius, *Goethes Briefwechsel mit seiner Frau*, vol. 1, letter-diary from Lauchstädt, 27 June–4 July 1803, 399: "eine bürgerliche Gesellschaft."
162. See, e.g., Goethe, Vulpius, *Goethes Briefwechsel mit seiner Frau*, vol. 1, letter from Lauchstädt, 11 July 1803, 414–415; letter from Lauchstädt, 12–13 July 1803, 418. This did not markedly change after Christiane's marriage to Goethe: she still belonged to a small, middle-class spa circle and a larger circle that included nobles. See, e.g., Goethe, Vulpius, *Goethes Briefwechsel mit seiner Frau*, vol. 2, letter from Lauchstädt, 15 July 1810, 172, 174.
163. Goethe, Vulpius, *Goethes Briefwechsel mit seiner Frau*, vol. 1, letter from Lauchstädt, 11 July 1803, 414: "artiger" – "als gegen andere Leute."
164. Goethe, Vulpius, *Goethes Briefwechsel mit seiner Frau*, vol. 1, letter from Lauchstädt, 11 July 1803, 414, 415: "so viel Weimarer" – "mit ansehen" – "erstaunt."
165. [Schulz], *Reise eines Liefländers*, 1795, 77: "ein paar Postzüge, eine diamantene Hutschleife."
166. See Goethe, Vulpius, *Goethes Briefwechsel mit seiner Frau*, vol. 1, letter-diary from Lauchstädt, 27 June–4 July 1803, 401; letter from Lauchstädt, 12–13 July 1803, 419.
167. Damm, *Christiane und Goethe*, 368.
168. Goethe, Vulpius, *Goethes Briefwechsel mit seiner Frau*, vol. 1, letter-diary from Lauchstädt, 4–10 July 1803, 413: "mir ist, als finge ich erst an zu leben."
169. Goethe, Vulpius, *Goethes Briefwechsel mit seiner Frau*, vol. 1, letter from Lauchstädt, 23 July 1803, 429: "Die Adelichen fangen an, allerhand dummes Zeug zu machen; man erzählt allerlei, was sie gegen die Bürgerlichen haben. Ich selbst weiß nichts, gegen mich sind sie alle artig." See also 410.
170. See Introduction to Part III.
171. See Kuhnert, *Urbanität*, 128–136. In Karl Philipp Moritz's autobiographical novel *Anton Reiser*, Anton and his father live far away from the center of Pyrmont because they cannot afford an accommodation closer to the spa district with its healing well. See Moritz, *Anton Reiser*, 29–30.
172. Marcard puts the start time for the peasants at 3 am, while Frankenau and Käppel put it at 4 am. See Marcard, *Beschreibung von Pyrmont*, vol. 1, 1784, 56; Frankenau, *Pyrmont*, 1799, 62; [Käppel], *Pyrmonts Merkwürdigkeiten*, 1800, 46.
173. See Frankenau, *Pyrmont*, 1799, 26–27, 63–64; Piepenbring, *Bemerkungen über die Schrift des Herrn Doctor Frankenau*, 1801, 17; Kuhnert, *Urbanität*, 137. On the poor in Hessian spas, see Vanja, "Arme Hessen."
174. See Marcard, *Beschreibung von Pyrmont*, vol. 1, 1784, 56; Piepenbring, *Bemerkungen über die Schrift des Herrn Doctor Frankenau*, 1801, 18.
175. The aforementioned "servant of a merchant from Prague" was another typical member of this group.
176. See Kuhnert, *Urbanität*, 136; see also Chapter 1.

177. See Kuhnert, *Urbanität*, 137, 134–138, quote 135: "'honette Personen' des mittleren Standes."
178. For example the so-called "Building for the Jews" (*Judenbau*) in Wilhelms-bad. See also [Merveilleux], *Amusemens des eaux de Schwalbach*, 1739, 19; Kuhnert, *Urbanität*, 202.
179. See Kuhnert, *Urbanität*, 204. Hannah Lotte Lund and Natalie Naimark-Goldberg have shown the possibilities and limitations that Jewish women experienced in their interactions at the spas. See Lund, *Der Berliner "jüdische Salon,"* 275–328; Naimark-Goldberg, "Health."
180. See, e.g., Frankenau, *Pyrmont*, 1799, 54; *Reise nach den Badeörtern*, 1798, 124; "Badechronik," *JLM* (May 1798), 291. See also Naimark-Goldberg, "Health," 77–78.
181. Göckingk, "Von dem Kurbrunnen bei Brückenau," 1782, 337–338: "Es war bei meiner Anwesenheit ein Jude da, der sich zwar für einen Christen ausgab, auch einen andern Namen angenommen hatte, jedermann wußt aber, daß er ein Jude war. Indeß that niemand als wenn er es wüßte, sondern begegnete ihm höflich, ja freundschaftlich, denn der Jude war ein Mann, der zu leben wußte. Man wird aus diesem einzigen Zuge schon schliessen, daß in diesem Bade eines katolischen geistlichen Fürsten viel Toleranz herschen müsse, und würklich ist es auch so."
182. [Giseke], "Fortsetzung der Briefe über Carlsbad," 1793, 813–814: "Sollten die jetzigen Nationen einmal, gleich den alten Römern und Griechen unterge-hen, und unsre europäische Sprachen sich als todte Sprachen erhalten, so wird man, wenn mitten in Deutschland und überall französische Inschriften gefunden werden, glauben, daß Frankreich eine Universalmonarchie gehabt, und sich Alles unterworfen habe." Little did Giseke know that this was an almost prophetic statement and that much of Germany would indeed soon be under French rule.
183. "Badechronik," *JLM* (November 1798), 627: "Auch fand ich dort zu meiner großen Freude die deutsche Sprache herrschend. Denn wenn auch unter manchen die ersten Complimente französisch abgelegt wurden, so wurde doch nachher die Unterredung deutsch fortgeführt. Dies deucht mich, muß doch jeden Teutschen freuen, wenn er übrigens auch noch so sehr überzeugt ist, daß die französische Sprache äußerst bequem ist, im Fach der Diploma-tik, um sich politisch zu hintergehen, oder wenn man . . . sprechen will und sich nichts zu sagen hat."
184. [Schulz], *Reise eines Liefländers*, 1795, 98: "Es kommen nämlich hierher nicht Kranke schlechtweg, sondern: Kranke von der Böhmischen Nation und Kranke von der Sächsischen; jetzt kommen noch Kranke von der Kurländischen und von der Polnischen Nation. Jede dieser Nationen will die erste seyn."
185. Goethe, Vulpius, *Goethes Briefwechsel mit seiner Frau*, vol. 1, letter from Karlsbad, 28 July 1806, 470: "Gestern begegneten mir Frau von Brösigke und ihre Tochter, die von Egerbrunn herüberkamen, wo es auch nicht zum heiteresten hergehen soll, weil die Östreicher und Polen zwei Parteien machen, die gegeneinander wirken, beide aber weder einen Sachsen, noch einen Preußen unter sich aufnehmen." See also Schopenhauer, "Das Bade-leben in Karlsbad während der Monate Julius und August im Jahre 1815," 289–290.
186. Kalckreuth, "Vertraute Rückrufe des Reisenden," 942: "die Engländer," "die Russen," "Franzosen," "Polen," "der Deutsche."
187. Würgler, *Medien*, 126: "Einer der wirkungsvollsten Effekte der Zensur dürfte die Selbstzensur gewesen sein, der sich Autoren und Autorinnen

präventiv unterwarfen. Der Mechanismus der Selbstzensur ist nur selten konkret nachzuweisen." See also Fulbrook, Rublack, "In Relation," 271: "the cultural force of self-silencing."

188. Ryba, *Karlsbad*, 1828, 201: "In Karlsbad wählt sich Jeder seine Gesellschaft selbst nach eignem Geschmacke, nach dem Grade seiner Bildung, und wechselt damit nach Gefallen. Einige halten sich nur an Leute ihres Ranges, andre an Menschen, die ihrem Geiste näher verwandt sind."

189. This is a reference to Don Quixote.

190. Hlawácek, *Karlsbad*, 1838, 118: "Das darf natürlich nicht übel genommen werden, wenn man etwa nicht so ganz leichten Zutritt zu den Cercles der höheren Stände findet, und wir bemerken, dass jeder, der mit dem Ton dieser Stände nicht auf's Innigste vertraut ist, ihnen auch ferne bleiben möge, wenn er dort nicht die Rolle des Ritters von der traurigen Gestalt spielen will; wer aber im Besitze dieses Tones ist, findet dort sicher Zutritt, wenn er auch nicht der *gentry* entstammt. Uebrigens wird kein Stand sich zu beklagen haben, dass er in Karlsbad isolirt stehe. Jeder findet hier Menschen genug, die seines Gleichen sind." (Italics in the original.)

191. Blackbourn, "'Taking the Waters'," 450, see 449–450.

192. See Zadoff, *Next Year in Marienbad*.

Conclusion

This history of the German spa in the long eighteenth century has revealed the cultural and social significance of the spa that went far beyond the search for bodily healing. The published discourse and the personal narratives of spa visitors show the central role of the spa in laying the groundwork for the modern tourist experience as well as in multiplying Enlightenment ideas about social equality. Furthermore, this study has focused on gradual changes in discourses and perceptions during the long eighteenth century, especially during the watershed period (*Sattelzeit*) of the late eighteenth and early nineteenth centuries. The dissemination of new perceptions of nature and of new social ideals and practices through the spa discourse made apparent the "meandering" emergence of cultural and social modernity. This process was characterized by gradual and uneven change to a much higher degree than grand narratives have often implied.

New elite perceptions of mountains and the seacoast had developed in Europe in the early to mid-eighteenth century, and spas and seaside resorts were instrumental in propagating these new cultural ideas in the German lands during the late eighteenth and early nineteenth centuries. As spatial heterotopias, spas became early tourist destinations. Authors of spa publications guided their readers' perception of the interior spaces of spas and seaside resorts as well as the surrounding landscape and the seacoast. In addition to directing the "tourist gaze,"[1] the published discourse informed spa visitors how to move in these spaces and prepared them for the daily routine of leisure activities at these resorts.

Spas were increasingly frequented by the rising bourgeoisie, and thus demands for recognition and equal treatment by the nobility became a defining feature of the published discourse from the middle of the eighteenth century onward. The prevailing discursive regime of the late eighteenth and early nineteenth centuries was "bourgeois" in the sense that it constructed a bourgeois identity in relation to the nobility. It was "enlightened" in the sense that it referenced Enlightenment principles like freedom and equality and embraced enlightened members of the nobility. Contemporaries' experiences at the spa showed the possibilities and limitations of demands for bourgeois equality. Even though the spa as a whole never became the ideal social heterotopia that the published discourse wanted it to be, the spa's role in disseminating new social ideas and as a meeting place for the enlightened elite was significant. As such, the German spa was an important eighteenth-century "arena of sociability,"[2] on par with Masonic lodges, coffeehouses, salons, reading societies, and other spaces of the Enlightenment public sphere.

The transformations of the spa between the late Middle Ages and the early eighteenth century laid the foundation for the spa's cultural and social significance from the mid-eighteenth century onward. Medical treatment at spas changed considerably over the course of the early modern era. While bathing as a curative practice continued throughout the period and beyond, the practices of drinking the healing waters and showering were added in the late sixteenth century. The establishment of spas with cold mineral waters in addition to hot springs caused the number of spas to grow, and drinking the waters became the most common spa practice during the seventeenth century. Typical early modern spa visits were more focused on healing than leisure, but this changed over the course of the eighteenth century. Improved conditions for travel – new roadways, stagecoaches – led to an increase in spa visits. As the bourgeoisie became more prosperous, members of the middle class were able to frequent spas in ever higher numbers. As a result, existing spas expanded and the number of spas increased. By the late eighteenth century, spas were furnished with elaborate leisure facilities.

The success of individual spas was determined by two major factors: first, the party responsible for taking the initiative in the development and expansion of a spa and, second, the number and social makeup of the spa visitors. Spa developers ranged from private individuals and urban magistrates to princes. Most eighteenth-century German spas were either created or expanded by princes, who also provided tax relief and commissioned advertising material, among other measures. It is significant that the majority of spas in eighteenth-century Germany were owned by rulers of small and mid-sized territories. Owning a spa heightened the prestige of the prince who could serve as host to other rulers of higher rank. Therefore, many spas served as summer residences for their owners.

The number of guests per season was a clear indicator of a spa's success among the spa-going public and defined its place in the hierarchy of spas. During the eighteenth and early nineteenth centuries, the number of spa visitors ranged from under 50 individuals to over 1,000 "parties." Usually, there was a correlation between the social rank of the spa guests and the spa's catchment area: many visitors from the high nobility and a large European catchment area went hand in hand. Even though guest lists were unreliable, we have enough information to identify a hierarchy of *teutsche* spas with Karlsbad and Pyrmont at the top, followed by Aachen, Schwalbach, and Lauchstädt. The spas' role as early tourist spaces and social heterotopias in the late eighteenth and early nineteenth centuries laid the basis for the exponential growth in the number of guests at some spas from the second decade of the nineteenth century onward. Spas like Baden-Baden, Ems, and Wiesbaden that were only middling spas during the eighteenth century thus rose to international fame in the nineteenth century.

Eighteenth-century spas were at the center of various circles of communication. Spas proved to be essential to the maintenance of social and information networks in Germany because members of the nobility and the bourgeoisie from different parts of a region or even from the entire country frequented fashionable spas. In contrast to Enlightenment societies like Masonic lodges, salons, and reading societies that were mostly oriented toward a local audience, spas served as important meeting places for the social elites of a larger geographical area. Friends met at spas, and spa guests established new personal and professional contacts during their annual visits. In addition, Pyrmont and other spas were gathering places for Freemasons, and some spas even had Masonic lodges, thus establishing a heterotopia within a heterotopia.

Face-to-face communication at spas ranged from secret and confidential to open and public. Secret diplomatic meetings between two rulers or their agents were common at spas, as were interactions between strangers in the public spaces of the spa. Spa visitors constantly moved between private, confidential conversations and engagement with the larger spa society. Letters exchanged between spa visitors and friends and family at home or at other spas significantly broadened this circle of communication. The spa was thus at the center of concentric circles of private and public communication. As fundamentally public spaces, however, spas also revealed the precarious nature of the confidential conversations that were made possible by face-to-face interactions. What many visitors regarded as one of the major advantages of spas was, at the same time, a source of scandals in eighteenth-century German society.

Spas became deeply intertwined with the print culture of the late Enlightenment era. Visitors expected to have access to newspapers, journals, and books at spas, and spas were in turn increasingly represented in these media. Starting in the mid-eighteenth century, spas figured in both nonfictional and fictional texts like spa guides, novels, novellas, comedies, poems, travelogues, and fictional travel narratives, as well as in frequent journal articles, for instance in the *Journal of Luxury and Fashions* (*Journal des Luxus und der Moden*). During the late eighteenth and early nineteenth centuries, a "tourist" strand of spa publications developed that described spas primarily as spaces of leisure, social interaction, and enjoyment of the landscape.

As spas were integrated into the Enlightenment public sphere, knowledge about spas as early tourist spaces became widespread by the late eighteenth and early nineteenth centuries. Reviews of spa guides appeared in journals, and authors published competing spa guides. "Middlebrow" fiction built on common knowledge about spas to make their main protagonists the subject of ridicule and laughter. And "highbrow" authors like Gotthold Ephraim Lessing and Jean Paul also relied on their readers' extensive knowledge about spas to evoke an entire tableau of spa experiences through just a few hints. Jean Paul's novella *Dr. Katzenberger's Spa Trip* (*Dr. Katzenbergers Badereise*) references contemporary knowledge about the spa as, among other things, a meeting place, a space of princely representation, and a marriage market.

Until the middle of the eighteenth century, the ideal spa was in a town or city. In line with contemporary perceptions of "civilized" and "wild" spaces, the spa had to be an urbanized space, surrounded by a "tamed" landscape with substantial evidence of human cultivation. While healing springs could be found in different kinds of landscapes in early modern central Europe – from rugged mountains to lowland plains – a spa needed to attract visitors to be successful. Therefore, spa guides sought to interpret a spa's interior space and surrounding landscape for prospective guests, either playing up its urban character and the cultivated fields and gently rolling hills around it or playing down its "untamed" and rugged surroundings. Before the late 1770s, "nature" entered the interior space of a spa only in a very limited fashion, in the form of tree-lined avenues and French gardens.

In the 1780s, the interior spaces of German spas changed considerably, in line with the transformation of formal French gardens into English landscape gardens. These gardens sought to recreate the natural landscape and transform spas into "rural" spaces. An ideal spa was now expected to offer an avenue *and* a landscape garden. Spa guides stated that, while an avenue was seen as a space for social interaction, landscape gardens provided walkers with the choice to be either alone or in company. Eighteenth-century spas thus multiplied Enlightenment ideas about landscape gardens as spaces that symbolized "freedom." At the same time, spas sought to attract visitors by offering urban amenities and leisure facilities. An ideal spa provided spaces for reading, dancing, gambling, and dining. It had a coffeehouse, a theater, a bookstore, a casino, and more. It provided pump rooms – facilities for drinking the healing water as part of the spa's morning ritual – and bathhouses. On the one hand, spas thus increasingly catered to the rising bourgeoisie. On the other hand, spas continued to be aristocratic spaces and spaces of representation for the ruling prince. The potential contradiction that resulted from these competing expectations of the spa was not lost on contemporaries who described spas as "court, town, and countryside."[3] Increasingly, writers called for spas to be more "rural," but during the 1780s the prevailing consensus was that spas could successfully merge urbanity and rurality – "art" and "nature" – to become perfect spaces for leisure.

The 1780s thus constitute a transitional period in terms of the concept of the spa as a spatial heterotopia. High and rugged hills and mountains were still regarded as undesirable, and spa guides continued to emphasize a landscape ideal of "meadows and pastures dotted with cattle," as Marcard wrote in his description of Pyrmont in 1784.[4] Spa visitors were rarely encouraged to leave the confines of the spa, and if nature walks in the surrounding countryside were offered as a possibility, these were still described as "wild." In light of this representation of the landscape, it is not surprising that neither the densely built small town of Wiesbaden nor Ems, a spa situated in a narrow valley of the river Lahn, was regarded as attractive during this time.

The expanding spa discourse of the 1790s and the early nineteenth century caused a shift in the expectations of the surrounding landscape. The spa played an important role in popularizing the new landscape perception – often labeled in shorthand as the "discovery of the Alps" – that some members of the elite like Albrecht von Haller had already begun to embrace in the first half of the eighteenth century. The published spa discourse thus became an important multiplier of the appreciation for mountainous regions which were now described as "wild and romantic" (*wildromantisch*) and "sublime." Spa guides were instrumental in propagating this new perception of nature to a wider public – and thereby normalizing it. Spa guests were encouraged to leave the confines of the spa and not only to "walk" but also to "hike" in nature. This fundamentally changed the perception of a desirable tourist area and desirable leisure activities.

In consequence, contemporaries' attitudes toward individual spas also shifted. Karlsbad was a striking example of a spa that successfully redefined itself from an urban space to a rural retreat situated in a narrow valley with "magnificent" cliffs – a complete reversal of the early modern spatial ideal of the spa. Capitalizing on the surrounding landscape, a new group of spas in the mountainous regions of central and southern Germany, especially in Saxon Switzerland, the Giant Mountains in Silesia, and the Black Forest, entered the collective consciousness of German spa visitors. While most spas found ways to conform to the new expectations, others came to be regarded as outdated. In some cases spa visitors reflected on the landscape perception in personal narratives about spa visits, but these instances are rare and thus highlight the gradual and largely unconscious nature of this cultural shift.

Following shortly upon the change in the perception of mountains, the "discovery of the seaside"[5] constituted another fundamental change to the map of fashionable German leisure resorts at the very end of the eighteenth century. "The discovery of the seaside" denotes a new elite conceptualization of the sea. It replaced the early modern image of the sea and the seacoast as ugly and threatening with a positive perception of the seaside as "picturesque," "sublime," and as a place to linger. These ideas came from England and arrived in the German discourse rather suddenly, when in 1793 Georg Christoph Lichtenberg published an article entitled "Why Does Germany Not Yet Have a Large Public Seaside Resort?" ("Warum hat Deutschland noch kein großes öffentliches Seebad?").[6] Lichtenberg's personal connections to Samuel Gottlieb Vogel, the first spa physician of Doberan-Heiligendamm on the Baltic coast, and Friedrich Wilhelm von Halem, the founder of the North Sea resort of Norderney, were instrumental in the resulting process of establishing seaside resorts in the German lands.

An analysis of these new foundations reveals that seaside resorts were closely modeled on spas and were for a long time held to the same expectations as spas. In fact, Doberan-Heiligendamm was a composite: Doberan was an existing spa where visitors lodged and pursued leisure activities and from where they made trips to the emerging seaside resort at Heiligendamm. As a published discourse on seaside resorts developed at the beginning of the nineteenth century, a gradual and sometimes laborious process of popularizing the new perception of the sea and the seacoast began. At the end of this process, an eighteenth-century elite concept had been slowly transformed into a modern tourist attitude.

Visits to spas and later to seaside resorts that lasted several weeks became an annual ritual for members of the nobility and the upper middle class. Spa guests' daily routine, while incorporating health practices and also, controversially, bourgeois mental labor and gambling, was mostly structured by communal meals and leisure activities. By the early nineteenth century, these activities encompassed a wide range of options including dancing at balls, attending theater and music performances, walking in the avenue and the English landscape garden, and, increasingly, hiking in the surrounding countryside or strolling on the beach. By mixing communal practices, which occurred at specific times of the day in shared spaces, with time periods that could be filled with more individualized activities, spas and seaside resorts provided visitors with a stabilizing routine. Just like modern all-inclusive resorts, cruise ships, or packaged trips, this routine transformed a space and time that were potentially open and unregulated into a space and time that felt predictable and welcoming. This routine also allowed for personal expression. Spa guides and diaries described this heterochrony – this "everyday life outside of everyday life" – in minute detail.

In sum, Part II of this study has revealed the gradual, long-term transformation of the spa as a spatial heterotopia. It took substantial time for the new landscape ideals that were initially propagated by elite authors – the appreciation for mountains and the seacoast – to break through and become part of the modern discourse of desirable tourist spaces and vacation spots. The published spa discourse served as a powerful multiplier of these new perceptions of natural environments, but the process was by no means linear or straightforward. The boundaries of the discourse on the spa as a spatial heterotopia shifted in slow motion; there was no discursive rupture. Rather, "old" and "new" statements stood side by side in the published discourse for quite some time. These discursive twists and turns led to a meandering discourse that was not replaced by a comprehensive new discursive regime until the early nineteenth century. The new discourse influenced individual perceptions and, over time, shifted collective viewing habits and practices at spas.

At the end of this process, the spa as a spatial heterotopia embodied the values and expectations associated with modern vacations. During a visit of several weeks, guests enjoyed urban amenities in the interior spaces of the spa and at the same time immersed themselves in the surrounding landscape or seascape. These two aspects had to be kept in careful balance for a spa to be successful, as the prevailing discourse about this spatial heterotopia focused on its character as a "rural idyll." The spa visit was perceived as an important break from everyday life, but the seemingly endless possibilities were tamed by a daily routine and guided excursions into the great outdoors. The spa visitors' expectations and memories were channeled by an extensive published discourse about these leisure spaces.

Social separation was the norm at the early modern spa, and differences in social rank between the nobility and the bourgeoisie were manifested in access to spaces and participation in leisure activities. Spa guides and personal accounts described the spa as catering to and dominated by the nobility. The bourgeoisie observed – but did not participate in – noble amusements, and members of the middle class, especially learned men, formed their own circles. Around 1750, a gradual change occurred that led to higher levels of interaction between the nobility and the bourgeoisie. Contemporary travelogues and personal narratives not only document this change but also attest to the enduring social boundaries between the two groups.

In the late eighteenth century the spa became a flashpoint of demands for equality between the nobility and the bourgeoisie. More and more members of the bourgeoisie could afford regular spa visits, which increased their numbers at the spas. But the bourgeoisie's influence went beyond their physical presence at the spas and extended into the published discourse. Spas, which were usually founded by princes and dominated socially by the nobility, were flooded by demands for bourgeois equality. Ludwig Friedrich Christoph Schmid's remark, "spa guests are like Freemasons, immediately acquainted and familiar,"[7] put this in a nutshell: members of the bourgeoisie expected to be accepted as equals by members of the nobility at the spa. The published spa discourse soon became preoccupied with Enlightenment ideas of, and demands for, the formation of new social practices and a new social order. These statements confirmed bourgeois self-confidence and strengthened bourgeois identity.

"Spa freedom" became a catchword of this debate, and references to the "freedom and equality of life at the spa" abounded. These terms encapsulated the idea of the spa as a space where social boundaries could be overcome once and for all. As a result, contemporaries carefully evaluated the so-called tone at each spa. "Tone" became a shorthand to denote a spa's social atmosphere. The published discourse began to focus on whether the nobility was willing to interact and share leisure spaces like assembly rooms with the bourgeoisie or instead insisted on maintaining social separation. Accordingly, a spa had either a "good" or a "bad" social tone.

The published discourse discussed in great detail the possibilities and limitations of the spa as a socially integrative space in the late eighteenth and early nineteenth centuries. Three types of discursive statement appeared across different genres of spa publications, and these views are surprisingly consistent with how spa visitors reflected on their experiences in personal narratives. First, some authors actively – and sometimes aggressively – argued for bourgeois equality vis-à-vis the nobility. The nobility was blamed for refusing social integration, and writers focused on the different ways in which the nobility slighted the bourgeoisie at the spa. This led to demands for social recognition by the nobility. In this context, authors discussed test cases for social integration, from access to leisure spaces and seating arrangements at communal tables to the choice of dance partners at balls and clothing as a signifier of social rank. Second, some authors searched for compromise, either by making the case that enlightened members of the nobility were ready to form a new elite with the bourgeoisie and that backward-looking nobles could be safely ignored or by constructing individual spas as exclusive heterotopias for the middle class. And third, some authors sought to hold the bourgeoisie partially responsible for the perceived lack of social integration by claiming that members of the middle class were often too timid in their interactions with the nobility.

Despite these differences, all three discursive statements emphasized the Enlightenment demand for social equality. Even when the bourgeoisie was criticized, the nobility remained the primary target of the published spa discourse. The published discourse usually employed crude generalizations – the enlightened bourgeoisie versus the proud, arrogant, and decidedly "unenlightened" nobility. The nobility was described as obsessed with birthright and lineage, while the rare enlightened nobleman (usually not a noblewoman!) was depicted in the same terms as the bourgeois – defined by his accomplishments, not by his birth. All of this made for excellent propaganda. But even in their personal narratives, contemporaries often described their fellow spa guests by applying the categories of the published discourse, and nobles were therefore seen as either "enlightened" or "proud" (and therefore "unenlightened") according to their conduct toward bourgeois spa visitors. This reveals a powerful "regime of truth"[8] encompassing both personal perceptions and the published spa discourse.

The limitations of the spa as a social heterotopia quickly became apparent. Spas continued to be spaces of princely representation. And even if a spa catered to a majority of guests from the bourgeoisie, most German spas survived only because of material support from their princely owners. The spa discourse thus stylized ruling princes as enlightened father figures who allegedly served only the common good and shared the bourgeoisie's values. The highest member of the aristocracy was explicitly excluded from any criticism because he was regarded as a powerful ally, even when the spa discourse disparaged members of the nobility.

The published discourse had created outsized, and ultimately unrealistic, goals and expectations for the spa as a whole. However, smaller circles of friends and acquaintances who met regularly at a spa succeeded in overcoming social boundaries, at least temporarily. Personal narratives showed that the spa allowed for noble-bourgeois interactions that were less constrained by social rank. "Being at a spa and being at court" indeed made for different experiences in the late eighteenth and early nineteenth centuries. Thus, the spa of the transitional period furthered the creation of an enlightened educated elite consisting of members of the nobility and the bourgeoisie.

The corollaries of the spa as a social heterotopia for this enlightened educated elite were mechanisms of social exclusion toward other social groups, especially the lower middle and lower classes. The gradual formation of European nation states also left its mark on the spas. Contemporaries increasingly noted the development of national identities and the formation of spa circles based on national origin. By the 1820s, the published discourse no longer made demands for social equality but signaled the acceptance of differences in social rank at the spa. However, the eighteenth century and the transitional period had left their imprint: the spa had become a meeting place for the circles of "the higher classes" of the nobility and the upper middle class, and it had created the ideal of a social heterotopia as a powerful legacy.

All in all, Part III of this study has shown the role played by the spa as a social heterotopia in the transformation of the early modern society of estates during the watershed period of the late eighteenth and early nineteenth centuries. The spa served both as an actual meeting place for the nobility and the bourgeoisie and as a "projection space" for the enlightened public sphere. As an actual space of "social extraterritoriality,"[9] the spa, alongside other institutions of Enlightenment sociability, created (limited) opportunities for the interaction of the enlightened nobility and the educated bourgeoisie. The spa thus provided this new social elite with a space to practice "new forms of sociability and communication."[10] As a projection space of the public sphere, the spa discourse took up Enlightenment ideas about social equality and successfully multiplied them. The published spa discourse began to discuss questions of noble-bourgeois interactions in the middle of the eighteenth century. Between the 1770s and the late 1810s it kept up a consistent drumbeat of demands for social integration. This demonstrates the enduring potency and influence of the Enlightenment that reached into the nineteenth century.

Most of the time, the published spa discourse operated through stereotypes and constructed a dichotomy between "the nobility" on the one hand and "the bourgeoisie" (*Bürger, Bürgerliche*) on the other. These demarcations did not even remotely reflect the actual social differentiations in late eighteenth-century German society.[11] Rather, as Pierre Bourdieu has observed, such "representations" enabled "agents to discover within themselves common properties that lie beyond the diversity of particular situations which isolate, divide and demobilize, and to construct their social identity."[12] By employing a binary social distinction, the published spa discourse appealed directly to the bourgeoisie and helped create a bourgeois identity vis-à-vis the nobility. At the same time, spa publications used the prevailing discourse about enlightened "freedom and equality" to broaden their appeal to a wider audience, namely to the enlightened nobility that shared the bourgeoisie's values and participated in the formation of a new enlightened educated elite.

This enlightened educated elite met in groups of friends and acquaintances at the spa and practiced noble-bourgeois integration within these circles. This is not without a certain irony because the term "circle" carried predominantly negative connotations in the published discourse. The formation of circles was usually seen as preventing noble-bourgeois interaction. Spa visitors, however, perceived social circles as generally positive and socially integrative experiences. While the spa as a whole could not fulfill the expectations of the published discourse, spa circles of enlightened sociability could do so, and as a result, spa guests were never completely disillusioned: *some* of their hopes associated with the spa as a social heterotopia – "a harmonious mingling of all estates, religions, and clothes,"[13] as Göckingk put it – became a lived reality. Goethe, who was not only a frequent spa visitor but also immersed himself in spa publications, expressed these very thoughts when he wrote to Countess Josephine O'Donnell in 1813: "I have always found, dear friend, that a spa visit can be compared with life in general. One arrives, as a newcomer, with all kinds of hopes and demands, some things remain unfulfilled, others are fulfilled beyond all expectations, some unexpected good and bad things happen, and in the end one reluctantly makes one's last exit."[14]

Notes

1. Urry, Larsen, *Tourist Gaze.*
2. Melton, *Rise of the Public*, 1.
3. Marcard, *Beschreibung von Pyrmont*, vol. 1, 1784, 61: "Hof, Stadt und Land."
4. Marcard, *Beschreibung von Pyrmont*, vol. 1, 1784, 322: "Wiesen, und mit Vieh bedeckten Weiden."

5. Corbin, *Lure of the Sea.*
6. Lichtenberg, "Warum hat Deutschland noch kein großes öffentliches Seebad? [1793]."
7. Schmid, *"Wer an seinem Schöpfer sündiget . . .",* entry of 30 June 1765, 31: "Badgäste sind wie Freymäurer gleich bekannt und vertraut."
8. Foucault, "Truth and Power," 131.
9. Möller, *Fürstenstaat,* 480: "sozialen Exterritorialität."
10. Maurice, *Freimaurerei,* 7: "neuer Geselligkeits- und Kommunikationsformen."
11. See Frey, "'Offene Gesellschaft'"; Langewiesche, "Bürgerliche Adelskritik." However, the creation of "bourgeois identity" via the "bourgeois media society" has received little attention in research so far. In this respect Frie correctly characterizes "nobility" as a delimitation and "projection" of the bourgeoisie. See Frie, "Adel und bürgerliche Werte," 414.
12. Bourdieu, *Language and Symbolic Power,* 130.
13. Göckingk, "Von dem Kurbrunnen bei Brückenau," 1782, 338: "eine harmonische Vermischung aller Stände, Religionen und Kleider."
14. Goethe, *Briefe – Tagebücher – Gespräche,* 11912 (i.e. Goethe-WA-IV, vol. 23, 425): "Wie ich immer gefunden habe, verehrte Freundinn, so läßt sich eine Badezeit mit dem Leben überhaupt vergleichen. Man kommt, als Neuling, mit allerley Hoffnungen und Forderungen an, manches bleibt unerfüllt, anderes erfüllt sich über alle Erwartung, manches unerwartete Gute und Böse ereignet sich und zuletzt tritt man ungern ab."

Map

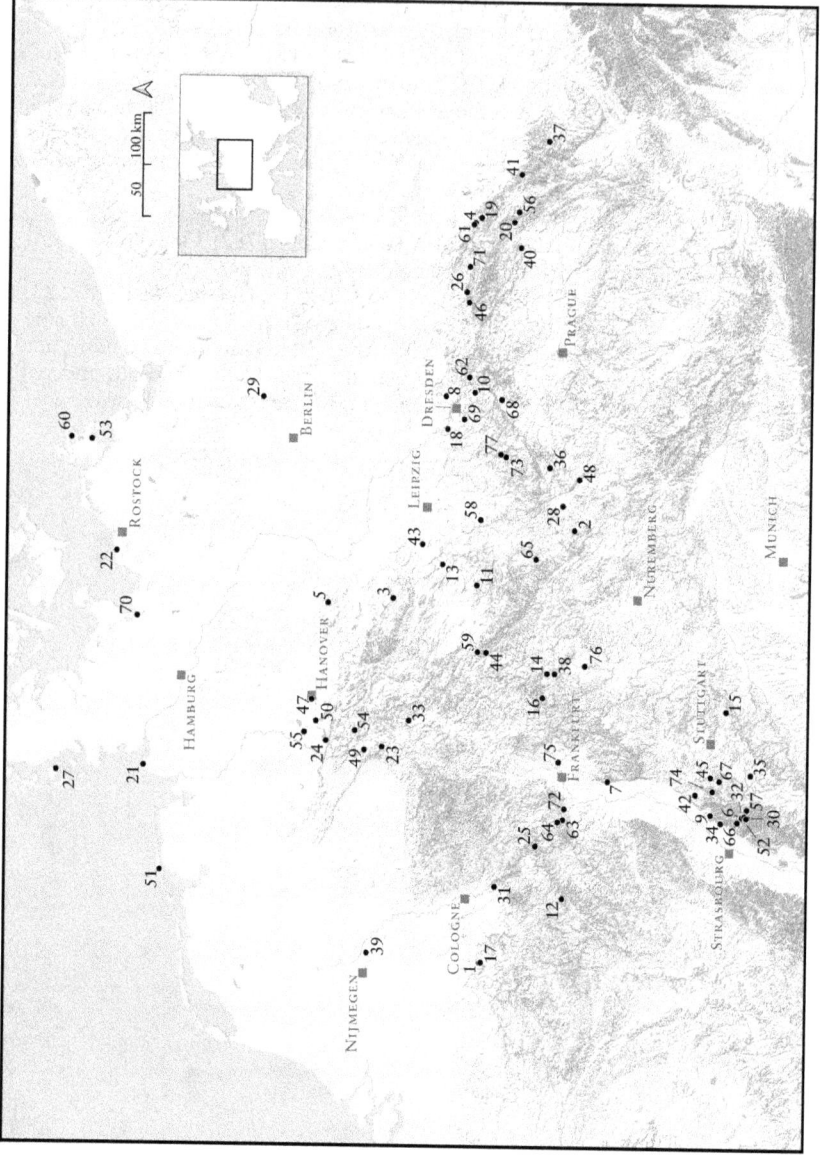

Teutsche Spas in the Published Spa Discourse, c. 1700–c. 1820

Map 295

1 Aachen
2 Alexandersbad (also Sichersreuth)
3 Alexisbad
4 Altwasser (Silesia, today Stary Zdrój in Poland)
5 Amalienbad (near Helmstedt)
6 Antogast (Renchtal)
7 Auerbach (today Fürstenlager Auerbach)
8 Augustusbad (also Radeberg)
9 Baden (today Baden-Baden)
10 Berggießhübel (also Gießhübel)
11 Berka
12 Bertrich
13 Bibra
14 Bocklet
15 Boll
16 Brückenau
17 Burtscheid (near Aachen)
18 Buschbad (near Meißen)
19 Charlottenbrunn (Silesia, today Jedlina-Zdrój in Poland)
20 Cudowa (also Kudowa, Silesia, today Kudowa-Zdrój in Poland)
21 Cuxhaven (also Ritzebüttel, North Sea)
22 Doberan (also Heiligendamm, Baltic Sea)
23 Driburg
24 Eilsen
25 Ems
26 Flinsberg (Silesia, today Świeradów-Zdrój in Poland)
27 Föhr (also Wilhelminen-Seebad, North Sea island)

28 Franzensbad (also Franzensbrunn or Eger, Bohemia, today Františkovy Lázně in the Czech Republic)
29 Freienwalde
30 Freiersbach (Renchtal)
31 Godesberg
32 Griesbach (Renchtal)
33 Hofgeismar
34 Huber Bad (also Hub, near Ottersweier)
35 Imnau
36 Karlsbad (also Carlsbad, Bohemia, today Karlovy Vary in the Czech Republic)
37 Karlsbrunn (also Carlsbrunn or Hinnewieder, Bohemia, today Karlova Studánka in the Czech Republic)
38 Kissingen
39 Kleve (also Cleve)
40 Kukus (Bohemia, today Kuks in the Czech Republic)
41 Landeck (Silesia, today Lądek-Zdrój in Poland)
42 Langensteinbach
43 Lauchstädt
44 Liebenstein
45 Liebenzell
46 Liebwerda (Bohemia, today Lázně Libverda in the Czech Republic)
47 Limmer (also Limmerbrunnen)
48 Marienbad (Bohemia, today Mariánské Lázně in the Czech Republic)
49 Meinberg

50 Nenndorf
51 Norderney (North Sea island)
52 Peterstal (Renchtal)
53 Putbus (on the island of Rügen, Baltic Sea)
54 Pyrmont
55 Rehburg
56 Reinerz (Silesia, today Duszniki-Zdrój in Poland)
57 Rippoldsau
58 Ronneburg
59 Ruhla
60 Sagard (on the island of Rügen, Baltic Sea)
61 Salzbrunn (Silesia, today Szczawno-Zdrój in Poland)
62 Schandau
63 Schlangenbad
64 Schwalbach (also Langen-Schwalbach)
65 Steben
66 Sulzbach (Renchtal)
67 Teinach (also Deinach)
68 Teplitz (also Töplitz, Bohemia, today Teplice in the Czech Republic)
69 Tharandt
70 Travemünde (Baltic Sea)
71 Warmbrunn (Silesia, today Cieplice Śląskie-Zdrój in Poland)
72 Wiesbaden
73 Wiesenbad
74 Wildbad
75 Wilhelmsbad (near Hanau)
76 Wipfeld (also Ludwigsbad)
77 Wolkenstein

Bibliography

Primary Sources

The journal commonly known as *Journal des Luxus und der Moden*, which was published between 1786 and 1827, had different titles over the years: 1786: *Journal der Moden*; 1787–1812: *Journal des Luxus und der Moden*; 1813: *Journal für Luxus, Mode und Gegenstände der Kunst*; 1814–1826: *Journal für Literatur, Kunst, Luxus und Mode*; 1827: *Journal für Literatur, Kunst und geselliges Leben*. In the notes of this book, the abbreviation *JLM* is used throughout.

For titles that were published anonymously, but an author has been identified, the author's name is provided in brackets.

Multiple titles by the same author and series of journal articles are in chronological order.

Abendroth, Amandus August, ed. *Ritzebüttel und das Seebad zu Cuxhaven.* Hamburg: Perthes & Besser, 1818.

Abendroth, Amandus August, ed. *Ritzebüttel und das Seebad zu Cuxhaven: Zweiter Theil enthaltend Veränderungen und Verbesserungen seit 1816 bis 1836.* Hamburg: Perthes, Besser & Maucke, 1837.

"Abentheuer einer kleinen Seereise nach Doberan." *Journal des Luxus und der Moden* 19 (June 1804): 276–281.

"Abgeschaffte Mißbräuche und öffentliche Verschönerung in Baden." *Journal von und für Deutschland* 2 (1788): 56–58.

Adelung, Johann Christoph, ed. *Grammatisch-kritisches Wörterbuch der hochdeutschen Mundart.* Vienna: Bauer, 1811. https://lexika.digitale-sammlungen. de/adelung/online/angebot.

"Allgemeine Bad-Uniforme für Damen, entworfen und angenommen von einer Gesellschaft Damen im Brückenauer Baade, im Sommer 1791." *Journal der Moden* 7 (April 1792): 206–208.

"Allgemeiner Modenbericht: Neuester geschmackvoller Badeanzug." *Journal des Luxus und der Moden* 18 (July 1803): 395–399.

"Anfragen und Anzeigen [Badeuniform für Damen]." *Journal des Luxus und der Moden* 12 (October 1797): 521–522.

"Anzeige [Godesberg]." *Bönnisches Intelligenzblatt* 2 (11 January 1791): 9–11.

Aufgefangene Grillen bey der Brunnen-Cur zu Langen-Schwalbach. N.p.: n.p., 1737.

August von Sachsen-Gotha-Altenburg. "Reisetagebuch: Pyrmont-Aufenthalt vom 30. Juni 1778 bis zum 27. Juli 1778." Forschungsbibliothek Gotha, Chart. B 1535.

"Baad-Reglement Bertrich." Landeshauptarchiv Koblenz, 1 C 2718.

"Badechronik: Die Bäder zu Warmbrunn in Schlesien." *Journal des Luxus und der Moden* 12 (April 1797): 169–176.

"Badechronik: Sächsische Bäder, 1. Lauchstädt, 2. Tharand." *Journal des Luxus und der Moden* 12 (May 1797): 248–254.

"Badechronik: Notiz Schlessicher Bäder. Der Brunnen zu Flinsberg." *Journal des Luxus und der Moden* 12 (June 1797): 292–296.

"Badechronik: 1. Seebad in Dobberan, 2. Aus Pyrmont." *Journal des Luxus und der Moden* 12 (September 1797): 452–456.

"Badechronik: 1. Schreiben aus Karlsbad, im August 1797, 2. Ronneburger Bad." *Journal des Luxus und der Moden* 12 (October 1797): 512–517.

"Badechronik: 1. Carlsbad, 2. Ueber Pyrmont." *Journal des Luxus und der Moden* 12 (November 1797): 544–559.

"Badechronik: 1. Eger, 2. Nenndorf." *Journal des Luxus und der Moden* 12 (December 1797): 599–605.

"Badechronik: 1. Gesang an die Nymphe des Karlsbades, 2. Die Bäder bei Landeck, in der Grafschaft Glatz, 3. Lauchstädt." *Journal des Luxus und der Moden* 13 (January 1798): 15–30.

"Badechronik: Der Gesundbrunnen zu Bibra." *Journal des Luxus und der Moden* 13 (February 1798): 87–91.

"Badechronik: Geismar." *Journal des Luxus und der Moden* 13 (March 1798): 188–193.

"Badechronik: Berichtigung wegen Pyrmont." *Journal des Luxus und der Moden* 13 (April 1798): 249.

"Badechronik: Ueber die Hazard-Spiele im Bade zu Flinsberg in Schlesien." *Journal des Luxus und der Moden* 13 (May 1798): 289–294.

"Badechronik: 1. Pyrmont im Jahr 1797, 2. Amalienbad bey Helmstädt." *Journal des Luxus und der Moden* 13 (September 1798): 497–512.

"Badechronik: 1. Radeberg und Tharand, 2. Eger, 3. Nenndorf." *Journal des Luxus und der Moden* 13 (October 1798): 586–592.

"Badechronik: 1. Freienwalde, 2. Carlsbad und Töplitz." *Journal des Luxus und der Moden* 13 (November 1798): 623–632.

"Badechronik: Ueber Sichersreut in Franken." *Journal des Luxus und der Moden* 13 (December 1798): 673–682.

"Badechronik: 1. Ueber Pyrmont 1798, 2. Das Buschbad, bey Meißen." *Journal des Luxus und der Moden* 14 (February 1799): 72–81.

"Badechronik: Ueber das Seebad zu Doberan am heiligen Damme an der Ostsee." *Journal des Luxus und der Moden* 14 (March 1799): 134–146.

"Badechronik: 1. Bericht aus Carlsbad. Den 24. July 1799, 2. Epigrammen in Carlsbad und Eger gemacht im July 1799." *Journal des Luxus und der Moden* 14 (September 1799): 461–468.

"Badechronik: 1. Gesundbrunnen zu Liebenstein, 2. Reise nach den Badeörtern Karlsbad, Eger und Töplitz." *Journal des Luxus und der Moden* 14 (October 1799): 496–515.

"Badechronik: Bemerkungen über die böhmischen Bäder, Karlsbad und Eger (Auszüge aus Briefen), 1. Karlsbad, 2. Eger." *Journal des Luxus und der Moden* 14 (November 1799): 549–565.

"Badechronik: Altwasser bey Schweidnitz in Schlesien." *Journal des Luxus und der Moden* 14 (December 1799): 622–625.

"Badechronik: 1. Neue Beschreibung von Eger und Schwalbach, 2. Ueber Dobberan im Jahr 1799." *Journal des Luxus und der Moden* 15 (February 1800): 73–80.

"Badechronik: 1. Töplitz, 2. Glückliche Aussichten fürs Liebensteiner Bad in Franken." *Journal des Luxus und der Moden* 15 (May 1800): 235–244.

"Badechronik: 1. Ueber die neueingerichteten Bäder zu Sagard, auf der Insel Rügen, 2. Neues Badereglement in den Preußischen Staaten." *Journal des Luxus und der Moden* 15 (June 1800): 293–300.

"Badechronik: Über das Liebensteiner Bad in Franken." *Journal des Luxus und der Moden* 15 (October 1800): 513–518.

"Badechronik: 1. Hofgeismar, 2. Das Buschbad bei Meißen, 3. Carlsbad und Eger (Auszug aus einem Brief)." *Journal des Luxus und der Moden* 15 (November 1800): 584–592.

"Badechronik: 1. Neue Anlagen in Karlsbad, 2. Seebad zu Doberan im Mecklenburg-Schwerinschen." *Journal des Luxus und der Moden* 16 (January 1801): 10–20.

"Badechronik: Ueber Carlsbad (Auszug eines Briefes vom 14ten Juli 1801)." *Journal des Luxus und der Moden* 16 (August 1801): 437–438.

"Badechronik: 1. Liebenstein, 2. Pyrmont, 3. Die Bäder um Dresden: Tharand, Das Seifersdorferthal." *Journal des Luxus und der Moden* 16 (September 1801): 489–497.

"Badechronik: 1. Carlsbad, 2. Pyrmont, 3. Liebenstein." *Journal des Luxus und der Moden* 17 (September 1802): 527–534.

"Badechronik: 1. Ueber Pyrmont, 2. Liebenstein, 3. Dobberan." *Journal des Luxus und der Moden* 17 (October 1802): 580–588.

"Badechronik: Scene aus dem Carlsbad im Jahre 1802, in einem Briefe." *Journal des Luxus und der Moden* 17 (November 1802): 620–628.

"Badechronik: 1. Ueber Liebenstein, 2. Ueber Warmbrunn." *Journal des Luxus und der Moden* 18 (October 1803): 538–547.

"Badechronik: 1. Ueber Pyrmont. Mlle Kirchgeßner. Feten in Pyrmont, 2. Wallfahrt nach Lauchstädt zu Mara's Gesängen im Julius 1803, 3. Naturschönheiten von Baaden in Oesterreich." *Journal des Luxus und der Moden* 18 (November 1803): 610–620.

"Badechronik: 1. Liebenwerda, 2. Ostfriesisches Seebad auf der Insel Nordernei, 3. See-Badeanstalt in Yarmouth." *Journal des Luxus und der Moden* 18 (December 1803): 652–662.

"Badechronik: Schilderung der Sächsischen und Böhmischen Bäder Radeberg, Schandau, Gießhübel und Töplitz im Sommer 1804." *Journal des Luxus und der Moden* 19 (August 1804): 401–408.

"Badechronik: 1. Karlsbad, im August 1804, 2. Das Bad zu Liebenstein im Sachsen-Meiningischen im Sommer 1804." *Journal des Luxus und der Moden* 19 (September 1804): 438–456.

"Badechronik: 1. Liebenstein und die Todenfeier Herzog Georgs im Sommer 1804, 2. Erinnerungen an Karlsbad, Eger und Töplitz." *Journal des Luxus und der Moden* 19 (October 1804): 487–495.

"Badechronik: 1. Liebenstein und Brückenau, 2. Amalienbad bei Helmstädt." *Journal des Luxus und der Moden* 20 (August 1805): 550–555.

"Badechronik: Das Augustusbad bei Radeberg." *Journal des Luxus und der Moden* 20 (October 1805): 677–684.

"Bade-Chronik von Teutschland vom Jahre 1805: 1. Über den diesjährigen Besuch der Bäder in Teutschland, 2. Auszug das Tagebuchs meiner Reise durch die Bäder Wiesbaden, Schlangenbad, Langenschwalbach, Ems, Aachen und Spaa im Monat Junius und August 1805, 3. Über das Bad zu Sagard auf Rügen." *Journal des Luxus und der Moden* 20 (December 1805): 769–806.

"Badechronik: Pyrmont im Sommer 1806." *Journal des Luxus und der Moden* 21 (October 1806): 645–647.

"Bade-Chronik: Schreiben eines Reisenden über Karlsbad und Alexandersbad, September 1807." *Journal des Luxus und der Moden* 22 (November 1807): 721–728.

"Bade-Chronik: 1. Das Bad zu Liebenstein im Julius 1808, 2. Bruchstück einer Reise von Frankfurt nach Wisbaden, Langenschwalbach, Schlangenbad und Brückenau, nebst Nachrichten von diesen Bädern im Monat August 1808." *Journal des Luxus und der Moden* 23 (September 1808): 620–638.

"Bade-Chronik: 1. Pyrmont im Jahr 1808, 2. Töplitz im September 1808, 3. Doberan und Hofgeismar." *Journal des Luxus und der Moden* 23 (October 1808): 688–704.

"Bade-Chronik 1809: Baden bei Carlsruhe." *Journal des Luxus und der Moden* 24 (August 1809): 518–521.

"Bade-Chronik: Liebenstein im Jahre 1809." *Journal des Luxus und der Moden* 24 (September 1809): 573–575.

"Bade-Chronik: 1. Pyrmont im Julius und August 1809, 2. Töplitz im August 1809, 3. Die neue Reilsche Bade-Anstalt in Halle, 4. Drieburg und Hof-Geismar im Sommer 1809." *Journal des Luxus und der Moden* 24 (October 1809): 615–633.

"Bade-Chronik: Das Seebad Doberan im Sommer 1809." *Journal des Luxus und der Moden* 24 (November 1809): 715–718.

"Bade-Chronik: Baden bei Rastatt." *Journal des Luxus und der Moden* 25 (July 1810): 446–447.

"Bade-Chronik: Frühreise durch die Bäder längs dem Rhein und der Lahn im Jahr 1810." *Journal des Luxus und der Moden* 25 (August 1810): 507–509.

"Bade-Chronik: Ueber die erste Säkular-Feier des Lauchstädter Gesundbrunnen. Am 23. Julius 1810." *Journal des Luxus und der Moden* 25 (September 1810): 548–557.

"Bade-Chronik: 1. Karlsbad und Töplitz im Sommer 1810. Anwesenheit der Kaiserin von Oesterreich, 2. Die diesjährige Curzeit im Wildbad." *Journal des Luxus und der Moden* 25 (October 1810): 606–626.

"Bade-Chronik: Pyrmont im Julius und August 1810." *Journal des Luxus und der Moden* 25 (November 1810): 723–728.

"Bade-Chronik: Die Bäder zu Eilsen bei Bückeburg." *Journal des Luxus und der Moden* 26 (July 1811): 441–446.

"Bade-Chronik: Baden bei Rastatt im Julius 1811." *Journal des Luxus und der Moden* 26 (August 1811): 507–508.

"Bade-Chronik: 1. Ems und Schwalbach im Julius 1811. Erster Brief: Ems, Zweiter Brief: Schwalbach, 2. Liebenstein am Thüringer Walde." *Journal des Luxus und der Moden* 26 (November 1811): 712–723.

"Bade-Chronik: Töplitz im Jahre 1811." *Journal des Luxus und der Moden* 26 (December 1811): 772–778.

"Badechronik: 1. Carlsbad im Sommer 1812. Ankunft der Kaiserin von Frankreich und des Kaisers von Oesterreich, 2. Baden, im Großherzogthum Baden, und seine Umgebungen im Sommer 1812." *Journal des Luxus und der Moden* 27 (August 1812): 540–547.

"Bade-Chronik: Pyrmont im Sommer 1812." *Journal des Luxus und der Moden* 27 (September 1812): 624–628.

"Bade-Chronik: Das Ronneburger Bad im Herzogthum Altenburg." *Journal des Luxus und der Moden* 27 (October 1812): 669–676.

"Badechronik: Das Schwefelbad zu Eilsen im Jahre 1812." *Journal für Luxus, Mode und Gegenstände der Kunst* 28 (January 1813): 45–49.

"Badechronik: Ueber das neuanzulegende Schwefelbad in Berka an der Ilm." *Journal für Luxus, Mode und Gegenstände der Kunst* 28 (March 1813): 155–157.

"Badechronik: 1. Das neue Bad zu Berka an der Ilm. Weitere Nachrichten davon, 2. Das Alexis-Bad." *Journal für Luxus, Mode und Gegenstände der Kunst* 28 (May 1813): 275–290.

"Bade-Chronik: Das Wiesenbad bei Annaberg in Sachsen." *Journal für Luxus, Mode und Gegenstände der Kunst* 28 (September 1813): 579–588.

"Bade-Chronik: Die Bäder am Rhein, im Sommer 1813." *Journal für Literatur, Kunst, Luxus und Mode* 29 (February 1814): 124–127.

"Bade-Chronik: 1. Teplitz im Julius 1814, 2. Carlsbad, zu Anfang des Julius 1814, 3. Schwäbische Bade-Chronik des Jahres 1813: Die Hub, 4. Das Bad zu Berka an der Ilm im Sommer 1814, 5. Bade-Literatur." *Journal für Literatur, Kunst, Luxus und Mode* 29 (August 1814): 516–531.

"Bade-Chronik des Jahres 1814: 1. Baden, im Großherzogthume, im Sommer 1814, 2. Die Würtembergischen Bäder und Gesundbrunnen." *Journal für Literatur, Kunst, Luxus und Mode* 29 (September 1814): 571–587.

"Bade-Chronik: Carlsbad und Franzensbrunn im Junius 1815." *Journal für Literatur, Kunst, Luxus und Mode* 30 (July 1815): 437–442.

"Bade-Chronik: Der Franzensbrunnen bei Eger." *Journal für Literatur, Kunst, Luxus und Mode* 30 (September 1815): 559–565.

"Bade-Chronik: 1. Das Badeleben in Carlsbad während der Monate Julius und August in diesem Jahre, 2. Neues Schwefelbad zu Stockhausen bei Sondershausen." *Journal für Literatur, Kunst, Luxus und Mode* 30 (November 1815): 655–674.

"Bade-Chronik: Lauchstädt gegen das Ende des Monats Julius 1819." *Journal für Literatur, Kunst, Luxus und Mode* 34 (July 1819): 467–469.

"Badeordnung für Baden-Baden 1596." Reprint in Mehring, Gebhard. *Badenfahrt: Württembergische Mineralbäder und Sauerbrunnen vom Mittelalter bis zum Beginn des 19. Jahrhunderts*, 161–164. Stuttgart: Kohlhammer, 1914.

"Badeordnung für Boll 1599." Reprint in Mehring, Gebhard. *Badenfahrt: Württembergische Mineralbäder und Sauerbrunnen vom Mittelalter bis zum Beginn des 19. Jahrhunderts*, 172–178. Stuttgart: Kohlhammer, 1914.

"Badeordnung für Griesbach 1605." Reprint in Weech, Friedrich von. "Zur Geschichte der Renchbäder Antogast, Freiersbach, Griesbach und Petersthal." *Zeitschrift für die Geschichte des Oberrheins* 28 (1874): 444–450.

"Badeordnung von Liebenzell, c. 1530." Reprint in Mehring, Gebhard. *Baden-fahrt: Württembergische Mineralbäder und Sauerbrunnen vom Mittelalter bis zum Beginn des 19. Jahrhunderts*, 164–165. Stuttgart: Kohlhammer, 1914.

"Badeordnung von Wildbad 1549." Reprint in Mehring, Gebhard. *Badenfahrt: Württembergische Mineralbäder und Sauerbrunnen vom Mittelalter bis zum Beginn des 19. Jahrhunderts*, 165–166. Stuttgart: Kohlhammer, 1914.

"Bade- und Reise-Epoque: Wanderung durch die Bäder von Driburg, Pirmont und Geismar 1807." *Journal des Luxus und der Moden* 22 (September 1807): 584–588.

"Bad Liebenstein, d. 15 July 1802." *Journal des Luxus und der Moden* 17 (August 1802): 465–466.

Baggesen, Jens. *Das Labyrinth oder Reise durch Deutschland in die Schweiz 1789*. Munich: Beck, 1986.

Bauhin, Johann. *Ein New Badbuch/ Vnd Historische Beschreibung/ Von der wunderbaren Krafft vnd würckung/ des WunderBrunnen vnd Heilsamen Bads zu Boll/ nicht weit vom Sawrbrunnen zu Göppingen/ im Hertzogthumb Würtemberg*. 4 vols. Stuttgart: Fürster, 1602.

Becker, Sophie. *Vor hundert Jahren: Elise von der Reckes Reisen durch Deutschland 1784–1786 nach dem Tagebuch ihrer Begleiterin Sophie Becker*. Edited by G. Karo and M. Geyer. Stuttgart: Spemann, 1884.

Becker, W.G. "Reise von Dreßden nach Tepliz in Böhmen: An den Geheimen Kriegsrath Müller in Leipzig." *Göttingisches Magazin der Wissenschaften und Litteratur* 3 (1783): 530–562.

Becker, W.G. "Kurze Beschreibung von Teplitz mit seinen Bädern, und den umliegenden Gegenden." In *Taschenbuch zum geselligen Vergnügen von W.G. Becker für 1794: Vierter Jahrgang*. 2nd, improved ed., 80–98. Leipzig: Gleditsch, 1813.

Beermann, Sigismund. *Einige Historische Nachrichten und Anmerckungen Von der Graffschafft Pyrmont und Ihren berühmten Saur-Brunnen/ Denen Brunnen-Gästen zu einiger Nachricht und Zeit-Verkürtzung*. Frankfurt a.M.: Hauenstein, 1706.

"Bemerkungen eines Badegastes in Franzensbrun bei Eger." *Neues Journal der practischen Arzneykunde und Wundazneykunst* 8, no. 3 (1803): 112–132.

"Bemerkungen über Nendorf und Rehburg." *Neues fortgesetztes Westphälisches Magazin zur Geographie, Historie und Statistik* 1, no. 3 (1798): 365–374.

"Berichtigung der Briefe über Lauchstädt." *Journal von und für Deutschland* 5 (1788): 221–223.

"Bertrich: alte Anlagen, Pläne von Kirn 1776; Kurgarten, erster Entwurf von Kirn, 1776; Gutachten Hofrat Wallmenich, 1782; neuer Bebauungsplan Kirn 1788." Landeshauptarchiv Koblenz, 1 C 2717.

"Bertrich: Skizze von Seitz, alte Badegebäude, vor 1780; Plan für Reihenhäuser in der Allee; Plan für Vergnügungspark von Kirn." Landeshauptarchiv Koblenz, 1 C 2719.

"Beschreibung der Brunnenanlagen bey dem Gesundbrunnen zu Driburg." *Journal des Luxus und der Moden* 6 (April 1791): 205–215.

Beschreibung des im Oesterreich-Schlesischen Antheil gelegenen Bades Carlsbrunn oder Hinnewieder und seiner Umgebungen: Als Anleitung für die diesen Ort besuchenden Badegäste und Naturfreunde. Breslau: Korn, 1812.

Blondel, François. *Außfürliche Erklärung vnd Augenscheinliche Wunderwirckung Deren Heylsamen Badt- und Trinckwässern zu Aach.* Aachen: Clemens, 1688.

Böckmann, Johann Lorenz. *Journal einer in Gefolge der Durchlaucht Printzen Friedrichs von Baaden gemachten Reise von Carlsruhe nach Deinach und von dort wieder zurück vom 4ten August biß zum 12ten September geführt von Joh. Lor. Böckmann Hof Rath und Prof. zu Carlsruhe Im Jahre 1785.* Reprint. Calw: Oelschläger, n.d.

Boclo, Ludwig. *Ludwig Boclo's Beschreibung einer Schülerwanderung im Jahre 1813.* Edited by Wilhelm Diehl. Friedberg: Printed by the editor, 1911.

Böttger, Christoph Henrich, ed. *Beschreibung der Gesundbrunnen und Bäder bey Hofgeismar, in Zwo Preisschriften.* Kassel: Schmiedt, 1772.

Böttiger, Karl August. *Literarische Zustände und Zeitgenossen: Begegnungen und Gespräche im klassischen Weimar.* Edited by Klaus von Gerlach and René Sternke. Berlin: Aufbau-Verlag, 2005.

Brandt, J.H. "Gartenbemerkungen auf einer Reise nach Pyrmont." In *Gartenkalender auf das Jahr 1782,* edited by C.C.L. Hirschfeld, 195–204. Altona: Eckhardt, 1782.

Briefe eines Reisenden an seinen Freund Ueber den Aufenthalte beim Godesberger Gesundbrunnen. Godesberg: n.p., 1793.

Brun, Friederika. "I. Blicke ins Main- und Rheinthal und Aufenthalt im Schlangenbade, in den Jahren 1801 und 1805." In *Episoden aus Reisen durch das südliche Deutschlands, die westliche Schweiz, Genf und Italien in den Jahren 1801, 1802, 1803: Nebst Anhängen vom Jahr 1805.* Vol. 1, 3–52. Zurich: Orell, Füßli & Co., 1806.

Bucholtz, Bergrath Dr. in Weimar. "Etwas über den Kißinger Gesundbrunnen in Francken." *Journal des Luxus und der Moden* 8 (Mai 1793): 241–248 and 8 (June 1793): 299–305.

[Budberg, Waldemar von]. *Beschreibung eines Aufenthalts im Schlangenbade 1777.* Riga: Hartknoch, 1779.

Büren, Adolph [Volger, Friedrich]. *Vier Wochen in Pyrmont, oder: Wer's Glück hat, führt die Braut heim, Erzählung in Briefen.* Braunschweig: Meyer, 1824. Reprint, edited by Titus Malms. Bad Pyrmont: Uhlmann, 1989.

Bürger, Elise. *Lilien-Blätter und Zypressenzweige von Theodora.* Frankfurt a.M.: Heller & Rohm, 1826.

Buwinghausen-Wallmerode, Freiherr von. *Tagebuch des Herzoglich Württembergischen Generaladjutanten Freiherrn von Buwinghausen-Wallmerode über die "Land-Reisen" des Herzogs Karl Eugen von Württemberg in der Zeit von 1767 bis 1773.* Edited by Freiherr Ernst von Ziegesar. Stuttgart: Bonz, 1911.

Campe, Joachim Heinrich. *Reise von Braunschweig nach Karlsbad und durch Böhmen, in Briefen von Eduard und Karl.* Braunschweig: Schulbuchhandlung, 1806.

Chun, P.P. *Die Reise der Chunischen Zöglinge durch einige Gegenden am Main- und Rheinstrome und in die Bäder Wiesbaden und Schwalbach.* Frankfurt a.M.: Pech, 1791.

"Correspondenz-Nachrichten aus dem Badischen: Heidelberg, Mannheim, Schwezingen, Carlsruhe, Baden." *Journal des Luxus und der Moden* 27 (August 1812): 517–524.

Cunitz, A.J. *Über das Bad zu Ruhla.* Eisenach: Wittekindt, 1804.

Cupido im Bad, oder Die verliebten Begebenheiten einiger hoher Standes-Personen. Frankfurt a.M.: Hagen, 1719.

Das alte teutsche ehrliche und liebliche Pyrmont Theologisch Juristisch Historisch und Physicalisch kurz und gut beschrieben an einige Freunde von einem Moralisten. N.p.: n.p., 1752.

Das Buschbad bei Meissen. Dresden: Gerlach, 1802.

Das Pyrmonter Brunnenarchiv von 1782. Reprint of *Pyrmonter Brunnen-Archiv.* Vol. 1. Berlin: Stahlbaum, 1782. Edited by Siegrid Düll. Sankt Augustin: Academia Verlag, 1995.

Delius, Heinrich Friedrich von. *Untersuchungen und Nachrichten von den Gesundbrunnen und Bädern in Kißingen und Boklet im Fürstenthum Würzburg.* Erlangen: Walther, 1770.

Delius, Heinrich Friedrich von. *Nachricht von dem Gesund Brunnen bey Sichersreuth ohnweit Wonsiedel.* Bayreuth: Lübeckische Buchhandlung, 1774.

Deneken, Arnold Gerhard. "Bemerkungen bey dem Rehburger Gesundbrunnen im Jahre 1796." *Deutsche Monatsschrift* 3 (1796): 195–206.

Deneken, Arnold Gerhard. *Bemerkungen über die Brunnen-Oerter Rehburg und Driburg.* Hanover: Helwing, 1798.

Der Kommersch zu Lauchstädt, oder das schöne Abentheuer: Ein prosaisches Gedicht in sieben Gesängen. Lauchstädt: n.p., 1790.

Der Wüstling: Eine Geschichte aus Pyrmont. Nach dem Englischen. Berlin, n.p., 1788.

Deutschlands vorzüglichste Badeörter, in Hinsicht ihrer Lage, Beschaffenheit und Umgebungen, für diejenigen, welche sie mit Nutzen besuchen wollen. Vol. 1, *Carlsbad und Töplitz.* Pirna: Friese, c. 1804.

"Die Einweihung des neuen Saales in Wißbaden am Himmelfahrtstage den 31sten Mai." *Journal des Luxus und der Moden* 25 (June 1810): 377–378.

Die holländische Sauce: Eine lauchstädtsche Badgeschichte. Halle: Michaelis, 1782.

Dietrich, Ewald. *Clara und Mathilde: der Jungfrauen Reise in die sächsische Schweiz und nach Carlsbad, Eine idyllische Erzählung.* Meißen: Goedsche, 1822.

Dietrich, Ewald, and Friedrich Reichel. *Darstellung der Heilquellen und Cur- und Bade-Orte des Königreichs Sachsen.* Dresden: Walther, 1824.

Ditfurth, Franz Dietrich von. "Bericht über den Wilhelmsbader Konvent, 1782." Edited by Georg Kloß. *Freimaurer-Zeitung* 5 (1847): 33–39 and 6 (1847): 41–48.

Donop, Charlotte Wilhelmine Amalie von. *Die Schönheiten Pyrmonts besungen von Charlotten Wilhelminen Amalien von Donop.* Göttingen: Bossiegel, 1750.

Dr. Z** in Br** [Dr. Conrad Anton Zwierlein in Brückenau]. "Vorschlag zu einer allgemeinen Baad-Uniforme für Damen." *Journal des Luxus und der Moden* 3 (July 1788): 269–273.

Du Mênil, August Peter Julius. *Der Rehburger Brunnen als Cur- und Erholungsort.* Hanover: Helwing, 1829.

[Eichler, A.K.]. *Beschreibung von Teplitz und seinen pitoreskischen Umgebungen: Ein Taschenbuch für Brunnengäste und Reisende.* Leipzig: Hinrichs, 1811.

Eichler, A.K. *Beschreibung von Teplitz und seinen mahlerischen Umgebungen: . . . Ein Taschenbuch für Brunnengäste und Reisende.* 5th ed. Teplitz: Geržabek, Spengler & Helm, 1823.

Elisabeth Charlotte von Orleans. *Aus den Briefen an die Kurfürstin Sophie von Hannover.* Edited by Eduard Bodemann. Hildesheim: Olms, 2003.

"Etwas über Achen: In Briefen." *Deutsches Museum* 2 (1780): 509–520.

"Etwas vom Carlsbade." *Hannoverisches Magazin* 24 (1786): 1297–1312.

Faber, Georg. "Beschreibung einer Bade- und Rheinreise des Butzbacher Hofes im Jahr 1632." In *Philipp, Landgraf von Hessen-Butzbach: Eine Festgabe zur Dreihundertjahrfeier der Begründung der Landgrafschaft Hessen-Butzbach*, edited by Wilhelm Diehl, 62–74. Darmstadt: Printed by the editor, 1909.

Fenner, Heinrich. *Das Schlangenbad.* Marburg: Neue Akademische Buchhandlung, 1806.

Fenner, Justus. *Freimüthige Briefe über Schwalbach, dessen Quellen und Umgebungen.* Frankfurt a.M.: Jäger, 1807.

Ficker, Wilhelm Anton, ed. *Driburger Taschenbuch auf das Jahr 1811.* Paderborn: Wesener, 1811.

Flachs, Fabrizius [Krause, C.S.]. "Ueber Lauchstädt: Aus dem Tagebuch eines Reisenden 1784." *Deutsches Museum* 1 (1785): 423–430.

Florencourt, Wilhelm Ferdinand Chaßot von. *Sittliche Schilderungen entworfen auf einer Reise von Braunschweig, über Pyrmont, Rinteln etc. nach Cassel in Briefen an einen Freund.* Berlin: Felisch, 1801.

Frankenau, Rasmus. *Pyrmont und sein Gesundbrunnen im Sommer 1798: Ein Fragment zur Beherzigung und Belehrung für Badegäste, Kranke und Ärzte.* Altona: n.p., 1799.

Friedrich I. von Sachsen-Gotha und Altenburg. *Die Tagebücher 1667–1686.* Vol. 1, *Tagebücher 1667–1677.* Edited by Roswitha Jacobsen. Weimar: Hermann Böhlaus Nachfolger, 1998.

Friedrich I. von Sachsen-Gotha und Altenburg. *Die Tagebücher 1667–1686.* Vol. 2, *Tagebücher 1678–1686.* Edited by Roswitha Jacobsen. Weimar: Hermann Böhlaus Nachfolger, 2000.

Friedrich I. von Sachsen-Gotha und Altenburg. *Die Tagebücher 1667–1686.* Vol. 3, *Kommentar und Register.* Edited by Roswitha Jacobsen. Weimar: Hermann Böhlaus Nachfolger, 2003.

Fritzsche, Johann Gottlieb. *Das Augustusbad bei Radeberg und dessen Umgebungen: in romantischen Briefen an G.* Dresden: Gerlach, 1805.

"Gästeliste Bertrich 1790." Landeshauptarchiv Koblenz, 1 C 5774.

Gerning, Johann Isaak von. *Die Heilquellen am Taunus: Ein didactisches Gedicht in vier Gesängen.* Leipzig: Amsterdamer Kunst- und Industrie-Comptoir, 1814.

"Gesundbrunnen bei Helmstädt." *Journal für Literatur, Kunst, Luxus und Mode* 34 (February 1819): 122–125.

[Giseke, Ludwig]. "Neue Briefe über Carlsbad, vom Jahre 1792, Erster Brief: Zugänge zu Carlsbad." *Deutsches Magazin* 5 (1793): 361–368.

[Giseke, Ludwig]. "Neue Briefe über Carlsbad, vom Jahre 1792, Zweiter Brief: Beschreibung der Stadt, Dritter Brief: Geschichte und Verfassung der Stadt, Vierter Brief: Quellen von Carlsbad, Fünfter Brief: Docktor Becher, Carlsbader Salz, Cremor Thermarum, Bäder." *Deutsches Magazin* 5 (1793): 383–444.

[Giseke, Ludwig]. "Fortsetzung der Briefe über Carlsbad, Sechster Brief: Industrie Carlsbads, Siebenter Brief: Zustand der Bürger, Preise, Ton und Charakter des Orts, Achter Brief: Spatziergänge und Gegenden von Carlsbad, Neunter Brief: Aufenthalt in Töplitz, Schluß der Correspondenz." *Deutsches Magazin* 6 (1793): 785–830.

[Göckingk, L.F.G. von]. "Briefe eines Reisenden an Herrn Drost von LB." *Deutsches Museum* 2 (1778): 465–474.

Göckingk, L.F.G. von. "Von dem Kurbrunnen bei Brückenau im Fuldischen." *Deutsches Museum* 1 (1782): 328–355.

Göckingk, L.F.G. von. "Kurbrunnen bey Brückenau." *Journal von und für Deutschland* 1 (1784): 591–592.

Göckingk, L.F.G. von. "Lied am Sprudel zu singen." *Für Aeltere Litteratur und Neuere Lectüre* 3, no. 2 (1785): 115–117.

Goethe, Johann Wolfgang von. *Was wir bringen: Vorspiel, bey Eröffnung des neuen Schauspielhauses zu Lauchstädt*. Tübingen: Cotta, 1802.

Goethe, Johann Wolfgang von. *Briefe – Tagebücher – Gespräche*. Digitale Bibliothek. Berlin: Direct Media Publishing, 1998. CD-ROM.

Goethe, Johann Wolfgang von, and Christiane Vulpius. *Goethes Briefwechsel mit seiner Frau*. Vol. 1, *1792–1806*. Edited by Hans Gerhard Gräf. Frankfurt a.M.: Rütten & Loening, 1916.

Goethe, Johann Wolfgang von, and Christiane Vulpius. *Goethes Briefwechsel mit seiner Frau*. Vol. 2, *1807–1816*. Edited by Hans Gerhard Gräf. Frankfurt a.M.: Rütten & Loening, 1916.

Goldwitz, Sebastian. *Die Mineralquellen zu Kissingen und Boklet im Fränkischen Hochstifte Würzburg*. Würzburg: Rienner, 1795.

Gottschalck, Friedrich, and Georg Curtze. *Das Alexisbad*. Halle: Hemmerde & Schwetschke, 1819.

Gottsched, Johann Christoph. *Ode auf den berühmten Lauchstädter Gesundbrunn, an Ihro Königl. Hoheit, die Durchlauchtigste Churprinzessinn zu Sachsen, an Dero Hohem Jahrfeste 1763 den 18. des Heumondes, bey dem Gebrauche dieses Bades unterthänigst gerichtet, nebst einem Singgedichte auf eben dasselbe*. Leipzig: Breitkopf, 1763.

Götz, J.N. "Wilhelmsbad, im August 1784." *Journal von und für Deutschland* 2, no. 9 (1784): 161–165.

Götzinger, Wilhelm Lebrecht. *Schandau und seine Umgebungen oder Beschreibung der sogenannten Sächsischen Schweiz*. Dresden: Berger, 1812. Reprint. Dresden: Verlag der Kunst, 1991.

Grattenauer, Karl Wilhelm Friedrich. *Über Neutralität, Erhaltung und Sicherheit der Bäder und Heilquellen in Kriegszeiten, mit besonderer Beziehung auf Schlesien*. Breslau: Joh. Fr. d. Ä., 1807.

[Grävemeyer, Frau von]. "Auszüge aus dem Tagebuche eines Frauenzimmers von einer im Jul. und August 1779 gemachten Reise." *Deutsches Museum* 2 (1780): 547–550.

[Grävemeyer, Frau von]. "Fortgesezte Auszüge aus dem Tagebuche eines Frauenzimmers, von einer im Julius und August 1779 gemachten Reise." *Deutsches Museum* 2 (1781): 196–216.

Grimmelshausen, Hans Jacob von. *An Unabridged Translation of Simplicius Simplicissimus by Johann Jakob Christoffel Von Grimmelshausen*. Translated with an introduction and notes by Monte Adair. Lanham, MD: University Press of America, 1986.

Grimmelshausen, Hans Jacob von. *Simplicissimus Teutsch*. Edited by Dieter Breuer. Frankfurt a.M.: Deutscher Klassiker Verlag, 2005.

[Grundig, Christoph Gottlob]. *Mit nützlichen Nachrichten und Anmerkungen erläuterte Beschreibung seiner, im Jahr 1751 in das Käyser Carls-Bad gethanen Reise: Nebst einer geographischen und nach dem Grundriß sowohl, denn nach dem Prospect von der Lage und Gegend des Ortes entworfenen Kupferplatte;*

wie auch einer vollständigen Nachricht aller von dem Carlsbad bekannter Bücher und Schrifften. Schneeberg: Fulde, 1754.

[Gumprecht, Engelmann Gottlieb]. *Briefe über das Radeberger Bad enthaltend: die Beschreibung der Gebäude, des Bades Entstehung, Bestandtheile, Kräfte, Wirkung, Gebrauch, Oekonomie, Promenaden, Vergnügungen und Environs. Mit einem Kupfer.* Dresden: Meinhold, 1790.

[Günderode, Friedrich Justinian von]. *Beschreibung einer Reise durch den kleinen Theil des Schwarzwaldes, welcher unterschiedene Gesundbrunnen, Bäder und die Handelsstadt Calb enthält: Mit vielen die Verfassung des Würtemberger Landes und den Nationalkarakter der Einwohner betreffenden Bemerkungen durchwebt; In sechs Briefen an einen Freund.* Frankfurt a.M.: Eichenbergische Erben, 1781.

Halem, Friedrich Wilhelm von. *Ueber die Seebade-Anstalt auf der Ostfriesischen Insel Norderney.* Aurich: Winter, 1801.

Halem, Friedrich Wilhelm von. *Die Insel Norderney und ihr Seebad nach dem gegenwärtigen Standpucte.* Hanover: Hahn, 1822.

[Halem, G.A. von]. "Schreiben eines Reisenden." *Deutsches Museum* 2 (1783): 353–362.

Hancke, Gottfried Benjamin. *Beschreibung Des Im Königreich Böhmen An der Elbe gelegenen Kuckus-Bades.* Schweidnitz: Müller, c. 1720.

Harleß, Christian Friedrich. *Das Bad zu Bertrich im Großherzogthum Niederrhein nach seinen physikalisch-chemischen Verhältnissen und nach seinen Heilkräften beschrieben: Mit einer Übersicht der Merkwürdigkeiten der vulkanischen Eifel.* Koblenz: Hölscher, 1827.

Harrer, Hubert von. *Karlsbad und die umliegende Gegend zum Unterricht und Vergnügen für Fremde und Kurgäste beschrieben.* Prague: Barth, 1801.

[Hassencamp, Johann Matthaeus]. *Briefe eines Reisenden von Pyrmont, Cassel, Marburg, Würzburg und Wilhelmsbad.* 2 vols. Frankfurt a.M.: n.p., 1783.

[Hassencamp, Johann Matthaeus]. *Brief eines Reisenden von Hanau und Wilhelmsbad.* N.p.: n.p., 1785.

[Hassencamp, Johann Matthaeus]. "Hanau und Wilhelmsbad, aus dem Briefe eines Reisenden." *Der Teutsche Merkur* (1785): 246–258.

Heineken, Johann. *Eilzens Heilquellen und deren Umgebungen in einigen Briefen dargestellt.* Hanover: Hahn, 1808.

Heinsse, Carl Gottfried. *Beschreibung des Wolkensteiner Bades: zum Gebrauche für dasige Badegäste und Unterricht für alle, die eine Badekur brauchen wollen.* Freiberg: Craz, 1808.

Held, Hans Heinrich Ludwig von. *Ueber das Meerbad bei Colberg und die beste und wohlfeilste Art sich desselben mit Nutzen zu bedienen.* Berlin: Schmidt, 1804.

Henkel, Johann Friedrich. *Bethesda Portuosa, Das hülfreiche Wasser zum Langen Leben, insonderheit in dem Lauchstädter Brunnen bey Merseburg und in dem Schlacken-Bade zu Freyberg: Mit neuen Entdeckungen nach der Historie, Chymie und Medicin angewiesen; Die andere Auflage.* Leipzig: Walther, 1746.

[Hesler, Ernst Friedrich]. *Das Leben eines Farospielers.* Leipzig: Kummer, 1794.

Hettler, Johann Philipp. *Neueste Nachrichten über die Bade-Anstalten zu Wilhelmsbad und desselben mineralischen Quellen.* Frankfurt a.M.: Fleischer, 1794.

Heydekker, Friedrich Wilhelm. *Beschreibung des Gesundbrunnens und Bades zu Freyenwalde und vieler daselbst gemachten medizinischen Wahrnehmungen:*

Ein Handbuch für Brunnengäste und für alle die von der Beschaffenheit und dem Gebrauche desselben eine getreue und ausführliche Nachricht wünschen. Berlin: Maurer, 1795.

Hirschfeld, Christian Cai Lorenz. *Theory of Garden Art.* Edited and Translated by Linda B. Parshall. Philadelphia: University of Pennsylvania Press, 2001.

Hirschfeld, Christian Cai Lorenz. *Theorie der Gartenkunst.* 5 vols. Leipzig: Weidmanns Erben & Reich, 1779–1785. Reprint. Hildesheim: Olms, 2003.

Hlawácek, Eduard. *Karlsbad in medicinischer, pitoresker und geselliger Beziehung: Für Kurgäste.* Prague: Kronbergers Witwe & Weber, 1838.

Hoepffner, Eduard Heinrich. *Ein Wort zu seiner Zeit über die Mineralquellen und Bäder in Aachen.* Aachen: Mayer & Frank, 1819.

Hoffmann, D. *Reise nach Töplitz in dem Jahre 1794.* Zerbst: Füchsel, 1797.

Homburg, Georg Wilhelm. *Erklärung des Plans von den Anlagen des Schwefelbades zu Nenndorf: Nebst einem Verzeichniß aller in diesen Anlagen und in der damit verbundenen Baumschule vorkommenden in- und ausländischen Holzarten und Pflanzen.* 1st ed. 1801. 2nd, improved ed. Hanover: Hahn, 1817.

[Hoser, Joseph Karl Eduard]. *Beschreibung von Karlsbad: Mit einem illuminierten Kupfer.* Prague: Calve, 1797.

[Hoser, Joseph Karl Eduard]. *Beschreibung von Teplitz in Böhmen: Mit einem illuminirten Kupfer.* Prague: Calve, 1798.

Hoser, C.E. [Joseph Karl Eduard]. *Beschreibung von Franzensbrunn bey Eger: Mit einer Ansicht und Grundriss der Brunnenkolonie.* Prague: Calve, 1799.

Hufeland, Christoph Wilhelm. *Praktische Uebersicht der vorzüglichsten Heilquellen Teutschlands nach eigenen Erfahrungen.* Berlin: Verlag der Realschulbuchhandlung, 1815.

Hufeland, Christoph Wilhelm. *Praktische Uebersicht der vorzüglichsten Heilquellen Teutschlands nach eigenen Erfahrungen.* 3rd, revised ed. Berlin: Reimer, 1831.

Hufnagel, Wilhelm Friedrich. *Meine Reise von Frankfurt am Mayn nach Carlsbad und Franzensbrunn.* Erlangen: Palm, 1800.

Humboldt, Wilhelm von. *Wilhelm von Humboldts Briefe an eine Freundin.* Edited by Albert Leitzmann. 2 vols. Leipzig: Insel, 1909.

Hundeshagen, Bernhard. *Der Heilbrunnen und Badeort Godesberg bei Bonn am Rheine.* Cologne: Ritzefeld, 1833.

Ihling, I.K. *Der Gesundbrunnen zu Liebenstein: Ein Gedicht.* Meiningen: Hartmann, 1804.

Irgend Jemand [Löhr, Johann Andreas Christian]. *Freimüthige Blätter über Gebrauch und Einrichtung des Karlsbades für Kurgäste und für Karlsbader selbst.* Leipzig: Fleischer, 1819.

Jasander [Dietmann, Johann Maximilian]. *Amusemens des eaux de Bade en Autriche, das ist Angenehmer Zeitvertreib und Ergötzlichkeiten in dem Nieder-Oesterreichischen Baadner-Bad.* Nuremberg: Schmidt, 1747.

[Jormann, Johann Albrecht]. *Das Schwalbacher Sommer-wehrende Perpetuum Mobile. Das ist: Die Wahre Abbildungen Des Apollinis Traumende Betrachtungen/ Was nemblich vor Wunderbahrliche Grillen daselbsten Zeit-wehrender vieler Menschen brauchender Cur/ sich regen/ bewegen/ zu sehen und zu passiren pflegt.* N.p.: n.p., 1690.

[Jormann, Johann Albrecht]. *Das Schwalbacher Sommer-wehrende Perpetuum Mobile. Das ist: Die Wahre Abbildungen Des Apollinis Traumende*

Betrachtungen/ Was nemblich vor Wunderbahrliche Grillen daselbsten Zeit-
wehrender vieler Menschen brauchender Cur/ sich regen/ bewegen/ zu sehen
und zu passiren pflegt. N.p.: n.p., 1701.

Kalckreuth, Friedrich Graf. "Vertraute Rückrufe des Reisenden wider Willen."
Zeitung für die elegante Welt 236 (2 December 1839): 941–943.

[Käppel, Gottfried]. *Pyrmonts Merkwürdigkeiten: Eine Skizze für Reisende und*
Kurgäste. Leipzig: Küchler, 1800.

Käppel, Gottfried. *Pyrmonts Merkwürdigkeiten: Eine Skizze für Reisende und*
Kurgäste. 2nd, augmented ed. Pyrmont: Helwing, 1810.

Karlsbad: Beschrieben zur Bequemlichkeit der hohen Gäste. Karlsbad: Malthe-
serkreuze, 1788.

Kerner, Justinus. *Das Wildbad im Königreich Würtemberg.* Tübingen: Heer-
brandt, 1813.

Kestner, Johann Christian. *Die wahre Brunnenfreiheit: Das Kurtagebuch des*
Johann Christian Kestner vom 9. bis 30. Juli 1765 in Bad Rehburg. Edited by
Alfred Schröcker. Hanover: Wehrhahn, 2005.

Ketelhodt, Friedrich Wilhelm von. *Das Tagebuch einer Reise der Schwarzburg-*
Rudolstädtischen Prinzen Ludwig Friedrich und Karl Günther durch Deutsch-
land, die Schweiz und Frankreich in den Jahren 1789 und 1790. Edited by
Joachim Rees and Winfried Siebers. Weimar: Hain, 2004.

[Klockenbring, F.A.]. "Auszug eines Schreibens aus Pyrmont." *Hannoverisches*
Magazin 8 (1770): 769–782.

Klüber, Johann Ludwig. *Beschreibung von Baden bei Rastatt und seiner Umge-*
bung. Vol. 1, *Baden, die Stadt. Mineralquellen, deren Gebrauch und Wirkung.*
Schloß. Römische Alterthümer. Literatur. Vol. 2, *Umgebung, nähere und ent-*
fernere. Tübingen: Cotta, 1810.

Knigge, Adolf Freiherr. *Ueber den Umgang mit Menschen: In drey Theilen.* 5th,
improved and augmented ed. Hanover: Ritscher, 1796. Reprint. Nendeln/
Liechtenstein: KTO, 1978.

Knigge, Baron. *Practical Philosophy of Social Life, or, the Art of Conversing with*
Men: After the German. Translated by P. Will. Lansingburgh: Penniman &
Bliss, 1805.

Koch, Johann Ernst Andreas. *Der Gesundbrunnen und das Bad zu Lauchstädt:*
historisch, physikalisch, chemisch und medicinisch beschrieben; Nebst einer
kurzen Topographie des Städtchens Lauchstädt. Leipzig: Schneider, 1790.

Koch, Johann Ernst Andreas. *Der Gesundbrunnen und das Bad zu Lauchstädt:*
Nebst einer kurzen Topographie des Städtchens Lauchstädt. Halle: Buchhandlungen des Waisenhauses, 1813.

Koromandel-Wedekind. *Der Brunnengast.* N.p.: n.p., 1744.

[Kortum, K.G.T.]. "Ueber Aachen und die Gesundbrunnen daselbst." *Magazin*
für Westphalen 1798: 53–93.

[Kotzebue, August von]. *Doctor Bahrdt mit der eisernen Stirn, oder Die deutsche*
Union gegen Zimmermann: Ein Schauspiel in vier Aufzügen, von Freyherrn
von Knigge. N.p.: n.p., 1790. Reprint. Leipzig: Zeitler, 1907.

Krieger, Joh. Fr. *Das Alexis-Bad im Unter-Harz mit seinen Umgebungen.* Magdeburg: Creutz, 1812.

Küttner, Carl Gottlob. *Reise durch Deutschland, Dänemark, Schweden, Norwe-*
gen und einen Theil von Italien, in den Jahren 1797, 1798, 1799. 4 parts.
Leipzig: Göschen, 1801.

[Lamprecht, Jacob Friedrich]. *Moralische und Satyrische Nachrichten aus dem Carlsbade, in einem Schreiben an den Herrn von H – abgelassen.* N.p.: n.p., 1736.

[Langer, E.T.]. "Review of [Hassencamp], *Briefe eines Reisenden von Pyrmont.*" *Allgemeine deutsche Bibliothek* 58 (1784): 604–605.

[La Roche, Sophie von]. "Eine Baad-Bekanntschaft." *Der Teutsche Merkur* 1 (1781): 149–176.

Lauchstädt, ein kleines Gemählde an Herrn D. H. in Z.: Ein Pendant zum dritten Bande der neuen Reisebemerkungen in und über Deutschland. N.p.: n.p., 1787.

Lavater, Johann Kaspar. *Reisetagebücher.* Part 2: *Reisetagebuch nach Süddeutschland 1778, Reisetagebuch in die Westschweiz 1785, Brieftagebuch von der Reise nach Kopenhagen 1793.* Edited by Horst Weigelt. Göttingen: Vandenhoeck & Ruprecht, 1997.

Lehndorff, Ernst Ahaverus Heinrich Graf von. *Aus den Tagebüchern des Grafen Lehndorff.* Edited by Haug v. Kuenheim. München: Deutscher Taschenbuch Verlag, 1982.

Lessing, Gotthold Ephraim. *Ernst und Falk: Mit den Fortsetzungen Johann Gottfried Herders und Friedrich Schlegels.* Edited by Ion Contiades. Frankfurt a.M.: Insel, 1968.

Lichtenberg, Georg Christoph. "Warum hat Deutschland noch kein großes öffentliches Seebad?" (Originally published in *Göttinger Taschen Calender* 1793: 92–109.) In *Schriften und Briefe.* Edited by Wolfgang Promies. Vol. 3, 95–102. 5th ed. Frankfurt a.M.: Zweitausendeins, 1994.

[Lichtenberg, Johann Heinrich]. *Nachricht von dem Auerbacher mineralischen Wasser mit vorläufigen Wahrnehmungen über dessen Wirkungen.* Darmstadt: Fürstliche Hof- und Canzley-Buchdruckerei, c. 1778.

Liste der angekommenen Kur- und Badegäste in der königl[ichen] Stadt Kaiser-Karlsbad im Jahre 1795. Karlsbad: Franieck, 1795.

L**s. *Bernhard und Allwine oder das Mährchen vom Rehburger Brunnen.* Göttingen: n.p., 1797.

Lüdemann, Wilhelm von. *Töplitz wie es ist, oder die beiden Grafen.* Dresden: Hilscher, 1829.

Luise, Königin von Preußen. *Briefe und Aufzeichnungen.* Edited by Malve Gräfin Rothkirch. Munich: Deutscher Kunstverlag, 1985.

Luise von Preussen, Fürstin Anton Radziwill. *Fünfundvierzig Jahre aus meinem Leben (1770–1815).* Edited by Fürstin Castellane-Radziwill. Braunschweig: Westermann, 1912.

[Marcard, Heinrich Matthias]. "Review of *Pyrmonter Brunnen-Archiv*, 1. Stück." *Allgemeine deutsche Bibliothek* 54 (1783): 306–308.

Marcard, Heinrich Matthias. *Beschreibung von Pyrmont.* Vol. 1. Leipzig: Weidmanns Erben & Reich, 1784.

Marcard, Heinrich Matthias. *Beschreibung von Pyrmont.* Vol. 2. Leipzig: Weidmanns Erben & Reich, 1785.

Marcard, Heinrich Matthias. *Kleines Pyrmonter Brunnenbuch, für Curgäste zu Hause und an der Quelle.* 2nd, revised and augmented ed. Pyrmont: Helwing, 1805.

Maskosky, Martin. *Im Namen JEsu! Das Göppingische Bethesda! Das ist kunstmässige Beschreibung des uralten heilsamen Sauerbrunnen bey der Hochfürstlichen Würtenbergischen Statt Göppingen!/ Von desselben Gelegenheit/*

Chimischer Probe/ heilsamer Wirkung und ordenlichem Gebrauche/ aus eigener Zwanzigjähriger Erfahrung zur Ehre GOttes und Nuzzen des Nächsten wolmeinend entworfen. Nördlingen: Hilbrandt, 1688.

[Mende, L.J.K.]. "Ueber den Besuch der Bäder und den Nutzen der Mineralwasser." *Monatsschrift für Deutsche* 2 (1801): 114–124.

Menke, Karl Theodor. *Pyrmont und seine Umgebungen, mit besonderer Hinsicht auf seine Mineralquellen: historisch – geographisch – physikalisch – medizinisch dargestellt.* Pyrmont: Uslar, 1818.

Merian, Matthäus, and Martin Zeiller. *Topographia Hassiae, Et Regionum Vicinarum: Das ist, Beschreibung und eigentliche Abbildung der vornehmsten Städte und Plätze in Hessen/ und denen benachbarten Landschaften.* Frankfurt a.M.: Meriansche Erben, 1665.

[Merveilleux, David François de]. *Amusemens des eaux de Schwalbach, des bains de Wisbaden et de Schlangenbad: Avec deux rélations curieuses, l'une de la neuvelle Jerusalem, et l'autre d'une partie de la tatarie independante.* Liège: Kints, 1738.

[Merveilleux, David François de]. *Amusemens des Eaux de Schwalbach, oder Zeitvertreibe bey den Wassern zu Schwalbach, denen Bädern zu Wisbaden, und dem Schlangenbade.* Lüttich: Kints, 1739.

[Merveilleux, David François de]. *Angenehmer Zeitvertreib in den Bädern zu Baaden, in der Schweitz, zu Schintznach und Pfeffers: Nebst der Beschreibung und Vergleichung ihrer Wasser mit den Bädern zu Schwalbach und andern des Reichs.* Danzig: n.p., 1739.

Mezler, Franz Xaver. *Vorläufige Nachrichten über den Kurort zu Imnau.* N.p.: n.p., 1795.

"Miscellen aus Heidelberg und Baaden." *Journal des Luxus und der Moden* 21 (November 1806): 735–736.

Mogalla, Georg Philipp. *Briefe über die Bäder zu Warmbrunn nebst einigen Bemerkungen über Flinsberg und Liebwerda.* Breslau: n.d., 1796.

Mogalla, Georg Philipp. *Die Bäder bey Landeck.* Breslau: Korn, 1799.

[Mogalla, Georg Philipp]. *Die Gesundbrunnen zu Cudowa und Reinerz.* Breslau: Korn, 1799.

[Möller, Christian F.]. *Der Adelsstolz im Bade zu Lauchstädt: Ein Lustspiel in drey Akten; Kann mit der Badeliste zugleich ausgegeben werden.* Philadelphia [*sic*]: n.p., 1791.

Monheim, Johann Peter Joseph. *Die Heilquellen von Aachen, Burtscheid, Spaa, Malmedy und Heilstein, in ihren historischen, geognostischen, physischen, chemischen und medizinischen Beziehungen.* Aachen: Mayer, 1829.

Montag, Karl Friedrich. *Das Schandauer Gesundheitsbad.* Pirna: Schuffenhauer, 1799.

Montaigne, Michel de. *The Journal of Montaigne's Travels in Italy by Way of Switzerland and Germany in 1580 and 1581.* Edited by W.G. Waters. 3 vols. London: Murray, 1903.

Montaigne, Michel de. *Tagebuch einer Reise durch Italien, die Schweiz und Deutschland in den Jahren 1580 und 1581.* Edited by Otto Flake. Frankfurt a.M.: Insel, 1988.

Morgenbesser, Johann Gottfried. *Nachricht an das Publikum die Gesundbrunnen zu Codowa, Reinertz, Altwasser, Charlottenbrunn, Salzbrunn und Flinsberg, in Schlesien betreffend.* Breslau: Wilhelm Gottlieb Korn, 1777.

Moritz, Karl Philipp. *Anton Reiser: Ein psychologischer Roman.* Edited by Horst Günther. Frankfurt a.M.: Insel, 1998.

Mosch, Carl Friedrich. *Die Bäder und Heilbrunnen Deutschlands und der Schweiz: Ein Taschenbuch für Brunnen- und Bade-Reisende.* 2 vols. Leipzig: Brockhaus, 1819.

Mosch, Carl Friedrich. *Die Bäder und Heilbrunnen Deutschland's und der Schweiz: Ein Taschenbuch für Brunnen- und Bade-Reisende.* 2 vols. 2nd ed. Leipzig: Brockhaus, 1821.

Mosch, Carl Friedrich. *Die Heilquellen Schlesiens und der Graffschaft Glaz.* Breslau: Korn, 1821.

Mosengeil, Friedrich. *Das Bad Liebenstein und seine Umgebungen.* Gotha: Ettinger, 1815.

[Moser, Johann Jacob]. *Brauchbare Nachrichten für diejenige, so sich des fürtrefflichen Würtembergischen Wildbades bedienen wollen: Zur Bequemlichkeit seiner Mit-Bad-Gäste gesammelt von einem dankbaren Bad-Gast.* Stuttgart: Cotta, 1758.

[Möser, Justus]. *Schreiben des Verfassers an seine Schwester über den angenehmen Aufenthalt zu Pyrmont: Ohne Kupfer, Zueignungen, Vorreden, Summarien, Noten, Registern und Druckfehlern.* 1746. Reprint in Erker, Brigitte. *Justus Möser in Pyrmont 1746–1793,* 24–31. Bad Pyrmont: Museumsverein im Schloss Pyrmont, 1991.

Möser, Justus. *Justus Möser: Briefwechsel.* Edited by William F. Sheldon. Hanover: Hahn, 1992.

"Nachricht von einem Gesundbrunnen bey Limmer im Hannöverschen." *Journal von und für Deutschland* 3, no. 4 (1786): 373–374.

"Nachtrag zur Bade-Chronik (Schwäbischen) vom Jahre 1814. Grießbach, Petersthal und Antogast, nebst Riepoltsau." *Journal für Literatur, Kunst, Luxus und Mode* 30 (January 1815): 49–54.

Neubeck, Valerius Wilhelm. *Die Gesundbrunnen: Ein Gedicht in vier Gesängen.* Leipzig: Göschen, 1798.

"Neuigkeiten aus Carlsruhe und Baden." *Journal des Luxus und der Moden* 25 (Dezember 1810): 796–798.

Neu-verbessert- und vermehrtes denckwürdiges Kayser Carls-Baad. Nuremberg: Albrecht, 1734 and 1736.

"Ordnung und Preise des Wihelmsbads [1779]." Reprint in Biehn, Heinz. *Wilhelmsbad und sein Theater,* after 26. Hanau: Comoedienhaus Wilhelmsbad Betriebsgesellschaft, 1969.

Osiander, Friedrich Benjamin. *Dank und Bitte an die Najade Nenndorf: Ein Gedicht mit Anmerkungen.* Göttingen: Huth, 1816.

P., W.L. von. "Bemerkungen auf einer Reise nach Lauchstädt nebst einigen Nachrichten vom dasigen Bade." *Journal von und für Deutschland* 5 (1788): 253–263.

Paul, Jean. *Dr. Katzenbergers Badereise: nebst einer Auswahl verbessertes Werkchen.* 2nd, revised ed. [1st ed. 1809]. Breslau: Max, 1823. Edited by Max Meier and Otto Mann. Stuttgart: Reclam, 1986.

Pauline zur Lippe. *Eine Fürstin unterwegs: Reisetagebücher der Fürstin Pauline zur Lippe 1799–1818.* Edited by Hermann Niebuhr. Detmold: Schriftleitung lippische Geschichtsquellen, 1990.

Pauline zur Lippe and Herzog Friedrich Christian von Augustenburg. *Briefe aus den Jahren 1790–1812.* Edited by Paul Rachel. Leipzig: Dieterich, 1903.

Paumgartner, Balthasar, and Magdalena. *Briefwechsel Balthasar Paumgartners des Jüngeren mit seiner Gattin Magdalena, geb. Behaim.* Edited by Georg Steinhausen. Tübingen: Litterarischer Verein in Stuttgart, 1895.

Pienitz, Christian Gotthelf. *Beschreibung des Augustusbades bey Radeberg: insbesondere für Kurgäste und zugleich als Wegweiser in den Umgebungen.* Dresden: Beger, 1814.

Piepenbring, Georg Heinrich. "Ueber Nenndorf und Pyrmont." *Oeconomische Nützlichkeiten* 4 (1792): 145–162.

Piepenbring, Georg Heinrich. *Bemerkungen über die Schrift des Herrn Doctor Frankenau Pyrmont betreffend: Zur Notiz für Aerzte, Brunnenärzte und Badegäste; . . . Zugleich ein Wort über die eben in Leipzig erschienenen Pyrmonter Merkwürdigkeiten.* N.p.: n.p., 1801.

Planer, Georg Andreas, and Johann Andreas Planer. *Ausführlicher Bericht von dem Deinacher-Sauer-Brunnen Im Hertzogthum Würtemberg/ Dessen Gehalt, Würckung, und so wohl innerlichem mit und ohne Milch, als auch äusserlichem Gebrauch, Samt Beygefügten merckwürdigen Observationibus.* Stuttgart: Cotta, 1740.

Polizey-Reglement für Meinberg, und andere diesen Brunnenort betreffende Nachrichten. Meinberg: n.p., 1796. Reprint. N.p.: n.p., 1950.

[Pöllnitz, Karl Ludwig Freiherr von]. *Amusemens des eaux de Spa: ouvrage utile a ceux qui vont boire ces eaux minérales sur les lieux.* 2 vols. Amsterdam: Mortier, 1734.

[Pöllnitz, Karl Ludwig Freiherr von]. *Amusemens des eaux de Spa, oder Vergnügungen und Ergötzlichkeiten bey denen Wassern zu Spaa.* Frankfurt: Rüdiger, 1735.

[Pöllnitz, Karl Ludwig Freiherr von]. *Vermakelyke tydkortingen bij het gebruik der wateren te Spa.* Amsterdam: Mortier, 1735.

[Pöllnitz, Karl Ludwig Freiherr von]. *Amusemens des eaux d'Aix la Chapelle, oder Zeit-Vertreib bey den Wassern zu Achen.* Berlin: Rüdiger, 1737.

[Pöllnitz, Karl Ludwig Freiherr von]. *Les Amusemens de Spa: or the Gallantries of the Spaw in Germany.* 2 vols. London: Ward & Chandler, 1737.

Pütter, Johann Stephan. *Selbstbiographie zur dankbaren Jubelfeier seiner 50jährigen Professorsstelle zu Göttingen.* Göttingen: Vandenhoeck & Ruprecht, 1798.

"Pyrmonter Gemälde nach dem Leben." *Journal des Luxus und der Moden* 15 (September 1800): 437–476.

Recke, Elisa von der. *Tagebuch einer Reise durch einen Teil Deutschlands und durch Italien in den Jahren 1804 bis 1806.* Edited by C.A. Böttiger. Berlin: Nicolai, 1815.

Recke, Elisa von der. *I. Aufzeichnungen und Briefe aus ihren Jugendtagen.* Edited by Paul Rachel. 2nd ed. Leipzig: Dieterich, 1902.

Recke, Elisa von der. *II. Tagebücher und Briefe aus ihren Wanderjahren.* Edited by Paul Rachel. Leipzig: Dieterich, 1902.

Recke, Elisa von der. *Mein Journal: Elisas neu aufgefundene Tagebücher aus den Jahren 1791 und 1793/95.* Edited by Johannes Werner. Leipzig: Koehler & Amelang, 1927.

Recke, Elisa von der. *Tagebücher und Selbstzeugnisse.* Edited by Christine von Träger. Munich: Beck, 1984.

Reglement den Gesundheits-Brunnen bey Hof-Geißmar betreffend. Kassel: n.p., 1765.

Reglement Wornach die Bürger und Hauß-auch Gast-Wirthe in der Stadt Lauchstädt sich zu achten haben. N.p.: n.p., 1780.

[Reichard, Heinrich August Ottokar]. *Geschichte meiner Reise nach Pirmont.* N.p.: n.p., 1773.

Reichard, Heinrich August Ottokar. *Der Passagier auf der Reise in Deutschland und einigen angränzenden Ländern, vorzüglich in Hinsicht auf seine Belehrung, Bequemlichkeit und Sicherheit: Ein Reisehandbuch für Jedermann.* Weimar: Gädicke, 1801.

Reise eines Gesunden in die Seebäder Swinemünde, Putbus und Dobberan. Berlin: Gädicke, 1823.

"Reise in die Bäder von Baden. (Von einer Dame.)." *Journal des Luxus und der Moden* 22 (August 1807): 509–518.

Reise nach den Badeörtern Karlsbad, Eger und Töplitz, im Jahr 1797: In Briefen. Leipzig: Voß, 1798.

Rem, Lucas. *Tagebuch des Lucas Rem aus den Jahren 1494–1541: Ein Beitrag zur Handelsgeschichte der Stadt Augsburg.* Edited by B. Greiff. Augsburg: Hartmann, 1861.

Reuß, F.A. [Franz Ambrosius]. *Die Mineralquellen zu Liebwerda in Böhmen.* Prague: Haase, 1811.

Reuß, Heinrich XXVI. Reichsgraf von. "Tagebuch einer Reise nach Karlsbad, 1768." Reprint in *Große Welt reist ins Bad: Nach Briefen, Erinnerungen und anderen Quellen,* edited by Heinz Biehn and Johanna Herzogenberg, 219–224. Munich: Prestel, 1960.

"Review of *Bernhard und Alwine, oder das Mährchen vom Rehburger Brunnen von L.-S,* 1797." *Neue allgemeine deutsche Bibliothek* 40 (1798): 25.

"Review of [Budberg], *Beschreibung eines Aufenthalts im Schlangenbade,* 1778 [sic]." *Allgemeine deutsche Bibliothek* 40, no. 1 (1780): 117–118.

"Review of Frankenau, *Pyrmont und sein Gesundbrunnen im Sommer 1798,* 1799." *Allgemeine Literatur-Zeitung* 21 (1800): 161–162.

"Review of Frankenau, *Pyrmont und sein Gesundbrunnen im Sommer 1798,* 1799." *Neue allgemeine deutsche Bibliothek: Anhang* (1803): 800–802.

"Review of Homburg, *Nähere Erklärung des Plans von den Anlagen des Schwefelbades zu Nenndorf,* 1801." *Neue allgemeine deutsche Bibliothek* 81, no. 1 (1803): 24.

"Review of [Hoser], *Beschreibung von Karlsbad,* 1797." *Neue allgemeine deutsche Bibliothek* 39 (1798): 438–439.

"Review of [Käppel], *Pyrmonts Merkwürdigkeiten,* 1800." *Neue allgemeine deutsche Bibliothek: Anhang* (1803): 802–803.

"Review of *Karlsbad: beschrieben zur Bequemlichkeit der hohen Gäste,* 1788." *Allgemeine deutsche Bibliothek* 95 (1790): 560.

"Review of Piepenbring, *Bemerkungen über die Schrift des Herrn Doctor Frankenau,* 1801." *Neue allgemeine deutsche Bibliothek* 72 (1802): 316–317.

"Review of [Schulz], *Reise eines Liefländers,* 1795." *Neue allgemeine deutsche Bibliothek* 26 (1796): 309–319.

Richel, A., ed. "Aachener Fremdenliste von 1768." *Zeitschrift des Aachener Geschichtsvereins* 22 (1900): 351–355.

Röper, F.L. *Geschichte und Anekdoten von Dobberan in Mecklenburg: Nebst einer umständlichen Beschreibung der dortigen Seebadeanstalten, und einem Grundrisse von Dobberan; Zur Belehrung für Fremde und Curgäste.* 2nd ed. Doberan: Röper, 1808.

Ryba, Joseph Ernest. *Karlsbad und seine Heilquellen: Ein Handbuch für Kurgäste, enthaltend eine ausführliche Anweisung zum Gebrauche der Mineralwässer von Karlsbad, nebst einer genauen Beschreibung dieses Brunenortes in physikalischer, historischer, topographischer und pittoresker Hinsicht.* Prague: Kronberger & Weber, 1828.

Salzmann, Christian Gotthilf. *Reisen der Salzmannischen Zöglinge.* Vol. 4. Leipzig: Crusius, 1787.

Sartori, Franz. *Taschenbuch für Carlsbads Curgäste wie auch für Liebhaber von dessen Naturschönheiten: Eine vollständige Beschreibung alles desjenigen, was Curbrauchende sowohl als wissbegierige Reisende von diesem Heilorte und seinen Umgebungen in topographischer, pittoresker, naturhistorischer, geschichtlicher und medicinischer Hinsicht zu wissen wünschen.* Vienna: Haas, 1817.

Sartori, Franz. *Taschenbuch für Marienbads Curgäste; oder vollständige Beschreibung dieses Heilortes und seiner Umgebungen in topographischer, pittoresker, geschichtlicher, naturhistorischer und medicinischer Hinsicht.* Vienna: Haas, 1819.

Schad, Moriz. *Das Lahnthal mit seinen Heilquellen Geilnau, Fachingen, Ems.* Nuremberg: Printed by the author, 1817.

[Schäfer, Andreas]. *Briefe eines Schweizers über das Wilhelmsbad bei Hanau.* Hanau: Schulz, 1780.

Schandau, seine Quellen und reizende Umgebungen: nebst einem Wegweiser nach dem Kuhstalle, dem Schneiderloche und den beiden Winterbergen; für Badekurgäste und Reisende. Dresden: Friese, c. 1804.

Scheidemantel, Friedrich Christian Gottlieb. *Anleitung zum vernünftigen Gebrauch aller Gesundbrunnen und Bäder Teutschland's.* Gotha: Ettinger, 1792.

Scherf, Johann Christian Friedrich. *Briefe für das Publikum über die Gesundheitswasser zu Meinberg.* Lemgo: Meyer, 1794.

"Schillers Denkfeier auf dem Weimarischen Hoftheater in Lauchstädt." *Journal des Luxus und der Moden* 20 (1805): 620.

Schmid, Ludwig Friedrich Christoph. *"Wer an seinem Schöpfer sündiget . . . ": Ludwig Friedrich Christoph Schmid über seinen Kuraufenthalt 1765 in Wiesbaden.* Edited by Jochen Dollwet. Wiesbaden: Stadtarchiv, 1994.

Schmidt, F.W.A. "An die Najade des Gesundbades zu Freienwalde." *Berlinische Monatsschrift* (1800): 59–60.

Schopenhauer, Adele. *Tagebücher der Adele Schopenhauer.* Leipzig: Insel, 1909.

Schopenhauer, Johanna. *Ausflucht an den Rhein und dessen nächste Umgebungen im Sommer des ersten friedlichen Jahres.* Leipzig: Brockhaus, 1818.

Schopenhauer, Johanna. "Die Brunnengäste." In *Erzählungen: Siebenter Teil,* 181–300. Frankfurt a.M.: Sauerländer, 1828.

Schopenhauer, Johanna. "Brief aus Karlsbad 1821." In *Johanna Schopenhauers Nachlass: Jugendleben und Wanderbilder,* edited by Adele Schopenhauer. Vol. 2, 309–315. Braunschweig: Westermann, 1839.

Schopenhauer, Johanna. "Das Badeleben in Karlsbad während der Monate Julius und August im Jahre 1815." (Originally printed in *JLM* 30 [November 1815].) Reprinted in *Johanna Schopenhauers Nachlass: Jugendleben und*

Wanderbilder, edited by Adele Schopenhauer. Vol. 2, 286–308. Braunschweig: Westermann, 1839.

Schopenhauer, Johanna. *A Lady Travels: The Diaries of Johanna Schopenhauer.* Edited and translated by Ruth Michaelis-Jena and Willy Merson. London: Routledge, 1988.

Schopenhauer, Johanna. *Im Wechsel der Zeiten, im Gedränge der Welt: Jugenderinnerungen, Tagebücher, Briefe.* Edited by Rolf Weber. Düsseldorf: Patmos, 2000.

Schreber, Daniel Gottfried. *Reise nach Carlsbad.* Leipzig: Dyck, 1771.

Schreiber, Aloys [Alois Wilhelm]. *Baaden in der Markgraffschaft mit seinen Bädern und Umgebungen.* Karlsruhe: Macklot, 1805.

Schreiber, Aloys [Alois Wilhelm]. *Baden im Großherzogthum mit seinen Heilquellen und Umgebungen neu beschrieben von Aloys Schreiber.* Heidelberg: Mohr & Zimmer, 1811.

Schreiber, Aloys [Alois Wilhelm]. *Grießbach mit seinen Umgebungen.* Karlsruhe: n.p., 1822.

Schreiber, Aloys [Alois Wilhelm]. *Handbuch für Reisende am Rhein von Schafhausen bis Holland, in die schönsten anliegenden Gegenden und an die dortigen Heilquellen.* 3rd ed. Heidelberg: Engelmann, 1822.

Schreiber, Aloys [Alois Wilhelm]. *Aachen, Spaa und Burtscheid: Handbuch für Fremde, Einheimische und Kurgäste.* Heidelberg: Engelmann, 1824.

Schuderoff, Jonathan. *Badebelustigungen.* Tübingen: Cotta, 1810.

[Schulz, Joachim Christoph Friedrich]. *Reise eines Liefländers von Riga nach Warschau, durch Südpreußen, über Breslau, Dresden, Karlsbad, Bayreuth, Nürnberg, Regensburg, München, Saltzburg, Linz, Wien und Klagenfurt, nach Botzen in Tyrol. Book 5: Enthaltend einen Abriß von Dresden, und die Reise von dort bis Saltzburg.* Berlin: Vieweg, 1795.

[Schulz, Joachim Christoph Friedrich]. "Geheime Szenen aus Bädern: I. Spaa, II. Karlsbad, III. Wilhelmsbad bey Hanau, IV. Wißbaden, V. Pyrmont." In *Kleine Prosaische Schriften vom Verfasser des Moriz.* Vol. 6, III, 94–142. Weimar: Hoffmann, 1800.

[Schütte, Johan Heinrich]. *Amusemens des eaux de Cleve, oder Vergnügungen und Ergötzlichkeiten bey denen Wassern zu Cleve: Zum Nutzen derjenigen, welche die angenehme Gegenden und Merkwürdigkeiten besehen, oder diese Mineral-Wasser gebrauchen wollen.* Lemgo: Meyer, 1748.

"Schwäbische Bade-Chronik des Jahres 1813: Bruckstücke aus den Bemerkungen eines Reisenden über Baden, die Hub, Griesbach, das Wildbad, im Sommer 1813." *Journal für Literatur, Kunst, Luxus und Mode* 29 (July 1814): 417–431.

[Schwarz, Sophie, née Becker, Sophie]. *Briefe einer Curländerinn auf einer Reise durch Deutschland.* Berlin: Vieweg, 1791.

Schweinitz, Anna Franziska von, ed. *Fürst und Föderalist: Tagebücher einer Reise von Dessau in die Schweiz 1783 und der Bund der Eidgenossen als Modell im Alten Reich.* Worms: Wernersche Verlagsgesellschaft, 2004.

Scultetus, Abraham. *Die Selbstbiographie des Heidelberger Theologen und Hofpredigers Abraham Scultetus (1566–1624).* Edited by Gustav Adolf Benrath. Karlsruhe: Evangelischer Presseverband für Baden, 1966.

Sickler, Friedrich. *Der Gesundbrunnen zu Liebenstein: Eine Schilderung.* Gotha: Ettinger, 1801.

Sponagel, Georg Christian. *Meine viertägigen Leiden im Bade Pyrmont: Eine Brunnen-Lectüre von G.C. Sponagel.* 1809. 3rd ed. Pyrmont: Uslar, 1824. Reprint. Börgerende-Rethwisch: n.p., n.d.

Sponagel, Georg Christian. *Des Vetters Feldzug in die Seebäder von Doberan: Von G.C. Sponagel, Verfasser der "Leiden in Pyrmont."* Hanover: Hahn, 1826. Reprint. Börgerende-Rethwisch: n.p., n.d.

[Springer, Johann Christoph Erich von]. *Auch einige Worte eines Nieder-Deutschen über die Hessischen Brunnen-Anstalten zu Nenndorf in der Graffschaft Schaumburg.* Helmstädt: Fleckeisen, 1795.

Springsfeld, Gottlob Carl. *Abhandlung vom Carlsbade, nebst einem Versuch einer Carlsbader Krankengeschichte.* Leipzig: Gleditsch, 1749.

Stöhr, August Leopold. *Kaiser Karlsbad und dieses weit berühmten Gesundheitsortes Denkwürdigkeiten, für Kurgäste, Nichtkurgäste und Karlsbader selbst.* Karlsbad: Franieck, 1810.

Stöhr, August Leopold. *Kaiser Karlsbad und dieses weit berühmten Gesundheitsortes Denkwürdigkeiten, für Kurgäste, Nichtkurgäste und Karlsbader selbst.* 2nd ed. Karlsbad: Franieck, 1812.

Stöhr, August Leopold. *Kaiser Karlsbad und dieses weit berühmten Gesundheitsortes Denkwürdigkeiten für Kurgäste, Nichtkurgäste und Karlsbader selbst.* 3rd ed. Karlsbad: Franieck, 1817.

"Teutsche Badechronik vom Jahr 1796, I. Nenndorf und Rehburg." *Journal des Luxus und der Moden* 11 (October 1796): 519–527.

"Teutsche Badechronik vom Jahr 1796, 2. Karlsbad. Briefe an einen der Herausgeber des J.d.M., Erster Brief." *Journal des Luxus und der Moden* 11 (November 1796): 553–559.

"Teutsche Badechronik vom Jahr 1796, 2. Karlsbad. Briefe an einen der Herausgeber des J.d.M., Zweyter Brief." *Journal des Luxus und der Moden* 11 (December 1796): 598–605.

Tharand: seine Bäder und Naturschönheiten; Freunden und Einheimischen zum Nutzen und Vergnügen dargestellt. Dresden: Friese, c. 1805.

"Theater im Amalienbad bei Helmstädt im Mai 1804." *Journal des Luxus und der Moden* 19 (August 1804): 400–401.

Tilling, Johann Christian. *Nachricht vom Carlsbade.* Leipzig: Walther, 1756.

Tralles, Balthasar Ludwig. *Das Kaiser-Carls-Bad in Böhmen in einer Ode entworfen: nebst einer Abhandlung von dem Gehalte und den Kräften dieses großen Heil-Mittels.* Breslau: Meyer, 1756.

Trampel, Johann Erhard. *Beschreibung des Bades zu Meinberg in der Graffschaft Lippe.* Lemgo: Meyer, 1770.

Trampel, Johann Erhard. *Wie muß der Kranke nach dem Brunnen reisen, wenn er Nutzen davon haben will?* Pyrmont: Helwing, 1806.

"Ueber den Luxus des Badereisens." *Journal des Luxus und der Moden* 4 (July 1789): 318–324.

"Ueber die Umgebungen von Töplitz: Aus dem Tagebuche eines Badegastes im Sommer 1811." *Journal des Luxus und der Moden* 27 (August 1812): 505–517.

"Ueber Pyrmont." *Journal des Luxus und der Moden* 15 (Oktober 1800): 505–506.

Unschuldiger Zeitvertreib im Carlsbad unter einer vereinten Gesellschaft. Frankfurt: n.p., 1751.

Unterhaltungen im Bade: oder Gesellschaftsscenen in verschiedenen Bädern Deutschlands gesammlet. Leipzig: Weygand, 1789.

Verzeichnis der im Sommer 1817 im Alexisbade angekommenen Badegäste und Fremden. Fürstin-Pauline-Bibliothek Ballenstedt, 19 O 87.

Vogel, Samuel Gottlieb. *Zur Nachricht und Belehrung für die Badegäste in Doberan im Jahr 1798.* Rostock: Adlers Erben, 1798.

Voigts, Jenny von. *Im Geist der Empfindsamkeit: Freundschaftsbriefe der Möser-tochter Jenny von Voigts an die Fürstin Luise von Anhalt-Dessau 1780–1808.* Edited by William and Ulrike Sheldon. Osnabrück: Verein für Geschichte und Landeskunde von Osnabrück, 1971.

"Vom gesellschaftlichen Leben in Pyrmont; (aus Herrn Marcard's Beschreibung von Pyrmont)." *Olla potrida* 2 (1785): 151–160.

"Vom LangenSchwalbacher Brunnen, Den 27. Nov. 1782." *Stats-Anzeiger* 2 (1782): 225–231.

"Von Schandau." *Zeitung für die elegante Welt* 122 (October 11, 1806): 983–984.

Waitz, August Christian. *Beschreibung der gegenwärtigen Verfassung des Curorts Hofgeismar.* Marburg: Akademische Buchhandlung, 1792.

Waitz, August Christian. "Nachrichten von einigen neuern Einrichtungen der Badeanstalt zu Nendorf unweit Hannover." *Neues Hannoversches Magazin* 21 (27 May 1811): 321–336 and 22 (3 June 1811): 337–344.

Warnstedt, Friedrich von. *Die Insel Föhr und das Wilhelminen See-Bad 1824.* Schleswig: Königliches Taubstummen-Institut, 1824.

"Warum auf dem Lande nicht ländlich? Ein Zeitvertreib in den Bädern zu Baaden." *Journal des Luxus und der Moden* 3 (Dezember 1788): 472–480.

[Wasserbach, Ernst Casimir]. *Perpetuum mobile Pyrmontanum aestivum, das ist: wahre Abbildung der Brunnen-Gesellschaft und des angenehmen Gekrümmels und Gewümmels, so bey dem Sauer-Brunnen zu Pyrmont in Westphalen diesen Sommer der Apoll im Traum wahrgenommen; Zur Zeit-Vertreibung und Veränderung bey der Brunnenkur mit schlechter Feder, weiln die poetischen Geister bey dem Wasser nichts dichten wollen, von Pyrmont zurückgeschrieben an einen aufrichtigen, deutschen Freund von einem kundbaren Westphälinger.* N.p.: n.p., 1719.

Weber, Christoph. *Nachrichten von der Lage, der Geschichte, dem Gehalte, dem Gebrauche und den Würkungen des Rehburger Gesund-Brunnens und Bades: in zwey Sendschreiben des Herrn Hofmedicus D. Christoph Weber zu Walsrode an einen seiner Freunde.* Hanover: Schmidt, 1773.

Weber, Christoph. *Fortgesetzte Nachrichten von der Lage, der Geschichte, dem Gehalte, dem Gebrauche und den Würkungen des Rehburger Gesund-Brunnens und Bades: Drittes Sendschreiben des Herrn Hofmedicus D. Christoph Weber zu Walsrode an einen seiner Freunde.* Hanover: Schmidt, 1773.

Weber, Christoph. *Fortgesetzte Nachrichten von der Lage, der Geschichte, dem Gehalte, dem Gebrauche und den Würkungen des Rehburger Gesund-Brunnens und Bades: Viertes Sendschreiben des Herrn Hofmedicus D. Christoph Weber zu Walsrode an einen seiner Freunde.* Hanover: Schmidt, 1777.

Weber, Christoph. *Fortgesetzte Nachrichten von der Lage, der Geschichte, dem Gehalte, dem Gebrauche und den Würkungen des Rehburger Gesund-Brunnens und Bades: Fünftes Sendschreiben des Herrn Hofmedicus D. Christoph Weber zu Walsrode an einen seiner Freunde.* Hanover: Schmidt, 1781.

[Weikard, Melchior Adam]. *Neueste Nachricht von den Mineralwässern bei Brückenau im Fuldischen.* Fulda: Stahel, 1780.

Weiz, F.A. "Schreiben des Hrn. D. Waitz in Naumburg an den Hrn. Grafen von W.: Ein Beytrag zur Geschichte des Gesundbrunnens in Biebra in Thüringen." *Journal von und für Deutschland* 5, nos. 1–6 (1788): 444–448.

Welcker, Johann Peter. *Gründliche Beschreibung des Schlangen-Bads: Worinnen Zugleich desselben vortreffliche Tugenden durch auserlesene eigene Observationes bestättigt werden.* 3rd ed. Idstein: Kürßner, 1747.

Wetzler, Johann Evangelist. *Ueber Gesundbrunnen und Heilbäder überhaupt, oder über deren Nutzen, Einrichtung und Gebrauch.* Mainz: Kupferberg, 1819.

Wetzler, Johann Evangelist. *Beschreibung der Gesundbrunnen und Bäder Wipfeld, Kissingen, Bocklet und Brückenau im Untermainkreise des Königreichs Baiern.* Mainz: Kupferberg, 1821.

Wetzler, Johann Evangelist. *Blicke auf Baierns Heilbrunnen und Bäder.* Munich: Thienemann, 1822.

Wetzler, Johann Evangelist. *Ueber Gesundbrunnen und Heilbäder insbesondere, oder Nachrichten über die vorzüglichsten Gesundbrunnen und Heilbäder in der nördlichen Schweiz, in Schwaben, in den Rhein- und Maingegenden, und in Franken.* Mainz: Kupferberg, 1822.

Wetzler, Johann Evangelist. *Die Gesundbrunnen und Bäder im Obermainkreise des Königreichs Baiern.* Nuremberg: Schrag, 1823.

Wetzler, Johann Evangelist. *Ueber Gesundbrunnen und Heilbäder insbesondere, oder Nachrichten über die vorzüglichsten Gesundbrunnen und Heilbäder in Böhmen.* Mainz: Kupferberg, 1825.

Wilhelm I. von Hessen. *Wir Wilhelm von Gottes Gnaden: Die Lebenserinnerungen Kurfürst Wilhelms I. von Hessen 1743–1821.* Edited by Rainer von Hessen. Frankfurt a.M.: Campus, 1996.

Wilhelmine von Bayreuth. *Eine preußische Königstochter: Glanz und Elend am Hofe des Soldatenkönigs in den Memoiren der Markgräfin Wilhelmine von Bayreuth.* Edited by Ingeborg Weber-Kellermann. Frankfurt a.M.: Insel, 1990.

Willebrand, Johann Peter. *Des Herrn Justizrath Johann Peter Willebrand freundschaftliche Nachrichten von einer Carlsbader Brunnenreise mit beygefügten Erinnerungen und Beylagen zum Druck befördert von J.H.K.* Leipzig: Hilscher, 1780.

Willich, Moritz von. *Vorläufer einer künftigen ausführlichen Beschreibung des Gesundbrunnens zu Sagard auf der Insel Rügen, nebst Anzeige von dessen Bestandtheilen und den bey und um denselben gemachten Anlagen.* Stralsund: Strucks Witwe, 1795.

Wipfeld am Main mit seinen Umgebungen, und der Schwefelquelle: Ein Taschenbuch für Bade-Gäste. Nuremberg: Stein, 1813.

[Zahn, Christian Jakob]. *Deinach: Luft, Lage, Vergnügungen, Bequemlichkeiten und Vortheile für die Gesundheit, die ein Aufenthalt bey diesem Brunnen gewähren kann.* Tübingen: Cotta, 1789.

[Zehmen, Carl Heinrich Ferdinand von]. *Der Badegast zu Teplitz: Ein topographisch medicinisches Taschenbuch für Einheimische u[nd] Fremde, welche außer einer sehr vollständigen Beschreibung von Teplitz und seinen Umgebungen die nothwendigsten Verhaltensregeln vor, während und nach dem Gebrauch des Bades, Nachrichten über alle nach Teplitz führende Straßen und nach einer ganz neuen Idee entworfene tabellarische Übersichten der Häuser ihrer*

Benennungen vermiethbaren Zimmer und Stallungen enthält. Prague: Enders, 1816.

Zentner, J. *Das Renchthal und seine Bäder: Griesbach, Peterthal, Antogast, Freiersbach und Sulzbach, im Kinzigkreise im Großherzogthum Baden, heilkundig, geschichtlich, topographisch, statistisch und landwirthschaftlich, mit einem botanischen und geologischen Anhange, dargestellt.* Freiburg i.Br.: Wagner, 1827.

"Zur Badechronik, Ueber Warmbrunn in Schlesien." *Journal des Luxus und der Moden* 18 (August 1803): 451–455.

"Zweiter Nachtrag zur Bade-Chronik des Jahres 1814: Der Sommer 1814 in den Heilbädern am Taunus und Rhein." *Journal für Literatur, Kunst, Luxus und Mode* 30 (February 1815): 88–91.

Zwierlein, Konrad Anton. *Abhandlung über die Gesundbrunnen bei Brückenau im Fürstenthume Fuld.* Fulda: Stahel, 1785.

Zwierlein, Konrad Anton. *Allgemeine Brunnenschrift für Badegäste und Aerzte: Nebst kurzer Beschreibung der berühmtesten Bäder und Gesundbrunnen Deutschlands.* Weißenfels: Severin, 1793.

Zwierlein, Konrad Anton. *Der Aesculap für Bad- und Brunnengäste.* Vienna: Schaumburg, 1800.

Secondary Sources

Adam, Wolfgang. "Freundschaft und Geselligkeit im 18. Jahrhundert." In *Der Freundschaftstempel im Gleimhaus in Halberstadt: Portraits des 18. Jahrhunderts, Bestandskatalog*, edited by Gleimhaus Halberstadt, 9–34. Leipzig: Seemann, 2000.

Agethen, Manfred. "Aufklärungsgesellschaften, Freimaurerei, Geheime Gesellschaften: Ein Forschungsbericht (1976–1986)." *Zeitschrift für Historische Forschung* 14 (1987): 439–463.

Agethen, Manfred. *Geheimbund und Utopie: Illuminaten, Freimaurer und deutsche Spätaufklärung.* Munich: Oldenbourg, 1987.

Albrecht, Wolfgang, and Hans-Joachim Kertschner, eds. *Wanderzwang – Wanderlust: Formen der Raum- und Sozialerfahrung zwischen Aufklärung und Frühindustrialisierung.* Tübingen: Niemeyer, 1999.

Allgemeine Deutsche Biographie. 56 vols. Leipzig: Duncker & Humblot, 1875–1912.

Appel, Rolf. *Lessing als Freimaurer.* Hamburg: Verlag der Lessing-Gesellschaft Hamburg, 1997.

Aretin, Karl Otmar Freiherr von. *Das Alte Reich 1648–1806.* Vol. 3, *Das Reich und der österreichisch-preußische Dualismus (1745–1806).* Stuttgart: Klett-Cotta, 1997.

Arndt, Johannes. "'Monarch' oder der 'bloße Edelmann'? Der deutsche Kleinpotentat im 18. Jahrhundert." In *Die frühneuzeitliche Monarchie und ihr Erbe: Festschrift für Heinz Duchhardt zum 60. Geburtstag*, edited by Ronald G. Asch, Johannes Arndt, and Matthias Schnettger, 59–90. Münster: Waxmann, 2003.

Asch, Ronald G., ed. *Der europäische Adel im Ancien Régime: Von der Krise der ständischen Monarchien bis zur Revolution (ca. 1600–1789).* Cologne: Böhlau, 2001.

Asch, Ronald, G. "Zwischen defensiver Legitimation und kultureller Hegemonie: Strategien adliger Selbstbehauptung in der frühen Neuzeit." *zeitenblicke* 4, no. 2 (2005). www.zeitenblicke.de/2005/2/Asch.

Asch, Ronald, G. "Staatsbildung und adlige Führungsschichten in der Frühen Neuzeit: Auf dem Weg zur Auflösung der ständischen Identität des Adels?" *Geschichte und Gesellschaft* 33 (2007): 375–397.

Baberowski, Jörg. *Der Sinn der Geschichte: Geschichtstheorien von Hegel bis Foucault.* Munich: Beck, 2005.

Bahlcke, Joachim, Winfried Eberhard, and Miloslav Polívka, eds. *Handbuch der historischen Stätten: Böhmen und Mähren.* Stuttgart: Kröner, 1998.

Baldyga, Natalya, ed. *The Hamburg Dramaturgy by G.E. Lessing: A New and Complete Annotated English Translation.* Translated by Wendy Arons and Sara Figal. London: Routledge, 2019.

Bauer, Joachim, and Gerhard Müller. *"Des Maurers Wandeln, es gleicht dem Leben": Tempelmalerei, Aufklärung und Politik im klassischen Weimar.* Rudolstadt: Hain, 2000.

Behringer, Wolfgang. *Im Zeichen des Merkur: Reichspost und Kommunikationsrevolution in der Frühen Neuzeit.* Göttingen: Vandenhoeck & Ruprecht, 2003.

Bending, Stephen, ed. *A Cultural History of Gardens in the Age of Enlightenment.* London: Bloomsbury Academic, 2016.

Benedict, Barbara M. "Consumptive Communities: Commodifying Nature in Spa Society." *The Eighteenth Century* 36 (1995): 203–219.

Benedikt, Heinrich. *Franz Anton Graf von Sporck (1662–1738): Zur Kultur der Barockzeit in Böhmen.* Vienna: Manz, 1923.

Bergdolt, Klaus. *Wellbeing: A Cultural History of Healthy Living.* Cambridge, UK and Malden, MA: Polity Press, 2008.

Berger, Joachim. *Anna Amalia von Sachsen-Weimar-Eisenach (1739–1807): Denk- und Handlungsräume einer "aufgeklärten" Herzogin.* Heidelberg: Winter, 2003.

Berger, Joachim. "Repräsentationsstrategien deutscher Fürstinnen in der Spätaufklärung." In *Hof – Geschlecht – Kultur: Luise von Anhalt-Dessau (1750–1811) und die Fürstinnen ihrer Zeit,* edited by Wilhelm Haefs and Holger Zaunstöck, 273–292. Göttingen: Wallstein, 2004.

Bernhard, Andreas. "Bad Aachen." In *Kurstädte in Deutschland: Zur Geschichte einer Baugattung,* edited by Rolf Bothe, 121–184. Berlin: Frölich & Kaufmann, 1984.

Biehn, Heinz, and Johanna Herzogenberg. *Große Welt reist ins Bad: Nach Briefen, Erinnerungen und anderen Quellen.* Munich: Prestel, 1960.

Bitz, Matthias. "Die Bäder und Sauerbrunnen im 17. und 18. Jahrhundert." In *Barock in Baden-Württemberg: Ausstellungskatalog.* Vol. 2, 183–191. Bruchsal: Badisches Landesmuseum Karlsruhe, 1981.

Bitz, Matthias. *Badewesen in Südwestdeutschland 1550 bis 1840: Zum Wandel von Gesellschaft und Architektur.* Idstein: Schulz-Kirchner, 1989.

Blackbourn, David. *The Long Nineteenth Century: A History of Germany, 1780–1918.* Oxford: Oxford University Press, 1998.

Blackbourn, David. "'Taking the Waters': Meeting Places of the Fashionable World." In *The Mechanics of Internationalism: Culture, Society, and Politics from the 1840s to the First World War,* edited by Martin H. Geyer and Johannes Paulmann, 435–457. Oxford: Oxford University Press, 2001.

Blackbourn, David. "Fashionable Spa Towns in Nineteenth-Century Europe." In *Water, Leisure, and Culture: European Historical Perspectives*, edited by Susan C. Anderson and Bruce H. Tabb, 9–21. Oxford: Berg, 2002.

Blanning, T.C.W. *The Culture of Power and the Power of Culture: Old Regime Europe 1660–1789*. Oxford: Oxford University Press, 2003.

Bleymehl-Eiler, Martina. "'Das Paradies der Kurgäste' – Die Bäder Wiesbaden, Langenschwalbach und Schlangenbad im 17. und 18. Jahrhundert." In *Badeorte und Bäderreisen in Antike, Mittelalter und Neuzeit*, edited by Michael Matheus, 53–80. Stuttgart: Steiner, 2001.

Bödeker, Hans Erich. "Das Kaffeehaus als Institution aufklärerischer Geselligkeit." In *Sociabilité et Société Bourgeoise en France, en Allemagne et en Suisse, 1750–1850 / Geselligkeit, Vereinswesen und bürgerliche Gesellschaft in Frankreich, Deutschland und der Schweiz 1750–1850*, edited by Étienne François, 65–80. Paris: Ed. Recherche sur les Civilisations, 1986.

Bödeker, Hans Erich. "Aufklärung als Kommunikationsprozeß." *Aufklärung* 2, no. 2 (1988): 89–111.

Bödeker, Hans Erich. "Die 'gebildeten Stände' im späten 18. und frühen 19. Jahrhundert: Zugehörigkeit und Abgrenzungen; Mentalitäten und Handlungspotentiale." In *Bildungsbürgertum im 19. Jahrhundert*. Part 4, *Politischer Einfluß und gesellschaftliche Formation*, edited by Jürgen Kocka, 21–52. Stuttgart: Klett-Cotta, 1989.

Bödeker, Hans Erich. "Reisebeschreibungen im historischen Diskurs der Aufklärung." In *Aufklärung und Geschichte: Studien zur deutschen Geschichtswissenschaft im 18. Jahrhundert*, edited by Hans Erich Bödeker, Georg G. Iggers, Jonathan B. Knudsen, and Peter H. Reill, 276–298. Göttingen: Vandenhoeck & Ruprecht, 1992.

Boerlin-Brodbeck, Yvonne. "Die 'Entdeckung' der Alpen in der Landschaftsmalerei des 18. Jahrhunderts." In *"Landschaft" und Landschaften im achtzehnten Jahrhundert: Tagung der Deutschen Gesellschaft für die Erforschung des 18. Jahrhunderts, Herzog August Bibliothek Wolfenbüttel 20.-23. November 1991*, edited by Heinke Wunderlich, 253–270. Heidelberg: Universitätsverlag Winter, 1995.

Boisseuil, Didier, and Hartmut Wulfram, eds. *Die Renaissance der Heilquellen in Italien und Europa von 1200 bis 1600 / Il Rinascimento delle fonti termali in Italia e in Europa dal 1200 al 1600*. Frankfurt a.M.: Peter Lang, 2012.

Borchert, Angela, and Ralf Dressel, eds. *Das Journal des Luxus und der Moden: Kultur um 1800*. Heidelberg: Universitätsverlag Winter, 2004.

Borgstedt, Angela. *Das Zeitalter der Aufklärung*. Darmstadt: Wissenschaftliche Buchgesellschaft, 2004.

Borsay, Peter. "Health and Leisure Resorts 1700–1840." In *The Cambridge Urban History of Britain*. Vol. 2, *1540–1840*, edited by Peter Clark, 775–803. Cambridge, UK: Cambridge University Press, 2000.

Bothe, Rolf. "Bad Driburg." In *Privat-Heilbad Bad Driburg: 200 Jahre im Familienbesitz 1781–1981*, edited by Peter Bonk, 42–57. Bad Driburg: Gräfliche Kurverwaltung Bad Driburg, 1981.

Bothe, Rolf. "Bad Driburg." In *Kurstädte in Deutschland: Zur Geschichte einer Baugattung*, edited by Rolf Bothe, 297–312. Berlin: Frölich & Kaufmann, 1984.

Bothe, Rolf, ed. *Kurstädte in Deutschland: Zur Geschichte einer Baugattung*. Berlin: Frölich & Kaufmann, 1984.

Bott, Gerhard. *Der Gesundbrunnen zu Hofgeismar.* 2nd ed. Munich: Deutscher Kunstverlag, 1975.

Bott, Gerhard. *Heilübung und Amüsement: Das Wilhelmsbad des Erbprinzen.* Hanau: CoCon, 2007.

Bott, Gerhard, ed. *Briefe eines Schweizers über das Wilhelmsbad bei Hanau.* Hanau: CoCon Verlag, 2009.

Bourdieu, Pierre. *Language and Symbolic Power.* Cambridge, UK: Polity Press, 1991.

Bousack, Bruno. *Heiße Quellen: Geschichte und Geschichte aus Bad Aachen.* Aachen: Meyer & Meyer, 1996.

Braun, Rudolf. "Konzeptionelle Bemerkungen zum Obenbleiben: Adel im 19. Jahrhundert." In *Europäischer Adel 1750–1950*, edited by Hans-Ulrich Wehler, 87–95. Göttingen: Vandenhoeck & Ruprecht, 1990.

Bresgott, Hans-Christian. *Ostseeküste – Ostseebad: Von der Entdeckung des Nordens zur Entstehung der deutschen Ostseebäder im 19. Jahrhundert.* Konstanz: UVK, 2017.

Busch, Helmut. "Reisen zum Gesundwerden: Badereisen." In *Reisen und Reiseliteratur im Mittelalter und in der Frühen Neuzeit*, edited by Xenja von Ertzdorff and Dieter Neukirch, 475–494. Amsterdam: Brill Rodopi, 1992.

Büschel, Hubertus. *Untertanenliebe: Der Kult um deutsche Monarchen 1770–1830.* Göttingen: Vandenhoeck & Ruprecht, 2006.

Buttlar von, Adrian. *Der Landschaftsgarten.* Munich: DuMont, 1980.

Cilleßen, Wolfgang. "Modezeitschriften." In *Von Almanach bis Zeitung: Ein Handbuch der Medien in Deutschland 1700–1800*, edited by Ernst Fischer, Wilhelm Haefs, and York-Gothart Mix, 207–224. Munich: Beck, 1999.

Cilleßen, Wolfgang. *Exotismus und Kommerz: Bäder- und Vergnügungswesen im Paris des späten 18. Jahrhunderts.* Frankfurt a.M.: Peter Lang, 2000.

Clausmeyer-Ewers, Bettina, and Irmela Löw. *Staatspark Wilhelmsbad Hanau: Parkpflegewerk, Historische Analyse, Dokumentation, gartendenkmalpflegerische Zielplanung.* Regensburg: Schnell & Steiner, 2002.

Conert, Elke. *Wilhelmsbad: Garten der Empfindsamkeit.* Hanau: CoCon, 1997.

Corbin, Alain. *The Lure of the Sea: The Discovery of the Seaside in the Western World, 1750–1840.* London: Penguin, 1995.

Corfield, Penelope J. "The Rivals: Landed and Other Gentlemen." In *Land and Society in Britain, 1700–1914: Essays in Honour of F.M.L. Thompson*, edited by Negley Harte and Roland Quinault, 1–33. Manchester: Manchester University Press, 1996.

Damm, Sigrid. *Christiane und Goethe: Eine Recherche.* Frankfurt a.M.: Insel, 2001.

Daniel, Ute. *Hoftheater: Zur Geschichte des Theaters und der Höfe im 18. und 19. Jahrhundert.* Stuttgart: Klett-Cotta, 1995.

Daniel, Ute. *Kompendium Kulturgeschichte: Theorien, Praxis, Schlüsselwörter.* Frankfurt a.M.: Suhrkamp, 2001.

Daniel, Ute. "How Bourgeois Was the Public Sphere of the Eighteenth Century? or: Why it is Important to Historicize *Strukturwandel der Öffentlichkeit*." *Das Achtzehnte Jahrhundert* 26 (2002): 9–17.

Dann, Otto. "Die Lesegesellschaften des 18. Jahrhunderts und der gesellschaftliche Aufbruch des deutschen Bürgertums." In *"Die Bildung des Bürgers": Die Formierung der bürgerlichen Gesellschaft und die Gebildeten im 18. Jahrhundert*, edited by Ulrich Herrmann, 100–118. Weinheim: Beltz, 1982.

Daunicht, Richard, ed. *Lessing im Gespräch: Berichte und Urteile von Freunden und Zeitgenossen.* Munich: Fink, 1971.

Dehio – Handbuch der deutschen Kunstdenkmäler: Brandenburg. Munich: Deutscher Kunstverlag, 2000.

Dehio – Handbuch der deutschen Kunstdenkmäler: Bremen, Niedersachsen. 2nd ed. Munich: Deutscher Kunstverlag, 1992.

Dehio – Handbuch der deutschen Kunstdenkmäler: Hessen. 3rd ed. Munich: Deutscher Kunstverlag, 1982.

Dehio – Handbuch der deutschen Kunstdenkmäler: Mecklenburg-Vorpommern. Munich: Deutscher Kunstverlag, 2000.

Dehio – Handbuch der deutschen Kunstdenkmäler: Rheinland-Pfalz, Saarland. 2nd ed. Munich: Deutscher Kunstverlag, 1984.

Dehio – Handbuch der deutschen Kunstdenkmäler: Sachsen-Anhalt II. Regierungsbezirke Dessau und Halle. Munich: Deutscher Kunstverlag, 2002.

Demel, Walter. *Der europäische Adel: Vom Mittelalter bis zur Gegenwart.* Munich: Beck, 2005.

Dewald, Jonathan. *The European Nobility, 1400–1800.* Cambridge, UK: Cambridge University Press, 1996.

Diefenbacher, Jörg. *Die Schwalbacher Reise.* Mannheim: Printed by the author, 2002.

Döcker, Ulrike. "Zur Konstruktion des 'bürgerlichen Menschen': Verhaltensideale und Lebenspraxis im Prozeß der 'Verbürgerlichung'." *Österreichische Zeitschrift für Geschichtswissenschaften* 1, no. 3 (1990): 7–47.

Döcker, Ulrike. *Die Ordnung der bürgerlichen Welt: Verhaltensideale und soziale Praktiken im 19. Jahrhundert.* Frankfurt a.M.: Campus, 1994.

Dorgerloh, Annette. "Franz Anton Graf von Sporck und sein Kukus-Bad in Böhmen." In *Bäder und Kuren in der Aufklärung: Medizinaldiskurs und Freizeitvergnügen*, edited by Raingard Eßer and Thomas Fuchs, 113–128. Berlin: Berliner Wissenschafts-Verlag, 2003.

Droste, Konrad. *. . . der Gesundtheyt wegen und des Vergnuehgens halber . . . Bad Rehburg 1690–2003: Ein Beitrag zur Medizinalgeschichte der Mittelweser-Region.* 2nd, revised ed. Rehburg-Loccum: Landkreis Nienburg/Weser, 2003.

Duchhardt, Heinz. *Stein: Eine Biographie.* Münster: Aschendorff, 2007.

Duden, Barbara. *Geschichte unter der Haut: Ein Eisenacher Arzt und seine Patientinnen um 1730.* Stuttgart: Klett-Cotta, 1987.

Dülmen, Andrea van. *Das irdische Paradies: Bürgerliche Gartenkultur der Goethezeit.* Cologne: Böhlau, 1999.

Dülmen, Richard van. *Die Gesellschaft der Aufklärer: Zur bürgerlichen Emanzipation und aufklärerischen Kultur in Deutschland.* Frankfurt a.M.: Fischer, 1986.

Emich, Birgit. "Bildlichkeit und Intermedialität in der Frühen Neuzeit: Eine interdisziplinäre Spurensuche." *Zeitschrift für Historische Forschung* 35 (2008): 31–56.

Engel, Hermann. "Die 'Akzisestadt' Pyrmont von 1720." *Niedersächsisches Jahrbuch für Landesgeschichte* 45 (1973): 377–392.

Engel, Hermann, ed. *Kulturgeschichtliche Streifzüge durch das Pyrmonter Tal: Gesammelte Abhandlungen und Aufsätze zur Geschichte der Herrschaft, der Stadt und des Staatsbades Pyrmont.* Munich: Printed by the author, 1973.

Engel, Hermann. "Der Pyrmonter Fürstensommer von 1681: Eine Studie zu Politik und Diplomatie am Ende des 17. Jahrhunderts." *Geschichtsblätter für Waldeck* 71 (1983): 115–178.

Ennen, Edith. "Residenzen: Gegenstand und Aufgabe neuzeitlicher Städtefor-schung." In *Residenzen: Aspekte hauptstädtischer Zentralität von der Frühen Neuzeit bis zum Ende der Monarchie*, edited by Kurt Andermann, 189–198. Sigmaringen: Thorbecke, 1992.

Erdmann, Claudia. *Aachen im Jahre 1812: Wirtschafts- und sozialräumliche Differenzierung einer frühindustriellen Stadt.* Stuttgart: Steiner, 1986.

Erker, Brigitte. *Justus Möser in Pyrmont 1746–1793.* Bad Pyrmont: Museums-verein in Schloss Pyrmont, 1991.

Erker, Brigitte. "Friedrich Nicolai in Pyrmont: Kontakte und Geselligkeit eines Aufklärers." In *Badegäste der Aufklärungszeit in Pyrmont: Beiträge zur Sonderausstellung " . . . bis wir uns in Pyrmont sehen"; Justus Mösers Badeaufenthalte 1746–1793, im Museum im Schloß Bad Pyrmont vom 14. April bis 29. Mai 1994*, edited by Dieter Alfter, 50–72. Bad Pyrmont: Stadt Bad Pyrmont, 1994.

Erker, Brigitte. "'Brunnenfreiheit' in Pyrmont, Gesundheit und Geselligkeit im letzten Drittel des 18. Jahrhunderts." In *Bäder und Kuren in der Aufklärung: Medizinaldiskurs und Freizeitvergnügen*, edited by Raingard Eßer and Thomas Fuchs, 53–97. Berlin: Berliner Wissenschafts-Verlag, 2003.

Erker, Brigitte, and Winfried Siebers. "' . . . von Pyrmont ab mit häßlichen Materialien beladen': Das Bahrdt-Pasquill – Eine literarische Fehde zwischen Aufklärung und Gegenaufklärung." In *Badegäste der Aufklärungszeit in Pyrmont: Beiträge zur Sonderausstellung " . . . bis wir uns in Pyrmont sehen"; Justus Mösers Badeaufenthalte 1746–1793, im Museum im Schloß Bad Pyrmont vom 14. April bis 29. Mai 1994*, edited by Dieter Alfter, 73–90. Bad Pyrmont: Stadt Bad Pyrmont, 1994.

Erker, Brigitte, and Winfried Siebers. "Justus Möser und der Pyrmont-Ohsener Freundeskreis: Mit einem bisher ungedruckten Gemeinschaftsbrief." *Osnabrücker Mitteilungen* 101 (1996): 271–280.

Eßer, Raingard, and Thomas Fuchs, eds. *Bäder und Kuren in der Aufklärung: Medizinaldiskurs und Freizeitvergnügen.* Berlin: Berliner Wissenschafts-Verlag, 2003.

Eulner, Hans-Heinz. "Der Kur- und Badebetrieb am Wilhelmsbad in medizinhistorischer Sicht." *Hanauer Geschichtsblätter* 21 (1966): 125–164.

Faessler, Peter, ed. *Bodensee und Alpen: Die Entdeckung einer Landschaft in der Literatur.* Sigmaringen: Thorbecke, 1985.

Faulstich, Werner. *Medien zwischen Herrschaft und Revolte.* Göttingen: Vandenhoeck & Ruprecht, 1998.

Faulstich, Werner. *Die bürgerliche Mediengesellschaft (1700–1830).* Göttingen: Vandenhoeck & Ruprecht, 2002.

Fauser, Markus. *Einführung in die Kulturwissenschaft.* Darmstadt: Wissenschaftliche Buchgesellschaft, 2004.

Fehrenbach, Elisabeth. *Adel und Bürgertum im deutschen Vormärz.* Munich: Stiftung Historisches Kolleg, 1994.

Fehrenbach, Elisabeth, ed. *Adel und Bürgertum in Deutschland 1770–1848.* Munich: Oldenbourg, 1994.

Festschrift zur 74. Versammlung deutscher Naturforscher und Ärzte. Karlsbad: Haase, 1902.

Fischer, Ernst, Wilhelm Haefs, and York-Gothart Mix, eds. *Von Almanach bis Zeitung: Ein Handbuch der Medien in Deutschland 1700–1800.* Munich: Beck, 1999.

Flemming, Willi. *Der Wandel des Deutschen Naturgefühls vom 15. zum 18. Jahrhundert.* Halle: Niemeyer, 1931.

Föhl, Thomas. "Wildbad." In *Kurstädte in Deutschland: Zur Geschichte einer Baugattung*, edited by Rolf Bothe, 473–512. Berlin: Frölich & Kaufmann, 1984.

Foucault, Michel. "Of Other Spaces." *Diacritics: A Review of Contemporary Criticism* 16 (1986): 22–27.

Foucault, Michel. "Des espaces autres." In *Dits et écrits, 1954–1988.* Vol. 4, *1980–1988*, 752–762. Paris: Editions Gallimard, 1994.

Foucault, Michel. "Of Other Spaces: Utopias and Heterotopias." In *Rethinking Architecture: A Reader in Cultural Theory*, edited by Neil Leach, 350–356. London: Routledge, 1997.

Foucault, Michel. "Truth and Power." In *Essential Works of Foucault 1954–1984.* Vol. 3, *Power.* Edited by James D. Faubion, 111–133. New York: New Press, 2000.

Foucault, Michel. *The Archaeology of Knowledge and the Discourse on Language.* New York: Vintage Books, 2010.

Frevert, Ute. "Ausdrucksformen bürgerlicher Öffentlichkeit – zwei Beispiele aus dem späten 18. Jahrhundert." In *Bürgerliche Gesellschaft in Deutschland: Historische Einblicke, Fragen, Perspektiven.* Frankfurt a.M.: Fischer, 1990, 80–89.

Frey, Manuel. "'Offene Gesellschaft' und 'gemeinsame Klasse': Adel und Adelskritik im bürgerlichen Trivialroman zwischen 1780 und 1815." *Zeitschrift für Geschichtswissenschaft* 44 (1996): 502–525.

Frey, Manuel. *Der reinliche Bürger: Entstehung und Verbreitung bürgerlicher Tugenden in Deutschland, 1760–1860.* Göttingen: Vandenhoeck & Ruprecht, 1997.

Frie, Ewald. "Adel und bürgerliche Werte." In *Bürgerliche Werte um 1800: Entwurf – Vermittlung – Rezeption*, edited by Hans-Werner Hahn and Dieter Hein, 393–414. Cologne: Böhlau, 2005.

Friedeburg, Robert von, and Wolfgang Mager. "Learned Men and Merchants: The Growth of the Bürgertum." In *Germany: A New Social and Economic History.* Vol. 2, *1630–1800*, edited by Sheilagh Ogilvie, 164–195. London: Arnold, 1996.

Frieling, Kirsten O. *Ausdruck macht Eindruck: Bürgerliche Körperpraktiken in sozialer Kommunikation um 1800.* Frankfurt a.M.: Peter Lang, 2003.

Fuchs, Thomas. "'Dieses Wasser aber ist ein natürlich/warmes und artzneyisch Bad': Bürgerlichkeit und Baden am Beispiel Wiesbadens im späten 18. und frühen 19. Jahrhundert." In *Bäder und Kuren in der Aufklärung: Medizinaldiskurs und Freizeitvergnügen*, edited by Raingard Eßer and Thomas Fuchs, 99–111. Berlin: Berliner Wissenschafts-Verlag, 2003.

Fuhs, Burkhard. *Mondäne Orte einer vornehmen Gesellschaft: Kultur und Geschichte der Kurstädte 1700–1900.* Hildesheim: Olms, 1992.

Fulbrook, Mary, and Ulinka Rublack. "In Relation: The 'Social Self' and Ego-Documents." *German History* 28 (2010): 263–272.

Fürbeth, Frank. "Zur Bedeutung des Bäderwesens im Mittelalter und der frühen Neuzeit." In *Paracelsus und Salzburg*, edited by Heinz Dopsch and Peter F. Kramml, 463–487. Salzburg: Gesellschaft für Salzburger Landeskunde, 1994.

Fürbeth, Frank. "Bibliographie der deutschen oder im deutschen Raum erschienenen Bäderschriften des 15. und 16. Jahrhunderts." *Würzburger medizinhistorische Mitteilungen* 13 (1995): 217–252.

Gaber, Jörn. "Nachwort: Politische Spätaufklärung und vorromatischer Frühkonservatismus; Aspekte der Forschung." In *Die Entstehung der politischen*

Strömungen in Deutschland 1770–1815, edited by Fritz Valjavec, 543–592. Düsseldorf: Droste, 1978.

Gadebusch-Bondio, Mariacarla. "Dietetics." In *Encyclopedia of Early Modern History Online*, edited by Graeme Dunphy and Andrew Gow. First published online 2015. http://dx.doi.org/10.1163/2352-0272_emho_COM_018306.

Gall, Lothar, ed. *Vom alten zum neuen Bürgertum: Die mitteleuropäische Stadt im Umbruch 1780–1820*. Munich: Oldenbourg, 1991.

Gall, Lothar. *Von der ständischen zur bürgerlichen Gesellschaft*. Munich: Oldenbourg, 1993.

Gamper, Michael. *"Die Natur ist republikanisch": Zu den ästhetischen, anthropologischen und politischen Konzepten der deutschen Gartenliteratur im 18. Jahrhundert*. Würzburg: Königshausen & Neumann, 1998.

Geisthövel, Alexa. "Promenadenmischungen: Raum und Kommunikation in Hydropolen, 1830–1880." In *Ortsgespräche: Raum und Kommunikation im 19. und 20. Jahrhundert*, edited by Alexander C.T. Geppert, Uffa Jensen, and Jörn Weinhold, 203–229. Bielefeld: transcript, 2015.

Gemeinde Bad Boll, ed. *Bad Boll 1595–1995: Vom herzoglichen Wunderbad zum Kurort*. Weißenhorn: Konrad, 1995.

Genth, Adolph. *Kulturgeschichte der Stadt Schwalbach*. Wiesbaden: Schellenberg, 1858.

Genth, Adolph. *Nachtrag zu der Kulturgeschichte der Stadt Schwalbach*. Wiesbaden: Sändig, 1860.

Gestrich, Andreas. *Absolutismus und Öffentlichkeit: Politische Kommunikation in Deutschland zu Beginn des 18. Jahrhunderts*. Göttingen: Vandenhoeck & Ruprecht, 1994.

Göres, Jörn, ed. *"Was ich dort gelebt, genossen" – Goethes Badeaufenthalte 1785–1823: Ausstellungskatalog*. Königstein: Athenäum, 1982.

Gräf, Hans Gerhard. *Goethe in Berka an der Ilm*. Weimar: Kiepenheuer, 1911.

Greiner, Karl. "Zur Geschichte von Bad Teinach und Zavelstein." *Zeitschrift für Württembergische Landesgeschichte* 14 (1955): 67–99.

Groh, Ruth, and Dieter Groh. *Weltbild und Naturaneignung: Zur Kulturgeschichte der Natur*. 2nd ed. Frankfurt a.M.: Suhrkamp, 1996.

Gröschel, Claudia. *Staatspark Fürstenlager: Das Fürstenlager bei Bensheim-Auerbach; Sommerresidenz der Landgrafen und Großherzöge von Hessen-Darmstadt bis 1918*. Bad Homburg: Verlag Ausbildung und Wissen, 1996.

Günther, Dagmar. "'And Now for Something Completely Different': Prolegomena zur Autobiographie als Quelle der Geschichtswissenschaft." *Historische Zeitschrift* 272 (2001): 25–61.

Günther, Harri, ed. *Gärten der Goethe-Zeit*. Leipzig: Edition Leipzig, 1993.

Günther, Walther, Werner Jäckh, and Klaus Lubkoll, eds. *Bad Boll: Geschichte und Gegenwart*. Stuttgart: Steinkopf, 1980.

Günzel, Klaus. *Bäder-Residenzen: Kuren und Amouren, Diplomatie und Intrigen*. Stuttgart: Deutsche Verlags-Anstalt, 1998.

Gyr, Ueli. "Geschichte des Tourismus: Strukturen auf dem Weg zur Moderne." In *European History Online (EGO)*, edited by the Leibniz Institute of European History. Mainz, 2010. www.ieg-ego.eu/gyru-2010-de.

Habermas, Jürgen. *Strukturwandel der Öffentlichkeit: Untersuchungen zu einer Kategorie der bürgerlichen Gesellschaft*. 1962. Frankfurt a.M.: Suhrkamp, 1990.

Habermas, Jürgen. *The Structural Transformation of the Public Sphere: An Inquiry into the Category of Bourgeois Society.* Translated by Thomas Burger. Cambridge, MA: MIT Press, 1991.

Habermas, Rebekka. *Frauen und Männer des Bürgertums: Eine Familiengeschichte (1750–1850).* Göttingen: Vandenhoeck & Ruprecht, 2000.

Haefs, Wilhelm. "Zensur im Alten Reich des 18. Jahrhunderts – Konzepte, Perspektiven und Desiderata der Forschung." In *Zensur im Jahrhundert der Aufklärung: Geschichte – Theorie – Praxis*, edited by Wilhelm Haefs and York-Gothart Mix, 389–424. Göttingen: Wallstein, 2006.

Hahn, Hans-Werner, and Dieter Hein. "Bürgerliche Werte: Zur Einführung." In *Bürgerliche Werte um 1800: Entwurf – Vermittlung – Rezeption*, edited by Hans-Werner Hahn and Dieter Hein, 9–30. Cologne: Böhlau, 2005.

Haltern, Utz. "Die Gesellschaft der Bürger." *Geschichte und Gesellschaft* 19 (1993): 100–134.

Hammermayer, Ludwig. *Der Wilhelmsbader Freimaurer-Konvent von 1782: Ein Höhe- und Wendepunkt in der Geschichte der deutschen und europäischen Geheimgesellschaften.* Heidelberg: Schneider, 1980.

Hardtwig, Wolfgang. "Eliteanspruch und Geheimnis in den Geheimgesellschaften des 18. Jahrhunderts." In *Aufklärung und Geheimgesellschaften: Zur politischen Funktion der Sozialstruktur der Freimaurerlogen im 18. Jahrhundert*, edited by Helmut Reinalter, 63–86. Munich: Oldenbourg, 1989.

Hardtwig, Wolfgang. *Genossenschaft, Sekte, Verein in Deutschland: Vom Spätmittelalter bis zur Französischen Revolution.* Munich: Beck, 1997.

Haslinger, Peter. "Diskurs, Sprache, Zeit, Identität: Plädoyer für eine erweiterte Diskursgeschichte." In *Das Gerede vom Diskurs – Diskursanalyse und Geschichte*, edited by Franz, X. Eder, 33–59. Innsbruck: StudienVerlag, 2005.

Heal, Bridget. "For Simple Folk and Connoisseurs: Lutheran Bible Illustration in the Renaissance and Baroque." In *The Cultural History of the Reformations: Theories and Applications*, edited by Susan C. Karant-Nunn and Ute Lotz-Heumann, 133–150. Wiesbaden: Harrassowitz, 2021.

Hedinger, Bärbel, ed. *Saison am Strand: Badeleben an Nord- und Ostsee 200 Jahre; Ausstellungskatalog.* Herford: Koehler, 1986.

Heimühle, Bernd. *Historische Kuranlagen und Goethe-Theater Bad Lauchstädt.* Halle: Ed. Stekofoto, 1996.

Hein, Dieter, and Andreas Schulz, eds. *Bürgerkultur im 19. Jahrhundert: Bildung, Kunst und Lebenswelt.* Munich: Beck, 1996.

Hessen, Rainer von. "Der Wilhelmsbader Freimaurerkonvent 1782: Aufklärung zwischen Vernunft und Offenbarung." In *Aufklärung in Hessen: Facetten ihrer Geschichte*, edited by Bernd Heidenreich, 10–23. Wiesbaden: Hessische Landeszentrale für Politische Bildung, 1999.

Hettling, Manfred. "Bürgerliche Kultur – Bürgerlichkeit als kulturelles System." In *Sozial- und Kulturgeschichte des Bürgertums: Eine Bilanz des Bielefelder Sonderforschungsbereichs (1986–1997)*, edited by Peter Lundgreen, 319–339. Göttingen: Vandenhoeck & Ruprecht, 2000.

Hettling, Manfred. "Soziale Figurationen und psychische Valenzen: Die Dynamik von Öffentlichkeit im 18. Jahrhundert." In *Figuren und Strukturen: Historische Essays für Hartmut Zwahr zum 65. Geburtstag*, edited by Manfred Hettling, Uwe Schirmer, and Susanne Schötz, 263–276. Munich: Saur, 2002.

Hettling, Manfred, and Stefan-Ludwig Hoffmann. "Der bürgerliche Wertehimmel: Zum Problem individueller Lebensführung im 19. Jahrhundert." *Geschichte und Gesellschaft* 23 (1997): 333–359.

Hettling, Manfred, and Stefan-Ludwig Hoffmann. "Zur Historisierung bürgerlicher Werte: Einleitung." In *Der bürgerliche Wertehimmel: Innenansichten des 19. Jahrhunderts*, edited by Manfred Hettling and Stefan-Ludwig Hoffmann, 7–21. Göttingen: Vandenhoeck & Ruprecht, 2000.

Heuvel, Christine van den. "'Warum hat Deutschland noch kein großes öffentliches Seebad?' Zu den Anfängen des Nordseebades Norderney." *Niedersächsisches Jahrbuch* 73 (2001): 133–167.

Hirsch, Erhard. "Hortus Oeconomicus: Nutzen, Schönheit, Bildung; Das Dessau-Wörlitzer Gartenreich als Landschaftsgestaltung der europäischen Aufklärung." In *"Landschaft" und Landschaften im achtzehnten Jahrhundert: Tagung der Deutschen Gesellschaft für die Erforschung des 18. Jahrhunderts, Herzog August Bibliothek Wolfenbüttel 20.-23. November 1991*, edited by Heinke Wunderlich, 179–207. Heidelberg: Universitätsverlag Winter, 1995.

Hirsch, Erhard. "'Kron'zeugen: Dessau-Wörlitz und die aufgeklärte Geschmacksrevolution: 'Landwirtschaft und Gärtnerei daselbst für Schulen in diesen Fächern'." In *Europa in der Frühen Neuzeit: Festschrift für Günter Mühlpfordt*. Vol. 5, *Aufklärung in Europa*, edited by Erich Donnert, 593–614. Cologne: Böhlau, 1999.

Hirsch, Erhard. "Utopia realisata: Utopie und Umsetzung; Aufgeklärt-humanistische Gartengestaltung in Anhalt-Dessau." In *Von der Geometrie zur Naturalisierung: Utopisches Denken im 18. Jahrhundert zwischen literarischer Fiktion und frühneuzeitlicher Gartenkunst*, edited by Richard Saage and Eva-Maria Seng, 151–179. Tübingen: Niemeyer, 1999.

Hirsch, Erhard. *Die Dessau-Wörlitzer Reformbewegung im Zeitalter der Aufklärung: Personen – Strukturen – Wirkungen.* Tübingen: Niemeyer, 2003.

Hirschberg, Leopold. *Der Taschengoedeke: Bibliographie deutscher Erstausgaben.* 2nd ed. Munich: Deutscher Taschenbuch Verlag, 1990.

Hoede, Roland. "Der Wilhelmsbader Konvent 1782: Freimaurerei zwischen Mystizismus und Aufklärung." *Quatuor Coronati* 37 (2000): 37–54.

Hohendahl, Peter Uwe, and Paul Michael Lützeler, eds. *Legitimationskrisen des deutschen Adels 1200–1900.* Stuttgart: Metzler, 1979.

Hölscher, Lucian. "Die Öffentlichkeit begegnet sich selbst: Zur Struktur öffentlichen Redens im 18. Jahrhundert zwischen Diskurs- und Sozialgeschichte." In *"Öffentlichkeit" im 18. Jahrhundert*, edited by Hans-Wolf Jäger, 11–31. Göttingen: Wallstein, 1997.

Im Hof, Ulrich. *Das gesellige Jahrhundert: Gesellschaft und Gesellschaften im Zeitalter der Aufklärung.* Munich: Beck, 1982.

Jancke, Gabriele, and Claudia Ulbrich, eds. *Vom Individuum zur Person: Neue Konzepte im Spannungsfeld von Autobiographietheorie und Selbstzeugnisforschung.* Göttingen: Wallstein, 2005.

Jeßing, Benedikt, Bernd Lutz, and Inge Wilds, eds. *Metzler Goethe Lexikon.* Stuttgart: Metzler, 1999.

Jöchner, Cornelia. "Geometrie oder Landschaft: Auflösung barocker Gartengrenzen am Karlsberg in Kassel; Fürstliche Landschaftsgestaltung an der Wende vom 17. zum 18. Jahrhundert." In *Frühneuzeitliche Hofkultur in Hessen und*

Thüringen, edited by Jörg Jochen Berns and Detlef Ignasiak, 142–166. Erlangen: Palm & Enke, 1993.

Johne, Willfried. *Bad Schandau*. Pirna: Tierbs, 2000.

Jost, Erdmut. *Landschaftsblick und Landschaftsbild: Wahrnehmung und Ästhetik im Reisebericht 1780–1820*. Freiburg i.Br.: Rombach, 2005.

Karell, Viktor. *Karlsbad im Wandel der Jahrhunderte*. Marburg: Quadriga, 1958.

Kaschuba, Wolfgang. "Erkundung der Moderne: Bürgerliches Reisen nach 1800." *Zeitschrift für Volkskunde* 87 (1991): 29–52.

Kaschuba, Wolfgang. "Deutsche Bürgerlichkeit nach 1800: Kultur als symbolische Praxis." In *Bürgertum im 19. Jahrhundert*. Vol. 3, *Verbürgerlichung, Rechte und Politik*, edited by Jürgen Kocka, 92–127. Göttingen: Vandenhoeck & Ruprecht, 1995.

Kaspar, Fred. *Brunnenkur und Sommerlust: Gesundbrunnen und Kleinbäder in Westfalen*. Bielefeld: Westfalen Verlag, 1993.

Kaspar, Fred. "Das Bad Driburg: Eine glückliche Schöpfung im Sinne der Aufklärung durch Caspar Heinrich von Sierstorpff." *Westfalen* 76 (1998): 76–99.

Kaspar, Fred. *Das Gräfliche Bad Driburg*. Münster: Westfälischer Heimatbund, 2004.

Kaufmann, Pius. *Gesellschaft im Bad: Die Entwicklung der Badefahrten und der "Naturbäder" im Gebiet der Schweiz und im angrenzenden südwestdeutschen Raum (1300–1610)*. Zurich: Chronos, 2009.

Kehn, Wolfgang. "Die Gartenkunst der deutschen Spätaufklärung als Problem der Geistes- und Literaturgeschichte." *Internationales Archiv für Sozialgeschichte der deutschen Literatur* 10 (1985): 195–224.

Kehn, Wolfgang. *Christian Cay Lorenz Hirschfeld 1742–1792: Eine Biographie*. Worms: Werner, 1992.

Kehn, Wolfgang. "Ästhetische Landschaftserfahrung und Landschaftsgestaltung in der Spätaufklärung: Der Beitrag von Christian Cay Lorenz Hirschfelds Gartentheorie." In *"Landschaft" und Landschaften im achtzehnten Jahrhundert: Tagung der Deutschen Gesellschaft für die Erforschung des 18. Jahrhunderts, Herzog August Bibliothek Wolfenbüttel 20.-23. November 1991*, edited by Heinke Wunderlich, 1–23. Heidelberg: Universitätsverlag Winter, 1995.

Kelsch, Wolfgang. "Der Freimaurer Lessing: Idee und Wirklichkeit einer freimaurerischen Utopie." In *Lessing in Braunschweig und Wolfenbüttel*, edited by Gerd Biegel, 52–61. Braunschweig: Braunschweigisches Landesmuseum, 1997.

Keyser, Erich, ed. *Hessisches Städtebuch*. Stuttgart: Kohlhammer: 1957.

Keyser, Erich, ed. *Württembergisches Städtebuch*. Stuttgart: Kohlhammer: 1961.

Kiesel, Helmuth, and Paul Münch. *Gesellschaft und Literatur im 18. Jahrhundert: Voraussetzungen und Entstehung des literarischen Markts in Deutschland*. Munich: Beck, 1977.

Kocka, Jürgen. "Bürgertum und Bürgerlichkeit als Probleme der deutschen Geschichte vom späten 18. zum frühen 20. Jahrhundert: Der Stand der Stadtbürger; eine frühneuzeitliche Tradition." In *Bürger und Bürgerlichkeit im 19. Jahrhundert*, edited by Jürgen Kocka, 21–63. Göttingen: Vandenhoeck & Ruprecht, 1987.

Kocka, Jürgen, ed. *Bürger und Bürgerlichkeit im 19. Jahrhundert*. Göttingen: Vandenhoeck & Ruprecht, 1987.

Köhler, Astrid. "Pyrmont von verschiedenen Seiten betretend: Zum literarischen Umgang mit der Heterotopie Badeort um 1800." *Publications of the English Goethe Society* 84 (2015): 48–62.

Kolbe, Wiebke. "Viel versprechende Strandwelten: Ein Werkstattbericht über den Umgang mit Bildquellen am Beispiel früher Seebäderplakate." *Werkstatt Geschichte* 36 (2004): 42–55.

Kolbe, Wiebke. "Strandurlaub als liminoider (Erfahrungs-) Raum der Moderne: Deutsche Seebäder im späten 20. Jahrhundert." In *Freizeit und Vergnügen vom 14. bis zum 20. Jahrhundert*, edited by Hans-Jörg Gilomen, Beatrice Schumacher, and Laurent Tissot, 187–199. Zurich: Chronos, 2005.

König, Gudrun M. "Das Picknick, der Spaziergang und die Landpartie – zu den Anfängen einer bürgerlichen Ausflugskultur." In *Ins Grüne: Ausflug und Picknick um 1900*, edited by Thomas Brune, 17–26. Stuttgart: Württembergisches Landesmuseum, 1992.

König, Gudrun M. *Eine Kulturgeschichte des Spazierganges: Spuren einer bürgerlichen Praktik 1780–1850*. Cologne: Böhlau, 1996.

König, Gudrun M. "Frei vom Gängelband? Zum Wandel bürgerlicher Bewegungsweisen." In *Körper – Verständnis – Erfahrung*, edited by Max Matter, 73–88. Marburg: Jonas, 1996.

Kos, Wolfgang, ed. *Die Eroberung der Landschaft: Semmering, Rax, Schneeberg; Katalog zur Niederösterreichischen Landesausstellung Schloss Gloggnitz 1992*. Vienna: Falter, 1992.

Koselleck, Reinhart. "Einleitung." In *Geschichtliche Grundbegriffe: Historisches Lexikon zur politisch-sozialen Sprache in Deutschland*. Vol. 1, edited by Otto Brunner, Werner Conze, and Reinhart Kosellek, XIII–XXVII. Stuttgart: Klett-Cotta, 1972.

Koselleck, Reinhart. "Das achtzehnte Jahrhundert als Beginn der Neuzeit." In *Epochenschwelle und Epochenbewußtsein*, edited by Reinhart Herzog and Reinhart Kosellek, 269–282. Munich: Fink, 1987.

Koselleck, Reinhart. *Kritik und Krise: Eine Studie zur Pathogenese der bürgerlichen Welt*. 1959. 8th ed. Frankfurt a.M.: Suhrkamp, 1997.

Kreutzmann, Marko. *Zwischen ständischer und bürgerlicher Lebenswelt: Adel in Sachsen-Weimar-Eisenach 1770 bis 1830*. Cologne: Böhlau, 2008.

Křížek, Vladimir. *Kulturgeschichte des Heilbades*. Stuttgart: Kohlhammer, 1990.

Kuhles, Doris, and Ulrike Standke, eds. *Journal des Luxus und der Moden 1786–1827: Analytische Bibliographie*. Munich: Saur, 2003.

Kuhnert, Reinhold P. *Urbanität auf dem Lande: Badereisen nach Pyrmont im 18. Jahrhundert*. Göttingen: Vandenhoeck & Ruprecht, 1984.

Kunisch, Johannes. "Die deutschen Führungsschichten im Zeitalter des Absolutismus." In *Deutsche Führungsschichten in der Neuzeit: Eine Zwischenbilanz*, edited by Hans Hubert Hofmann and Günther Franz, 111–141. Boppard am Rhein: Boldt, 1980.

Kunst, Hans-Joachim. "Delineatio des Canals und Fürstlichen Lustgartens zu Weimar." In *Frühneuzeitliche Hofkultur in Hessen und Thüringen*, edited by Jörg Jochen Berns und Detlef Ignasiak, 313–322. Erlangen: Palm & Enke, 1993.

Kurverwaltung Nordseeheilbad Juist, ed. *150 Jahre Seebad Juist: Eine Idee setzt sich durch*. N.p.: n.p., 1990.

Küster, Hansjörg, "Das Gartenreich Dessau-Wörlitz: Eine von Natur, Gestaltung und Ideen geprägte Landschaft." In *Landschaft um 1800: Aspekte der Wahrnehmung in Kunst, Literatur, Musik und Naturwissenschaft*, edited by Thomas Noll, Urte Stobbe, and Christian Scholl, 113–123. Göttingen: Wallstein, 2012.

Lampe, Joachim. *Aristokratie, Hofadel und Staatspatriziat in Kurhannover: Die Lebenskreise der höheren Beamten an den kurhannoverschen Zentral- und Hofbehörden, 1714–1760.* 2 vols. Göttingen: Vandenhoeck & Ruprecht, 1963.

Landwehr, Achim. *Geschichte des Sagbaren: Einführung in die Historische Diskursanalyse.* Tübingen: Edition diskord, 2001.

Landwehr, Achim, and Stefanie Stockhorst. *Einführung in die europäische Kulturgeschichte.* Paderborn: Schöningh, 2004.

Langewiesche, Dieter. "Bürgerliche Adelskritik zwischen Aufklärung und Reichsgründung in Enzyklopädien und Lexika." In *Adel und Bürgertum in Deutschland 1770–1848*, edited by Elisabeth Fehrenbach, 11–28. Munich: Oldenbourg, 1994.

Lauterbach, Iris. "Der europäische Landschaftsgarten, ca. 1710–1800." In *European History Online (EGO)*, edited by the Leibniz Institute of European History. Mainz, 2012. www.ieg-ego.eu/lauterbachi-2012-de.

Lempa, Heikki. "The Spa: Emotional Economy and Social Classes in Nineteenth-Century Pyrmont." *Central European History* 35 (2002): 37–73.

Lempa, Heikki. *Beyond the Gymnasium: Educating the Middle-Class Bodies in Classical Germany.* Lanham: Lexington Books, 2007.

Lempa, Heikki, "Emotions, Gender and the Body: The Case of Nineteenth-Century German Spa Towns." In *The Routledge History Handbook of Gender and the Urban Experience*, edited by Deborah Simonton, 362–373. London: Routledge, 2017.

Lennhoff, Eugen, Oskar Posner, and Dieter A. Binder. *Internationales Freimaurerlexikon.* Munich: Herbig, 2003.

Lietzmann, Hilda. "Des Reichsgrafen Franz Anton von Sporck Kukus-Bad: Ein Beitrag zur Kulturgeschichte Böhmens um 1700." *Archiv für Kulturgeschichte* 55 (1973): 138–165.

Löffler, Katrin. "Aufklärerische Kommunikationsformen in der Stadt Leipzig." In *Leipzig um 1800: Beiträge zur Sozial- und Kulturgeschichte*, edited by Thomas Topfstedt and Hartmut Zwahr, 17–42. Beucha: Sax, 1998.

Loleit, Simone. *Wahrheit, Lüge, Fiktion: Das Bad in der deutschsprachigen Literatur des 16. Jahrhunderts.* Bielefeld: transcript, 2008.

Lotz-Heumann, Ute. "Kurorte im Reich des 18. Jahrhunderts – ein Typus urbanen Lebens und Laboratorium der bürgerlichen Gesellschaft: Eine Problemskizze." In *Bäder und Kuren in der Aufklärung: Medizinaldiskurs und Freizeitvergnügen*, edited by Raingard Eßer and Thomas Fuchs, 15–35. Berlin: Berliner Wissenschafts-Verlag, 2003.

Lotz-Heumann, Ute. "Unterirdische Gänge, oberirdische Gänge, Spaziergänge: Freimaurerei und deutsche Kurorte im 18. Jahrhundert." *Aufklärung* 15 (2003): 159–186.

Lotz-Heumann, Ute. "Daheim und auf Reisen: Fürst Franz im Bade – Heterotopie und fürstliche Repräsentation an der Wende vom 18. zum 19. Jahrhundert." In *Das Leben des Fürsten: Studien zur Biografie von Leopold III. Friedrich Franz von Anhalt-Dessau (1740–1817)*, edited by Holger Zaunstöck, 109–120. Halle: Mitteldeutscher Verlag, 2008.

Lotz-Heumann, Ute. "Repräsentationen von Heilwassern und -quellen in der Frühen Neuzeit: Badeorte, lutherische Wunderquellen und katholische Wallfahrten." In Matthias Pohlig, Ute Lotz-Heumann, Vera Isaiasz, Ruth Schilling, Heike Bock, and Stefan Ehrenpreis. *Säkularisierungen in der Frühen Neuzeit: Methodische Probleme und empirische Fallstudien*, 277–330. Berlin: Duncker & Humblot, 2008.

Lotz-Heumann, Ute. "Wie kommt der Wandel in den Diskurs? Die Heterotopie Kurort in der Sattelzeit." In *Diskursiver Wandel*, edited by Achim Landwehr, 281–308. Wiesbaden: VS Verlag, 2010.

Löw, Martina. *Raumsoziologie*. Frankfurt a.m.: Suhrkamp, 2001.

Ludz, Peter Christian, ed. *Geheime Gesellschaften*. Heidelberg: Schneider, 1979.

Luhmann, Niklas. *Liebe als Passion: Zur Codierung von Intimität*. Frankfurt a.m.: Suhrkamp, 1982.

Lund, Hannah Lotte. *Der Berliner "jüdische Salon" um 1800: Emanzipation in der Debatte*. Berlin: de Gruyter, 2012.

Lundgreen, Peter, ed. *Sozial- und Kulturgeschichte des Bürgertums: Eine Bilanz des Bielefelder Sonderforschungsbereichs (1986–1997)*. Göttingen: Vandenhoeck & Ruprecht, 2000.

Luz, Wilhelm August. *Das Büchlein vom Bade*. Berlin-Grunewald: Herbig, 1958.

Mai, Andreas. "Touristische Räume im 19. Jahrhundert: Zur Entstehung und Ausbreitung von Sommerfrischen." *WerkstattGeschichte* 36 (2004): 7–23.

Martin, Alfred. *Deutsches Badewesen in vergangenen Tagen*. Jena: Eugen Diederichs, 1906.

Martus, Steffen. *Aufklärung: Das deutsche 18. Jahrhundert – Ein Epochenbild*. 2nd ed. Berlin: Rowohlt, 2015.

Maurer, Michael. *Die Biographie des Bürgers: Lebensformen und Denkweisen in der formativen Phase des deutschen Bürgertums (1680–1815)*. Göttingen: Vandenhoeck & Ruprecht, 1996.

Maurer, Michael. "Goethe als Prototyp: Zur sozialen Einordnung eines Bürgers von Adel." In *Goethe im sozialen und kulturellen Gefüge seiner Zeit*, edited by Jürgen Voss, 17–40. Bonn: Bouvier, 1999.

Maurer, Michael. "Reisen interdisziplinär – Ein Forschungsbericht in kulturgeschichtlicher Perspektive." In *Neue Impulse der Reiseforschung*, edited by Michael Maurer, 287–410. Berlin: Akademie Verlag, 1999.

Maurice, Florian. "'Staat im Staate' oder 'Schule der Untertanen'? Die Freimaurerei im Staat des aufgeklärten Absolutismus." In *Aufklärung und Geheimgesellschaften: Freimaurer, Illuminaten und Rosenkreuzer; Ideologie – Struktur und Wirkungen*, edited by Helmut Reinalter, 9–22. Bayreuth: Freimauerischen Forschungsgesellschaft, 1992.

Maurice, Florian. *Freimauerei um 1800: Ignaz Aurelius Feßler und die Reform der Großloge Royal York in Berlin*. Tübingen: Niemeyer, 1997.

McNeil, Peter. "The Appearance of Enlightenment: Refashioning the Elites." In *The Enlightenment World*, edited by Martin Fitzpatrick, Peter Jones, Christa Knellwolf, and Ian McCalman, 381–400. London: Routledge, 2007.

Mehrdorf, Wilhelm, and Luise Stemler. *Chronik von Bad Pyrmont*. Bad Pyrmont: Stadt Bad Pyrmont, 1967.

Mehring, Gebhard. *Badenfahrt: Württembergische Mineralbäder und Sauerbrunnen vom Mittelalter bis zum Beginn des 19. Jahrhunderts*. Stuttgart: Kohlhammer, 1914.

Melton, James Van Horn. *The Rise of the Public in Enlightenment Europe.* Cambridge, UK: Cambridge University Press, 2001.

Mensing, Wilhelm. *Der Freimaurer-Konvent von Wilhelmsbad vom 14.7. bis zum 1.9.1782 am Vorabend der französischen Revolution von 1789.* Bayreuth: Forschungsloge Quatuor Coronati, 1974.

Mensing, Wilhelm. "Der Illuminatismus auf dem Freimaurer-Konvent in Wilhelmsbad vom 14.7. bis zum 1.9.1782." *Zeitschrift für bayerische Landesgeschichte* 41 (1978): 271–291.

Mergel, Thomas. "Die Bürgertumsforschung nach 15 Jahren." *Archiv für Sozialgeschichte* 41 (2001): 515–538.

Michels, Norbert, ed. *Anhalt in alten Ansichten.* Halle: Mitteldeutscher Verlag, 2006.

Miller, Max, and Gerhard Taddey, eds. *Handbuch der historischen Stätten: Baden-Württemberg.* Stuttgart: Kröner, 1980.

Mintzker, Yair. *The Defortification of the German City, 1689–1866.* Cambridge, UK: Cambridge University Press, 2012.

Mittelstädt, Ina. *Wörlitz, Weimar, Muskau: Der Landschaftsgarten als Medium des Hochadels (1760–1840).* Cologne: Böhlau, 2015.

Möller, Horst. "Die Bruderschaft der Gold- und Rosenkreuzer: Struktur, Zielsetzung und Wirkung einer anti-aufklärerischen Geheimgesellschaft." In *Freimaurer und Geheimbünde im 18. Jahrhundert in Mitteleuropa*, edited by Helmut Reinalter, 199–239. Frankfurt a.M.: Suhrkamp, 1983.

Möller, Horst. "Aufklärung und Adel." In *Adel und Bürgertum in Deutschland 1770–1848*, edited by Elisabeth Fehrenbach, 1–9. Munich: Oldenbourg, 1994.

Möller, Horst. *Fürstenstaat und Bürgernation: Deutschland 1763–1815.* Berlin: Siedler, 1994.

Mörke, Olaf. "Social Structure." In *Germany: A New Social and Economic History*. Vol. 2, *1630–1800*, edited by Sheilagh Ogilvie, 134–163. London: Arnold, 1996.

Mühlphordt, Günter. "Europapolitik im Duodezformat: Die internationale Geheimgesellschaft 'Union' – Ein radikalaufklärerischer Bund der Intelligenz (1786–1796)." In *Freimaurer und Geheimbünde im 18. Jahrhundert in Mitteleuropa*, edited by Helmut Reinalter, 319–364. Frankfurt a.M.: Suhrkamp, 1983.

Müller, Susanne. *Die Welt des Baedeker: Eine Medienkulturgeschichte des Reiseführers 1830–1945.* Frankfurt a.M.: Campus, 2012.

Müller, Winfried. *Die Aufklärung.* Munich: Oldenbourg, 2002.

Münch, Paul. *Lebensformen in der Frühen Neuzeit 1500–1800.* Frankfurt a.M.: Ullstein, 1996.

Münch, Paul, ed. *"Erfahrung" als Kategorie der Frühneuzeitgeschichte.* Munich: Oldenbourg, 2001.

Naimark-Goldberg, Natalie. "Health, Leisure and Sociability at the Turn of the Nineteenth Century: Jewish Women in German Spas." *Leo Baeck Institute Year Book* 55 (2010): 63–91.

Neugebauer-Wölk, Monika. *Esoterische Bünde und bürgerliche Gesellschaft: Entwicklungslinien zur modernen Welt im Geheimbundwesen des 18. Jahrhunderts.* Göttingen: Wallstein, 1995.

Neugebauer-Wölk, Monika, ed. "Arkanwelten im 18. Jahrhundert: Zur Struktur des Politischen im Kontext von Aufklärung und frühmoderner Staatlichkeit." *Aufklärung* 15 (2003): 7–65.

Niedermeier, Michael. "Wörlitz als höfische Veranstaltung? Eros zwischen höfischer Selbstreflexion, pädagogischer Kontrolle und naturalisierter Utopie." In *Von der Geometrie zur Naturalisierung: Utopisches Denken im 18. Jahrhundert zwischen literarischer Fiktion und frühneuzeitlicher Gartenkunst*, edited by Richard Saage and Eva-Maria Seng, 180–208. Tübingen: Niemeyer, 1999.

Niedermeier, Michael. "'Die ganze Erde wird zu einem Garten': Gedächtniskonstruktion im frühen deutschen Landschaftsgarten zwischen Aufklärung und Geheimnis." In *Weimar – Archäologie eines Ortes*, edited by Georg Bollenbeck, Jochen Golz, Michael Knoche, and Ulrike Steierwald, 120–175. Weimar: Hermann Böhlaus Nachfolger, 2001.

Nipperdey, Thomas. "Verein als soziale Struktur in Deutschland im späten 18. und frühen 19. Jahrhundert: Eine Fallstudie zur Modernisierung I." In *Gesellschaft, Kultur, Theorie: Gesammelte Aufsätze zur neueren Geschichte*, edited by Helmut Berding, Jürgen Kocka, Hans-Christoph Schröder, and Hans-Ulrich Wehler, 174–205. Göttingen: Vandenhoeck & Ruprecht, 1976.

Nipperdey, Thomas. "Kommentar: 'Bürgerlich' als Kultur." In *Bürger und Bürgerlichkeit im 19. Jahrhundert*, edited by Jürgen Kocka, 143–148. Göttingen: Vandenhoeck & Ruprecht, 1987.

Nizze, Adolf. *Doberan-Heiligendamm: Geschichte des ersten deutschen Seebades*, 1936. Reprint. Wismar: Godewind, 2006.

Nohl, Günther, ed. *Berichte vom Meinberger Brunnen im Lande Lippe*. Bad Meinberg: Topp & Möller, 1967.

North, Michael. *"Material Delight and the Joy of Living": Cultural Consumption in the Age of Enlightenment in Germany*. London: Routledge, 2016.

Nowitzki, Hans-Peter. "Curriculum Vitae: Fundstücke und Nachträge zur Biographie Ernst Platners." *Aufklärung* 19 (2007): 343–378.

Oppenheim, Roy. *Die Entdeckung der Alpen*. Frankfurt a.M.: Büchergilde Gutenberg, 1977.

Outram, Dorinda. *The Enlightenment*. Cambridge, UK: Cambridge University Press, 1995.

Ozturk, Anthony. "Interlude: Geo-Poetics; The Alpine Sublime in Art and Literature, 1779–1860." In *Heights of Reflection: Mountains in the German Imagination from the Middle Ages to the Twenty-First Century*, edited by Sean Ireton and Caroline Schaumann, 77–97. Rochester, NY: Camden House, 2012.

Palmer, Richard. "'In This Our Lightye and Learned Tyme': Italian Baths in the Era of the Renaissance." In *The Medical History of Waters and Spas*, edited by Roy Porter, 14–22. London: Wellcome Institute for the History of Medicine, 1990.

Park, Katharine. "Natural Particulars: Medical Epistemology, Practice, and the Literature of Healing Springs. In *Natural Particulars: Nature and the Disciplines in Renaissance Europe*, edited by Anthony Grafton and Nancy Siraisi, 1–16. Cambridge, MA: MIT Press, 1999.

Paulmann, Johannes. *Pomp und Politik: Monarchenbegegnungen in Europa zwischen Ancien Régime und Erstem Weltkrieg*. Paderborn: Schöningh, 2000.

Porter, Roy, ed. *The Medical History of Waters and Spas*. London: Wellcome Institute for the History of Medicine, 1990.

Porter, Roy. *Die Kunst des Heilens: Eine medizinische Geschichte der Menschheit von der Antike bis heute*. Berlin: Spektrum, 2007.

Prignitz, Horst. *Vom Badekarren zum Strandkorb: Zur Geschichte des Badewesens an der Ostseeküste.* Leipzig: Koehler & Amelang, 1977.

Probst, Irmgard. *Die Balneologie des 16. Jahrhunderts im Spiegel der deutschen Badeschriften.* Münster: Institut für Geschichte der Medizin der Universität Münster, 1971.

Purdy, Daniel. *The Tyranny of Elegance: Consumer Cosmopolitanism in the Era of Goethe.* Baltimore: Johns Hopkins University Press, 1998.

Puschner, Uwe. "Lesegesellschaften." In *Kommunikation und Medien in Preußen vom 16. bis zum 19. Jahrhundert,* edited by Bernd Sösemann, 193–206. Stuttgart: Steiner, 2002.

Putschky, Carmen. "Wilhelmsbad, Hofgeismar und Nenndorf: Drei Kurorte Wilhelms I. von Hessen-Kassel." PhD diss. Philipps-Universität Marburg, 2000. http://archiv.ub.uni-marburg.de/diss/z2002/0396/pdf/dcp.pdf.

Raymond, Petra. *Von der Landschaft im Kopf zur Landschaft aus Sprache: Die Romantisierung der Alpen in den Reiseschilderungen und die Literarisierung des Gebirges in der Erzählprosa der Goethezeit.* Tübingen: Niemeyer, 1993.

Rees, Joachim, and Winfried Siebers, eds. *Erfahrungsraum Europa: Reisen politischer Funktionsträger des Alten Reichs 1750–1800; Ein kommentiertes Verzeichnis handschriftlicher Quellen.* Berlin: Berliner Wissenschafts-Verlag, 2005.

Reif, Heinz. *Adel im 19. und 20. Jahrhundert.* Munich: Oldenbourg, 1999.

Reinalter, Helmut, ed. *Freimaurer und Geheimbünde im 18. Jahrhundert in Mitteleuropa.* Frankfurt a.M.: Suhrkamp, 1983.

Reinalter, Helmut, ed. *Aufklärungsgesellschaften.* Frankfurt a.M.: Peter Lang, 1993.

Reinalter, Helmut. "Freimaurerei und Geheimgesellschaften." In *Aufklärungsgesellschaften,* edited by Helmut Reinalter, 83–96. Frankfurt a.M.: Peter Lang, 1993.

Reinhard, Wolfgang. *Lebensformen Europas: Eine historische Kulturanthropologie.* Munich: Beck, 2004.

Reinhold, Heinrich. *Bad Lauchstädt, seine literarischen Denkwürdigkeiten und sein Goethetheater.* Halle: Buchhandlungen des Waisenhauses, 1914.

Renner, Michael. "Ein Dichter auf Badereise: Leopold Gökingks Bad Brückenauer Impressionen 1781." *Zeitschrift für bayerische Landesgeschichte* 27 (1964): 600–620.

Rieck, Werner. "'Doctor Bahrdt mit der eisernen Stirn . . . ': Zimmermann und Kotzebue im Kampf gegen die Aufklärung." *Weimarer Beiträge* 12 (1966): 909–935.

Röhring, Micha. "1639–1989: 350 Jahre Gesundbrunnen bei Hofgeismar." *Jahrbuch des Landkreises Kassel* (1989): 123–128.

Rosseaux, Ulrich. *Städte in der Frühen Neuzeit.* Darmstadt: Wissenschaftliche Buchgesellschaft, 2006.

Rosseaux, Ulrich. *Freiräume: Unterhaltung, Vergnügen und Erholung in Dresden (1694–1830).* Cologne: Böhlau, 2007.

Rossel, K. "Kurfürst Augusts von Sachsen Badereise nach Langenschwalbach im Jahr 1584." *Annalen des Vereins für Nassauische Alterthumskunde und Geschichtsforschung* 6, no. 2 (1859/1860): 376–381.

Rumpel, Sabine. "Der Einfluß der Obrigkeit." In *Bad Boll 1595–1995: Vom herzoglichen Wunderbad zum Kurort,* edited by Gemeinde Boll, 78–86. Weißenhorn: Konrad, 1995.

Rumpel, Sabine. "Zwischen Kurvergnügen und Verkauf." In *Bad Boll 1595–1995: Vom herzoglichen Wunderbad zum Kurort*, edited by Gemeinde Boll, 119–136. Weißenhorn: Konrad, 1995.

Ruppert, Hans, ed. *Goethes Bibliothek: Katalog*. Weimar: Arion, 1958.

Sarasin, Philipp. "Subjekte, Diskurse, Körper: Überlegungen zu einer diskursanalytischen Kulturgeschichte." In *Kulturgeschichte heute*, edited by Wolfgang Hardtwig and Hans-Ulrich Wehler, 131–164. Göttingen: Vandenhoeck & Ruprecht, 1996.

Sarasin, Philipp. "Diskurstheorie und Geschichtswissenschaft." In *Handbuch Sozialwissenschaftliche Diskursanalyse*. Vol. 1, *Theorien und Methoden*, edited by Reiner Keller, Andreas Hirseland, Werner Schneider, and Willy Viehöver, 53–79. Opladen: Leske & Budrich, 2001.

Sarasin, Philipp. *Reizbare Maschinen: Eine Geschichte des Körpers 1765–1914*. Frankfurt a.M.: Suhrkamp, 2001.

Sarasin, Philipp. *Geschichtswissenschaft und Diskursanalyse*. Frankfurt a.M.: Suhrkamp, 2003.

Schaumann, Caroline. "From Meadows to Mountaintops: Albrecht von Haller's 'Die Alpen'." In *Heights of Reflection: Mountains in the German Imagination from the Middle Ages to the Twenty-First Century*, edited by Sean Ireton and Caroline Schaumann, 57–76. Rochester, NY: Camden House, 2012.

Schepers, Wolfgang. *Hirschfelds Theorie der Gartenkunst 1779–1785*. Worms: Werner, 1980.

Schiff, Gert. "Der Gründer von Kuks: Franz Anton Reichsgraf von Sporck, Die Tugenden und Laster, Erläuterungen zum Zyklus der Tugenden und Laster, Die Plastiken im Neuwald." *Kulturelle Monatsschrift* 23 (1963): 2, 11–12, 32, 45–46, 58, 60, 62.

Schilling, Heinz. "Wandlungs- und Differenzierungsprozesse innerhalb der bürgerlichen Oberschicht West- und Nordwestdeutschlands im 16. und 17. Jahrhundert." In *Schichtung und Entwicklung der Gesellschaft in Polen und Deutschland im 16. und 17. Jahrhundert: Parallelen, Verknüpfungen, Vergleiche*, edited by Marian Biskup and Klaus Zernack, 121–173. Wiesbaden: Steiner, 1983.

Schilling, Heinz. *Die Stadt in der Frühen Neuzeit*. Munich: Oldenbourg, 1993.

Schindler, Norbert. "Freimaurerkultur im 18. Jahrhundert: Zur sozialen Funktion des Geheimnisses in der entstehenden bürgerlichen Gesellschaft." In *Klassen und Kultur: Sozialanthropologische Perspektiven in der Geschichtsschreibung*, edited by Robert M. Berdahl et al., 205–262. Frankfurt a.M.: Syndikat, 1982.

Schlögl, Rudolf. "Die patriotisch-gemeinnützigen Gesellschaften: Organisation, Sozialstruktur, Tätigkeitsfelder." In *Aufklärungsgesellschaften*, edited by Helmut Reinalter, 61–81. Frankfurt a.M.: Peter Lang, 1993.

Schmidt, Alexander. "Das Überleben der 'Kleinen': Die Zäsur 1806 und die Politik Sachsen-Weimar-Eisenachs (1796–1813)." In *Das Jahr 1806 im europäischen Kontext: Balance, Hegemonie, und politische Kulturen*, edited by Hans-Werner Hahn, Andreas Klinger, and Georg Schmidt, 349–380. Cologne: Böhlau, 2008.

Schneider, Helmut J. "Institution und Intimität: Zur Vergeistigung des Sozietätsgedankens in Lessings Freimaurergesprächen." In *Europäische Sozietätsbewegung und demokratische Tradition: Die europäischen Akademien der Frühen Neuzeit zwischen Frührenaissance und Spätaufklärung*, edited by Klaus Garber and Heinz Wismann, 1668–1696. Tübingen: Niemeyer, 1996.

Schneider-Strittmatter, Hermann. *Langensteinbach: Das einstige Fürstenbad.* Karlsruhe: Langensteinbach Bürgermeisteramt, 1970.

Schultze, Johanna. *Die Auseinandersetzung zwischen Adel und Bürgertum in den deutschen Zeitschriften der letzten drei Jahrzehnte des 18. Jahrhunderts (1773–1806).* Berlin: Ebering, 1925. Reprint. Vaduz: Kraus, 1965.

Schüttler, Hermann. "Der Wilhelmsbader Freimaurerkonvent im Spiegel der Illuminaten." In *Geheime Gesellschaft: Weimar und die deutsche Freimaurerei; Katalog zur Ausstellung der Stiftung Weimarer Klassik im Schiller-Museum Weimar 21. Juni bis 31. Dezember 2002,* edited by Joachim Berger and Klaus-Jürgen Grün, 175–184. Munich: Hanser, 2002.

Seibert, Peter. *Der literarische Salon: Literatur und Geselligkeit zwischen Aufklärung und Vormärz.* Stuttgart: Metzler, 1993.

Seitz, Gabriele. *Wo Europa den Himmel berührt: Die Entdeckung der Alpen.* Frankfurt a.M.: Büchergilde Gutenberg, 1989.

Seng, Eva-Maria. "Die Wörlitzer Anlagen zwischen Englischem Landschaftsgarten und Bon-Sauvage-Utopie?" In *Von der Geometrie zur Naturalisierung: Utopisches Denken im 18. Jahrhundert zwischen literarischer Fiktion und frühneuzeitlicher Gartenkunst,* edited by Richard Saage and Eva-Maria Seng, 117–150. Tübingen: Niemeyer, 1999.

Siemann, Wolfram. "Zensur im Übergang zur Moderne: Die Bedeutung des 'langen 19. Jahrhunderts'." In *Zensur im Jahrhundert der Aufklärung: Geschichte – Theorie – Praxis,* edited by Wilhelm Haefs and York-Gothart Mix, 357–387. Göttingen: Wallstein, 2006.

Sommer, Hermann. *Zur Kur nach Ems: Ein Beitrag zur Geschichte der Badereise von 1830 bis 1914.* Stuttgart: Steiner, 1999.

Spode, Hasso. "Die paneuropäische Touristenklasse: Zum Potential der historischen Tourismusforschung." *Themenportal Europäische Geschichte,* 2006. www.europa.clio-online.de/essay/id/fdae-1358.

Steudel, J. "Geschichte der Bäder- und Klimaheilkunde." In *Handbuch der Bäder- und Klimaheilkunde,* edited by Walter Amelung and Arrien Evers, 1–18. Stuttgart: Schattauer, 1962.

Steward, Jill. "The Role of Inland Spas as Sites of Transnational Cultural Exchange in the Production of European Leisure Culture (1750–1870)." In *Leisure Cultures in Urban Europe, c. 1700–1870,* edited by Peter Borsay and Jan Hein Furnée, 234–259. Manchester: Manchester University Press, 2016.

Stobbe, Urte. "Konkurriende Wahrnehmungsmodelle gebildeter Reisender: Zur Diversifizierung der Gartenbetrachtung in der Reise- und Gartenliteratur." In *Landschaft um 1800: Aspekte der Wahrnehmung in Kunst, Literatur, Musik und Naturwissenschaft,* edited by Thomas Noll, Urte Stobbe, and Christian Scholl, 172–206. Göttingen: Wallstein, 2012.

Stoffel, Patrick. *Die Alpen: Wo die Natur zur Vernunft kam.* Göttingen: Wallstein, 2018.

Stolberg, Michael. *Homo patiens: Krankheits- und Körpererfahrung in der Frühen Neuzeit.* Cologne: Böhlau, 2003.

Stollberg-Rilinger, Barbara. "Zeremoniell als politisches Verfahren: Rangordnung und Rangstreit als Strukturmerkmale des frühneuzeitlichen Reichstags." In *Neue Studien zur frühneuzeitlichen Reichsgeschichte,* edited by Johannes Kunisch, 91–132. Berlin: Duncker & Humblot, 1997.

Stollberg-Rilinger, Barbara. "Ordnungsleistung und Konfliktträchtigkeit der höfischen Tafel." In *Zeichen und Raum: Ausstattung und höfisches Zeremoniell in den deutschen Schlössern der Frühen Neuzeit*, edited by Peter-Michael Hahn and Ulrich Schütte, 103–122. Munich: Deutscher Kunstverlag, 2006.

Strahlmann, Berend. "Heinrich Matthias Marcard: Leibmedicus des Herzogs Peter Friedrich Ludwig von Oldenburg." *Oldenburger Jahrbuch* 60 (1961): 57–120.

Struck, Wolf-Heino. *Wiesbaden in der Goethezeit*. Wiesbaden: Steiner, 1979.

Studt, Birgit. "Die Badenfahrt: Ein neues Muster der Badepraxis und Badegeselligkeit im deutschen Spätmittelalter." In *Badeorte und Bäderreisen in Antike, Mittelalter und Neuzeit*, edited by Michael Matheus, 33–52. Stuttgart: Steiner, 2001.

Stützel-Prüsener, Marlies. "Lesegesellschaften." In *Aufklärungsgesellschaften*, edited by Helmut Reinalter, 39–59. Frankfurt a.M.: Peter Lang, 1993.

Tausch, Harald. "Franz Anton von Sporcks 'Kuckus=Bad': Intermediale Aspekte von Gartenkunst und Literatur in einem böhmischen Badeort zwischen Barock und Frühaufklärung (J.Chr. Günther und Ph.B. Sinold)." In *Der andere Garten: Erinnern und Erfinden in Gärten von Institutionen*, edited by Natascha N. Hoefer and Anna Ananieva, 125–157. Göttingen: Vandenhoeck & Ruprecht, 2005.

Taute, Reinhold. *Der Wilhelmsbader Konvent und der Zusammenbruch der Strikten Observanz*. Berlin: Wunder, 1909.

Thielcke, Hans. *Die Bauten des Seebades Doberan-Heiligendamm um 1800 und ihr Baumeister Severin*. 1917. Reprint. Börgerende-Rethwisch: Godewind, 2005.

Thomas, Keith. *Man and the Natural World: Changing Attitudes in England 1500–1800*. London: Penguin, 1984.

Tilgner, Hilmar. *Lesegesellschaften an Mosel und Mittelrhein im Zeitalter des aufgeklärten Absolutismus: Ein Beitrag zur Sozialgeschichte der Aufklärung im Kurfürstentum Trier*. Stuttgart: Steiner, 2001.

Trauzettel, Ludwig. "Das Gartenreich von Wörlitz und Dessau: Fürst Franz, die Reformen und das Gartenreich." In *Gärten der Goethe-Zeit*, edited by Harri Günther, 45–75. Leipzig: Edition Leipzig, 1993.

Trepp, Anne-Charlott. *Sanfte Männlichkeit und selbständige Weiblichkeit: Frauen und Männer im Hamburger Bürgertum zwischen 1770 und 1840*. Göttingen: Vandenhoeck & Ruprecht, 1996.

Triendl-Zadoff, Mirjam. *Nächstes Jahr in Marienbad: Gegenwelten jüdischer Kulturen der Moderne*. Göttingen: Vandenhoeck & Ruprecht, 2007.

Trommsdorff, Hermann. *Die Freimaurerei in Pyrmont: Beiträge zur Kulturgeschichte Niedersachsens im 18. Jahrhundert; Festschrift zur Feier der Neugründung der Loge Freidrich zu den drei Quellen in Bad Pyrmont*. Göttingen: Hofer, 1928.

Umbach, Maiken. "The Politics of Sentimentality and the German *Fürstenbund*, 1779–1785." *Historical Journal* 41 (1998): 679–703.

Umbach, Maiken. "Visual Culture, Scientific Images and German Small-State Politics in the Late Enlightenment." *Past and Present* 158 (1998): 110–145.

Umbach, Maiken. *Federalism und Enlightenment in Germany 1740–1806*. London: Bloomsbury Academic, 2000.

Umbach, Maiken. "Culture and *Bürgerlichkeit* in Eighteenth-Century Germany." In *Culture of Power in Europe during the Long Eighteenth Century*, edited by Hamish Scott and Brendan Smith, 180–199. Cambridge, UK: Cambridge University Press, 2007.

Urry, John, and Jonas Larsen. *The Tourist Gaze 3.0.* Los Angeles: Sage, 2011.

Vanja, Christina. "Arme Hessen in Kurbädern des 18. Jahrhunderts." *Virus: Beiträge zur Sozialgeschichte der Medizin* 12 (2013): 11–25.

Vierhaus, Rudolf, ed. *Deutsche patriotische und gemeinnützige Gesellschaften.* Munich: Kraus, 1980.

Vierhaus, Rudolf, ed. *Bürger und Bürgerlichkeit im Zeitalter der Aufklärung.* Heidelberg: Schneider, 1981.

Vierhaus, Rudolf. "Umrisse einer Sozialgeschichte der Gebildeten in Deutschland." In *Deutschland im 18. Jahrhundert: Politische Verfassung, soziales Gefüge, geistige Bewegungen: Ausgewählte Aufsätze*, 167–182. Göttingen: Vandenhoeck & Ruprecht, 1987.

Vogel, Gerd-Helge. *Die Entstehung des ersten deutschen Seebades Doberan-Heiligendamm unter dem Baumeister Carl-Theodor Severin (1763–1836).* Niederjahna: Donatus, 2018.

Voges, Michael. *Aufklärung und Geheimnis: Untersuchungen zur Vermittlung von Literatur- und Sozialgeschichte am Beispiel der Aneignung des Geheimbundmaterials im Roman des späten 18. Jahrhunderts.* Tübingen: Hermann Böhlaus Nachfolger, 1987.

Wackenroder, Ernst, ed. *Die Kunstdenkmäler des Landkreises Cochem.* Munich: Deutscher Kunstverlag, 1984.

Walton, John K. "Coastal Resorts and Cultural Exchange in Europe, 1780–1870." In *Leisure Cultures in Urban Europe, c. 1700–1870*, edited by Peter Borsay and Jan Hein Furnée, 260–277. Manchester: Manchester University Press, 2016.

Warneken, Bernd Jürgen. "Bürgerliche Gehkultur in der Epoche der Französischen Revolution." *Zeitschrift für Volkskunde* 85 (1989): 177–187.

Wegner, Ewald. "Staatsbad Bocklet." In *Kurstädte in Deutschland: Zur Geschichte einer Baugattung*, edited by Rolf Bothe, 257–264. Berlin: Frölich & Kaufmann, 1984.

Wegner, Ewald. "Staatsbad Brückenau." In *Kurstädte in Deutschland: Zur Geschichte einer Baugattung*, edited by Rolf Bothe, 265–280. Berlin: Frölich & Kaufmann, 1984.

Wehler, Hans-Ulrich. *Deutsche Gesellschaftsgeschichte.* Vol. 1, *Vom Feudalismus des Alten Reiches bis zur Defensiven Modernisierung der Reformära 1700–1815.* 2nd ed. Munich: Beck, 1989.

Weinland, Martina. "Geschichte des Bades Nenndorf: Von seiner Gründung bis zum 20. Jahrhundert." In *Kurstädte in Deutschland: Zur Geschichte einer Baugattung*, edited by Rolf Bothe, 385–400. Berlin: Frölich & Kaufmann, 1984.

Weiss, Richard, ed. *Die Entdeckung der Alpen: Eine Sammlung schweizerischer und deutscher Alpenliteratur bis zum Jahr 1800.* Frauenfeld: Huber, 1934.

Whaley, Joachim. "The Transformation of the Aufklärung: From the Idea of Power to the Power of Ideas." In *Culture of Power in Europe during the Long Eighteenth Century*, edited by Hamish Scott and Brendan Smith, 158–179. Cambridge, UK: Cambridge University Press, 2007.

Wiedemann, Alfred. *Geschichte Godesbergs und seiner Umgebung*, 2nd, augmented ed. Bad Godesberg: Weidlich, 1930.

Wieland, Christian. "Selbstzivilisierung zur Statusbehauptung." *Geschichte und Gesellschaft* 33 (2007): 326–349.

Wilhelmy-Dollinger, Petra. "Emanzipation durch Geselligkeit: Die Salons jüdischer Frauen in Berlin zwischen 1780 und 1830." In *Bild und Selbstbild der Juden Berlins zwischen Aufklärung und Romantik*, edited by Marianne Awerbuch and Stefi Jersch-Wenzel, 121–138. Berlin: Colloquium, 1992.

Wilson, W. Daniel. *Unterirdische Gänge: Goethe, Freimaurerei und Politik*. Göttingen: Wallstein, 1999.

Winkler, Kurt. "Bad Kissingen." In *Kurstädte in Deutschland: Zur Geschichte einer Baugattung*, edited by Rolf Bothe, 361–384. Berlin: Frölich & Kaufmann, 1984.

Winterling, Aloys. *Der Hof der Kurfürsten von Köln 1688–1794: Eine Fallstudie zur Bedeutung "absolutistischer" Hofhaltung*. Bonn: Röhrscheid, 1986.

Wood, Karl E. *Health and Hazard: Spa Culture and the Social History of Medicine in the Nineteenth Century*. Newcastle: Cambridge Scholars Publishing, 2012.

Woźniakowski, Jacek. *Die Wildnis: Zur Deutungsgeschichte des Berges in der europäischen Neuzeit*. Frankfurt a.M.: Suhrkamp, 1987.

Würgler, Andreas. *Medien in der Frühen Neuzeit*. Munich: Oldenbourg, 2009.

Wurst, Karin. *Fabricating Pleasure: Fashion, Entertainment, and Cultural Consumption in Germany, 1780–1830*. Detroit: Wayne State University Press, 2005.

Zadoff, Mirjam. *Next Year in Marienbad: The Lost Worlds of Jewish Spa Culture*. Philadelphia: University of Pennsylvania Press, 2012.

Zaunstöck, Holger. *Sozietätslandschaft und Mitgliederstrukturen: Die mitteldeutschen Aufklärungsgesellschaften im 18. Jahrhundert*. Tübingen: Niemeyer, 1999.

Zaunstöck, Holger. "Die vernetzte Gesellschaft: Überlegungen zur Kommunikationsgeschichte des 18. Jahrhunderts." In *Geheime Gesellschaft: Weimar und die deutsche Freimaurerei; Katalog zur Ausstellung der Stiftung Weimarer Klassik im Schiller-Museum Weimar 21. Juni bis 31. Dezember 2002*, edited by Joachim Berger and Klaus Jürgen Grün, 147–153. Munich: Hanser, 2002.

Zaunstöck, Holger. "Zur Einleitung: Neue Wege der Sozietätengeschichte." In *Sozietäten, Netzwerke, Kommunikation: Neue Forschungen zur Vergesellschaftung im Jahrhundert der Aufklärung*, edited by Holger Zaunstöck and Markus Meumann, 1–10. Tübingen: Niemeyer, 2003.

Zaunstöck, Holger, and Markus Meumann, eds. *Sozietäten, Netzwerke, Kommunikation: Neue Forschungen zur Vergesellschaftung im Jahrhundert der Aufklärung*. Tübingen: Niemeyer, 2003.

Zeman, Herbert. "Vom Badereisen und vom Dichten – Goethe." In *Zwischen Aufklärung und Restauration: Sozialer Wandel in der deutschen Literatur (1700–1848); Festschrift für Wolfgang Martens zum 65. Geburtstag*, edited by Wolfgang Frühwald and Alberto Martino, 263–281. Tübingen: Niemeyer, 1989.

Zetzsche, Christian. *200 Jahre Freimaurerei in Pyrmont: Geschichte und Selbsterlebtes*. Langenhagen: Poppdruck, 1975.

Ziegler, Anke. *Deutsche Kurstädte im Wandel: Von den Anfängen bis zum Idealtypus im 19. Jahrhundert*. Frankfurt a.M.: Peter Lang, 2004.

Index

Page numbers in italics refer to figures.

Aachen 5, 25, 29, 44–45; drinking wells at 28; landscape and built space at 106–107, 112, 113; map of 106; patrons of 31–32; showers at 27
Adelholzen 114, 115
Adelsstolz im Bade zu Lauchstädt, Der 228, 230, 255
Alexandersbad 31, 34, 149, 252
Alexisbad 34, 42, 149, 150–152, 152
Alexius Friedrich Christian (duke of Anhalt-Bernburg) 34
Allgemeine Literatur-Zeitung 79
Allgemeines Preußisches Landrecht see General Prussian Land Law
Alps: "discovery" of 99–100; spa landscapes and regions compared to 142–143, 149
alte teutsche ehrliche und liebliche Pyrmont, Das 73
Altwasser 48, 57n161, 178n49
American Revolutionary War 39
Antogast 48, 178n47
Auerbach 36, 46
August (elector of Saxony) 44
Augustusbad 48, 57n159, 178n46
avenues 112–114, 116–119, 158, 286

Badeausschlag see bathing rash
Badefreiheit see spa freedom
Badegeschenke see spa gifts
Baden (in Swabia) see Baden-Baden
Baden (in Switzerland) 29, 72, 134, 200–201
Baden (near Vienna) 72
Baden-Baden 5, 25, 29, 31, 285; landscape and surroundings of 149, 153, 155, 156; patrons of 34–35; visitors to 42, 46

Badenweiler 35
Badeuniform see spa uniform
Baggesen, Jens 86n24, 130, 147, 170–171, 255
Bagni di Lucca 29, 200–201
Bagno Vignioni 25
Bahrdt, Karl Friedrich 67–68
Bahrdt pasquinade 66–68
balneology 20n53, 70–71, 76–77
Baltic Sea, seaside resorts on 157–158, 162–163
Bath (England) 249
bathing rash 25
baths, Roman 25
Bauhin, Johannes: New Badbuch (New Spa Book) 112, 114, 114
Becher, David 148, 208
Becker, Sophie 12; in circle of Dorothea (duchess of Courland) 256, 259–260; on daily routine at Karlsbad 172; at Masonic lodge in Brückenau 64–65
Beermann, Sigismund 70, 201, 202; Einige Historische Nachrichten und Anmerckungen Von der Graffschafft Pyrmont und Ihren berühmten Saur-Brunnen (Some Historical News and Notes about the County of Pyrmont and Its Famous Mineral Spring) 73
beggars 47
Bellomo, theater company of 45–46
Berggießhübel 48, 57n159, 178n46
Berka 30, 31, 34
Bertrich 31, 34, 42, 46, 124, 126, 127
Bertuch, Friedrich Justin 35–36, 63
bibles, illustrated 231
Bibra, Heinrich von (prince-bishop of Fulda) 251

Bilderbibeln see bibles, illustrated
Blondel, Franz: treatise on Aachen by
    44, 106–107
Bocklet 31, 34–35, 48, 126, *128*, 130
Bode, Johann Joachim Christoph 256,
    259–260
Bohemian spa cluster 48; as
    "Bohemian Switzerland" 149
Boll 31, 34, 112, *114*, 114
Böttiger, Karl August 258–259
bourgeoisie 193–195, 211; bourgeois
    identity 203–204, 228–229,
    237–239, 242–243; criticism of
    244–248; noble interactions with
    201–202, 204–211 (*see also* social
    tone; spa freedom); print media
    and 8; ruling princes and 253–254;
    social circles within 254–255; as
    visitors to spas 5–6, 200–203
*Briefe eines Reisenden an seinen
    Freund Ueber den Aufenthalte beim
    Godesberger Gesundbrunnen* 32
Briefe eines Schweizers 31
Brückenau 31, 48; beggars at 47;
    clergy as visitors to 46; Jewish
    visitor to 263–264; landscape and
    interior spaces of 126; Masonic
    lodge at 64; palace at 130, *131*;
    patrons of 34, 251; seating
    arrangements at 206–207; social
    tone of 215–216, 234–235
Brühl, Christina von (countess) 256
Brühl, Hans Moritz von (count)
    256–257
Brunhildisfelsen (Taunus) 155
Brunnenärzte see physicians, spa
Brunnenfreiheit see spa freedom
Brunnenkönig see spa king
Brunnenlisten see spa lists
Brunnentempel see spring temple
Bühren, Adolph: *Vier Wochen in
    Pyrmont* (*Four Weeks in Pyrmont*) 81
Burtscheid 107
Buschbad 48, 57n159, 178n46
Buwinghausen-Wallmerode,
    Alexander Baron (*Freiherr*) von 32
Buxhöwden, Friedrich von (count) 65

Campe, Joachim Heinrich 43, 63;
    Bahrdt pasquinade and 68; *Reise
    von Braunschweig nach Karlsbad
    (Travels from Braunschweig to
    Karlsbad)* 237, 240

Carl August (duke of Saxe-Weimar-
    Eisenach) 34, 63
Carlsbad *see* Karlsbad
censorship 8–9, 265
Charlottenbrunn 48, 57n161, 178n49
Cheb *see* Eger
Chryselius, Johann Wilhelm 120
Cieplice Śląskie-Zdrój *see* Warmbrunn
circles, social 254–261, 264–266,
    291–292
Claudius, Matthias 63
Clemens August (elector of Cologne)
    32–33
Cleve *see* Kleve
clothing 234–237, *236*, 241–242,
    269n42
Cobenzl, Ludwig von (count) 65
coffeehouses 68–69
communication, interpersonal
    58–60, 69, 285; at coffeehouses
    68–69; confidential 61–63, 65–68;
    diplomatic 65; at Freemason
    gatherings 63–65; letter-writing 60,
    173, 285
Congress of Ems 65
Congress of Vienna 14
Corbin, Alain: *The Lure of the Sea*
    100–101
Cudowa 48, 57n161, 178n49
cultural history 2–3, 99, 193
Cuxhaven 162, 164, 173

daily routine at spas 167, 170–174, 288
dancing 205, 218, 233–234
Daubersberg, castle 153, *154*
Deneken, Arnold Gerhard 7, 47, 70,
    217
Deutsche Monatsschrift 70, 144–145,
    217
Deutsches Magazin 14, 143, 229, 264
Deutsches Museum 235, 251
Deutsche Union see German Union
dietetics 71, 77, 169
discourse 10–11; personal narratives
    and 11–13
Ditfurth, Franz Dietrich von 67
Doberan *see* Doberan-Heiligendamm
Doberan-Heiligendamm 80, 158–164,
    161, 161–163, *163*, 166, 173, 288
Donop, Charlotte Wilhelmine Amalie
    von: *Die Schönheiten Pyrmonts
    (The Beauties of Pyrmont)* 73,
    205, 233

Dorothea (duchess of Courland),
  circle of 254–260
Doubravská hora *see* Daubersberg,
  castle
Dresden 34, 48, 155
dress *see* clothing
Driburg 32, 48–49, 145, 272n64
drinking cure 27–29, *28*, 284
Duszniki-Zdrój *see* Reinerz

Eberhard II (count of Württemberg) 25
Eclectic League 67
Eger 32
Ekklektischer Bund see Eclectic League
Elisabeth Charlotte (duchess of Orléans)
  36
Elisabeth Charlotte (electress of
  Brandenburg) 44
Ellenbogen 147
Ems 5, 29, 285; Congress of 65;
  landscape and built space at 104,
  108–109, *110*, 128–129, 149, 155,
  287; patrons of 35–36
engravings 10, 31, 74; landscape in
  111, 119, 152, 154–155; leisure
  activities advertised in 113–114;
  of maps 155; of spa clothing
  235–236; urban space accentuated
  in 108–109
enlightened educated elite 192; spas
  foster creation of 195, 239, 242,
  255, 291–292
Enlightenment 10; spa as multiplier
  of Enlightenment ideas 2, 218,
  283–284
equality *see* social equality at spas
exclusion, mechanisms of 15,
  261–266, 291

Ferdinand (duke of Brunswick-Lüneburg-
  Wolfenbüttel) 66
Ficker, Wilhelm Anton: *Driburger
  Taschenbuch* (*Driburg Pocketbook*)
  145, 243
fictional works, spas in 61–63, 74–76,
  78–84, 203, 285–286
Findlater, 7th Earl of (James Ogilvy) 43
Flinsberg 48, 57n161, 178n49
Florencourt, Wilhelm Ferdinand
  Chaßot von 242
Föhr 162, 164–166
Foucault, Michel 10–11, 13, 129
Frankenau, Rasmus 3, 74, 78–79

Františkovy Lázně *see* Franzensbad
Franz, Prince *see* Leopold III Friedrich
  Franz (prince, later duke of
  Anhalt-Dessau)
Franzensbad 43, 48; landscape and
  surroundings of 151, 153; patrons
  of 32; social tone of 216–217
Franzensbrunn *see* Franzensbad
Frederick, Prince (duke of York
  and Albany and prince-bishop of
  Osnabrück) 63
Frederick I (king of Prussia) 43
Frederick II (king of Prussia)
  43–44, 65
Frederick IV (king of Denmark) 44
Frederick Christian II (duke of
  Schleswig-Holstein-Sonderburg-
  Augustenburg) 254, 256
Frederick William II (king of Prussia)
  37, 65, 276n103
freedom *see* spa freedom
Freemasonry: Masonic sociability
  191–192, 231; spas and 58, 63–67,
  285
Freienwalde 31, 33, 46, 231, 234
Freiersbach 48, 178n47
French Revolution 14, 215
Friedrich Anton Ulrich (prince of
  Waldeck and Pyrmont) 33
Friedrich Franz (duke of
  Mecklenburg-Schwerin) 159
Friedrich Karl August (prince of
  Waldeck and Pyrmont) 37, 64,
  251, 253
Fürstenbund see League of Princes
Fürstenlager Auerbach *see* Auerbach

Galen 71
gambling at spas 44, 77, 132,
  168–169
gardens: English landscape 100,
  115–119, 123–126, 286; French
  formal 112–114, 286
Geiler, Johannes, von Kaysersberg
  104, 202
*General Gazette for Literature, The
  see Allgemeine Literatur-Zeitung*
General Prussian Land Law 194
gentry 242, 266
Georg Wilhelm (elector of
  Brandenburg) 44
*German Magazine see Deutsches
  Magazin*

German Monthly see Deutsche
  Monatsschrift
German Museum see Deutsches
  Museum
German Union 67
Gerning, Johann Isaak von: *Die
  Heilquellen am Taunus* (*The Spas at
  the Taunus Mountains*) 153, 155
Gesundbrunnen 27
Geßler, Karl Friedrich von (count) 256
Gießhübel *see* Berggießhübel
gifts *see* spa gifts
Giseke, Ludwig 169, 229–230, 232,
  264; "Briefe über Carlsbad" ("Letters
  about Karlsbad") 142–144
Göckingk, Leopold Friedrich
  Günther von 63, 256, 278n129; on
  Brückenau 47, 126, 130, 206–207,
  215–216, 234–235, 251, 263–264;
  on Lauchstädt 39, 229, 235; *Lied
  am Sprudel zu singen* (*Song to be
  Sung at the Hot Spring*) 257; on
  Pyrmont 229; on spa clothing and
  social tone 234–235; on spa as site
  of "harmonious mingling" 292
Godesberg 31, 34, 36, 126
Goethe, Christiane von 12, 94n155,
  172, 260–261
Goethe, Johann Wolfgang von 43, 63,
  256; on daily routine at Pyrmont
  172; library of 75; on national
  circles at Karlsbad 265; on outings
  at Wiesbaden 145; on spa visits
  generally 292; on work at the spa
  168–170
Gold- und Rosenkreuzer see Order of
  the Golden and Rosy Cross
Götzinger, Wilhelm Lebrecht: *Schandau
  und seine Umgebungen* (*Schandau
  and its Surroundings*) 150–151
Grand Landlodge 67
Grattenauer, Karl Wilhelm Friedrich
  214
Graupen 153, *154*
Grävemeyer, Eberhard and Marie von
  60–61
Griesbach 48, 153, 178n47
Grimmelshausen, Hans Jacob
  Christoph von: *Der Abentheuerliche
  Simplicissimus* (*Simplicius
  Simplicissimus*) 4, 30–31, 33
Große Landesloge see Grand Landlodge
Grundig, Christoph Gottlob:
  Beschreibung seiner . . . in das

Käyser Carls-Bad gethanen Reise
  (*Description of His . . . Journey to
  Imperial Karlsbad*) 73, 111–112,
  112, 201–202, 214
guest lists *see* spa lists
guidebooks 77–78
Gustav III (king of Sweden) 44

Hagenrode, monastery *152*, 152
Halem, Friedrich Wilhelm von 158,
  288; Norderney guidebook by
  164–165
Halle 45
Haller, Albrecht von 287; "Die
  Alpen" ("The Alps") 100
Hancke, Gottfried Benjamin: treatise
  on Kukus by 38
Harrer, Hubert von: *Karlsbad und die
  umliegende Gegend* (*Karlsbad and
  the Surrounding Area*) 146
Hassencamp, Johann Matthaeus:
  Briefe eines Reisenden (*Letters of a
  Traveler*) 239–240, 251
healing, spas as sites of: health
  benefits attributed 3; practices of
  25, 27–29; sickness at 7
Heiligendamm *see*
  Doberan-Heiligendamm
Heinrich XXVI (count of Reuß
  Younger Line) 148, 208
Henkel, Johann Friedrich: *Bethesda
  Portuosa* 107, 201
Herder, Johann Gottfried 63, 256
Herz, Henriette 192
heterochrony, spa as 14, 167–169,
  174, 288
heterotopia, spa as 13–15, 183–185,
  287–289, 291–292; temporal aspect
  of (*see* heterochrony, spa as)
hierarchy of German spas 41–49, 284
hiking 142–145, 165
Hirschfeld, Christian Kay Lorenz:
  Theorie der Gartenkunst (*Theory
  of Garden Art*) 100, 116–118,
  128–129, 132, 157, 251–252
Hofgeismar 30, 31, 36; garden at 117,
  123; as multifunctional recreation
  space 116; noble-bourgeois
  interactions at 132, 253–254; social
  tone of 216; visitors to 46; Wilhelm
  IX of Hanau and 34–35
*Hollandaise Sauce, The see
  holländische Sauce, Die*
holländische Sauce, Die 234

Hoser, Joseph Karl Eduard: Franzensbad spa guide by 7, 151, 216–217
Hrad Krupka *see* Rosenburg, castle
Hub *see* Huber Bad
Huber Bad 149
Hufeland, Christoph Wilhelm 1, 63; on dietetics 92n137; on Driburg's social tone 272n64; *Praktische Uebersicht der vorzüglichsten Heilquellen Teutschlands (Practical Overview of the Most Prominent Healing Springs in Germany)* 1, 155–156
humanists 104, 202
Humboldt, Wilhelm von 167

identity: bourgeois 203–204, 228–229, 237–239, 242–243, 245, 292; German 264; national 264–265, 291
Illuminati 67, 192
Imnau 34, 149–150, 172
inhabitants of spas 33
Innocent Pastimes in Karlsbad see Unschuldiger Zeitvertreib im Carlsbad

Jagemann, Karoline 260
Janus, Gerhard Otto 159
Jedlina-Zdrój *see* Charlottenbrunn
Jews at spas 263–264
Journal des Luxus und der Moden 76; "Badechronik" ("Spa Chronicle") in 5–7, 47, 74, 144, 264; on Baden in Switzerland 134; on Dorothea of Courland and her circle 255–256; on enlightened rulers 252–253; on Freienwalde 231, 234; on function of spas 6–7; as historical source 8; on Hofgeismar 216; on Karlsbad 14, 40–41, 146, 241, 254; on Kissingen 35; on Nenndorf 214–215; on Pyrmont 40; on Ronneburg 213; on Saxon Switzerland 155; on social hierarchy and the spa 212; spa freedom evoked in 214–215; spa uniform in 235–236, *236*; urban nature of spas criticized in 134; on Wilhelm IX of Hanau 252
Journal of Luxury and Fashions see Journal des Luxus und der Moden
Journey to the Spas of Karlsbad, Eger, and Teplitz see Reise nach den Badeörtern Karlsbad, Eger und Töplitz
Juist 159

Käppel, Gottfried: *Pyrmonts Merkwürdigkeiten (Pyrmont's Noteworthy Features)* 79, 171, 216, 244
Karl (prince of Hesse-Kassel) 66
Karl Eugen (duke of Württemberg) 32, 207
Karl Friedrich (margrave of Baden) 65
Karl-Joseph (prince of Ligne) 43
Karl Ludwig Friedrich (prince of Mecklenburg-Strelitz) 64
Karlovy Vary *see* Karlsbad
Karlsbad 5, 25, 29, 43–44, 48, 284; *Amusemens* publications and 73–74; burning of 32; daily routine at 170, 172; landscape and built space at 104, 111–112, 143–148, 287; language and national identity at 264–265; leisure activities at 121, 123; map of *112*; noble-bourgeois interactions at 201–202, 232, 237–238, 240–242; patrons of 31–32; social circles at 254, 257, 265–266; social tone of 216, 229; trumpet fanfares at 82; visitors to 40–43
Karlsbad Decrees 9, 65, 250, 265
Kaunitz, Wenzel Anton von 69
Kestner, Johann Christian 12, 71–72, 208–210, 214
Ketelhodt, Friedrich Wilhelm von: travel diary of 7, 56n138, 184n144
Kissingen 34–36, 48
Kleve 107
Klüber, Johann Ludwig: *Beschreibung von Baden bei Rastatt (Description of Baden near Rastatt)* 151, 155
Knigge, Adolph Baron (*Freiherr*) 63, 68; *Über den Umgang mit Menschen (Practical Philosophy of Social Life)* 168, 212
Koromandel-Wedekind: *Der Brunnengast (The Spa Guest)* 70, 73, 107, 205–206, 210
Kotzebue, August von 63, 256; *Doctor Bahrdt mit der eisernen Stirn (Doctor Bahrdt with the Iron Forehead)* 68
Krieger, Johann Friedrich: *Das Alexisbad im Unter-Harz (Alexisbad in the Lower Harz)* 150–152, 246
Krupka *see* Graupen
Kudowa *see* Cudowa
Kudowa-Zdrój *see* Cudowa
Kuks *see* Kukus
Kukus 37–38

Lądek-Zdrój *see* Landeck
Landeck 48, 57n161, 178n49
landscape perceptions 15, 99–101,
    286–287; early modern spa ideal
    and 104–114, 119; late eighteenth-
    century spa ideal and 142–156
Langen-Schwalbach *see* Schwalbach
Langensteinbach 34–35, 46, 65, 149
languages at spas 264
Lauchstädt 5, 31, 45–46, 284; castle
    at 130; landscape and urban nature
    of 107, 133–134; leisure spaces and
    activities at *120*, 120–121, *121*,
    122; medical efficacy of waters at
    3; noble-bourgeois interactions at
    201, 232, 255, 260–261; patrons
    of 34; pleasure as main purpose of
    7; social circles at 254–255; social
    tone of 229, 235
Lauchstädt, a Small Painting see
    Lauchstädt, ein kleines Gemählde
Lauchstädt, ein kleines Gemählde
    232, 254–255
Lavater, Johann Kaspar 253–254
League of Princes 65
Lehndorff, Ernst Ahasverus Heinrich
    von (count) 207
Leopold III Friedrich Franz (prince,
    later duke of Anhalt-Dessau) 4,
    65, 100
Lessing, Gotthold Ephraim 85n17,
    286; *Ernst und Falk* (*Ernst and*
    Falk) 61–63, 78, 85n17
Letters from a Traveler to his Friend
    about his Visit to the Godesberg
    Spa see Briefe eines Reisenden
    an seinen Freund Ueber den
    Aufenthalte beim Godesberger
    Gesundbrunnen
Letters of a Swiss see Briefe eines
    Schweizers
letter-writing 60, 173, 285
Leuck 29
Levin, Rahel 192
Lichtenberg, Georg Christoph:
    "Warum hat Deutschland noch kein
    großes öffentliches Seebad?" ("Why
    Does Germany Not Yet Have a
    Large Public Seaside Resort?")
    157–158, 160, 166, 288
Liebenstein 31, 34, 82, *83*
Liebenzell 149
Limmer 48
Limmerbrunnen *see* Limmer

Lindenthal, Freifrau von 252
Liselotte von der Pfalz *see* Elisabeth
    Charlotte (duchess of Orléans)
Loket *see* Ellenbogen
love, romantic 81
Ludwig X (landgrave of Hesse-
    Darmstadt) 36
Ludwigsbad *see* Wipfeld
Luise (duchess of Anhalt-Dessau) 60

Marcard, Heinrich Matthias 61,
    68; *Beschreibung von Pyrmont*
    (*Description of Pyrmont*) 61–62,
    78, 117–120, 130, 169–170,
    174, 213, 242, 248–249, 251,
    262–263, 287; *Kleines Pyrmonter*
    Brunnenbuch (*Little Book about*
    the Pyrmont Spa) 41, 79
Mariánské Lázně *see* Marienbad
Marienbad 48, 149
Masonic Congress of Wilhelmsbad
    66–67
Masonry *see* Freemasonry
Maulbronn 80–81
Mauvillon, Jacob 68
Meinberg 31, 34, 48–49, 126, 147, 216
Mendelssohn, Moses 263
Menke, Karl Theodor 79
Merian, Matthäus: *Topographia*
    Hassiae 108, 108–109, *109*, *110*,
    114, *115*
Merveilleux, David François
    de: *Amusemens des eaux de*
    Schwalbach (*Amusements at the*
    Waters of Schwalbach) 72, 136n14,
    204–206
middle classes *see* bourgeoisie
Mitterbacher, Bernhard 147
Moltke, Adam Gottlob Detlef von
    86n24, 255
Monatsschrift für Deutsche 168
Montaigne, Michel de 29, 200–201
Monthly for Germans see
    Monatsschrift für Deutsche
Moral and Satirical News from
    Karlsbad see Moralische und
    Satyrische Nachrichten aus dem
    Carlsbade
Moralische und Satyrische
    Nachrichten aus dem Carlsbade 73
Moritz, Karl Philipp: *Anton Reiser*
    280n171
Mosch, Carl Friedrich: *Die Bäder*
    und Heilbrunnen Deutschlands

und der Schweiz (*The Spas and Healing Springs of Germany and Switzerland*) 40, 152–153, 155, 162–164

Moser, Johann Jacob 111

Möser, Justus 7, 59–61, 249, 254; *Schreiben des Verfassers an seine Schwester* (*Letter by the Author to His Sister*) 7, 63–64, 66, 73, 169

mountains, perceptions of 142, 283, 287; German spa map reshaped by 148–149; in personal narratives 146–148; in spa discourse 142–146

Napoleonic Wars 4, 14, 29, 65, 264

national identity 264–265, 291

nature 15, 99–101, 286–287; art and 134, 149; gardens and 112–114; *see also* mountains, perceptions of; sea, perceptions of

Nenndorf 31, 34–35, 144

Neue allgemeine deutsche Bibliothek 79

Neu-verbessert- und vermehrtes denckwürdiges Kayser Carls-Baad 73, 111

New General German Library see Neue allgemeine deutsche Bibliothek

Newly Improved and Augmented Memorable Imperial Karlsbad see Neu-verbessert- und vermehrtes denckwürdiges Kayser Carls-Baad

Newspaper for the Elegant World see Zeitung für die elegante Welt

Nieuport (count) 148, 241, 256

Nicolai, Christoph Friedrich: Bahrdt pasquinade and 68; as Freemason spa guest 63; Justus Möser and 7, 60; in social circles 61, 254, 256, 258–259

nobility 194–195; bourgeois interactions with 202, 204–211 (*see also* social tone, spa freedom); discursive statements about 227–249; early modern spas geared toward and dominated by 200–203; public sphere and 192; in social circles 254–261; as visitors to spas 42–47

Noble Pride at the Spa of Lauchstädt see Adelsstolz im Bade zu Lauchstädt, Der

Norderney 158, 162, 164–165, 167

North Sea 157–158; islands of 164–167

Old, German, Honest, and Delightful Pyrmont, The see alte teutsche ehrliche und liebliche Pyrmont, Das

Order of Strict Observance 64, 66–67

Order of the Golden and Rosy Cross 67

outings 142, 145–147, 150–153, 160–162, 174

palaces at spas 37–38, 123–124, 130, *131*, 153, 160

Papen, Georg Friedrich 64

patrons of spas 30–31; princely 32–39; urban and private 31–32

Paul, Jean 286; *Dr. Katzenbergers Badereise* (*Dr. Katzenberger's Spa Trip*) 78, 80–82, 84, 286

Pauline (princess of Lippe) 173, 256–257

Pauline Christine Wilhelmine (princess of Anhalt-Bernburg) *see* Pauline (princess of Lippe)

Paumgartner, Balthasar 29, 200–201

Partien see outings

peasants 47, 262–263

Perpetuum Mobile Pyrmontanum 73

personal narratives 11–13

Peter I (tsar of Russia) 43

Peterstal 48, 178n47

Pfäfers 27, 29, 72, 104, *105*

physicians, spa 31; bathing recommendations of 25; on bringing work to spas 169; dietetic advice of 71; rivalry between 82; therapeutic claims of 3, 101

Pienitz, Christian Gotthelf: *Beschreibung des Augustusbades bey Radeberg* (*Description of Augustusbad near Radeberg*) 151

Piepenbring, George Heinrich: *Bemerkungen über die Schrift des Herrn Doctor Frankenau Pyrmont betreffend* (*Remarks on the Work by Doctor Frankenau Concerning Pyrmont*) 79, 270

Platner, Ernst 256–259

Plombières 25, 26, 29, 200–201

Plummers see Plombières

Pöllnitz, Karl Ludwig von 72; *Amusemens des eaux d'Aix la Chapelle* (*Amusements at the Waters of Aix la Chapelle*) 72, 107

Poltz (mayor of Karlsbad) 208

princes: as enlightened 250–254; as spa patrons 32–39, 130–133 print culture, spas and 8–10, 70, 285; *see also* guidebooks; publications, spa

prostitution 81

publications, spa 10, 74; *Amusemens* 72–74, 78; balneological 70–71; engravings in (*see* engravings); spa guides 6, 10, 74, 75–77; travelogues 74; as visual aids 144

public sphere 8, 69, 191–192, 291

Putbus 162

Pütter, Johann Stephan: bourgeois uncertainties and self-confidence of 238–239; as Freemason 63; interpersonal communication at Pyrmont and 59–60; landscape not perceived by 146; on Pyrmont bookshop 70; on ruling princes at Pyrmont 253; on Schwalbach 44; spa visits encouraged by royal ministry 168; on work at the spa 169

Pyrmont 1, 29, 31, 43, 284; *Amusemens* publications and 73; avenues in 62, 112, 117–119, 133, 165, 176n27; Bahrdt pasquinade and 66–68; castle at 130, *113, 118*; communal meals at 82, 83, 218, 238; daily routine at 170–172; diplomatic meetings at 65–66; early modern spa ideal and 107–108; as excise town 33; Freemasonry and 63–64, 66–67; gardens at 112, 117–119; heterotopic contradictions at 130, 133; interpersonal communication at 59–64, 68–69; landscape at 107–108, *113*, 119, 147, 287; map of *118*; noble-bourgeois interactions at 201, 205–206, 238–239, 244–245, 248–249; patrons of 33–34; princely representation at 36–37, 130; reference network about 78–79; scholarly interaction at 70, 202; services and activities offered at 119–120; social circles at 60–61, 254, 258; social exclusion at 262–263; social tone of 216, 229; in spa cluster with Meinberg and Driburg 49; spa lists of 40–41; visitors to 42, 47

Pyrmonter Brunnen-Archiv 68–69, 212

Pyrmonter Fürstensommer see Pyrmont Summer of Princes

Pyrmont-Ohsen circle 60–61

Pyrmont Spa Archive see Pyrmonter Brunnen-Archiv

Pyrmont Summer of Princes 65, 206

Recke, Elisa von der 147–148, 241–242, 254, 255–260

recreation, spas as space of 115–117; Bertrich 126; Bocklet 126; Brückenau 126; Ems 129; Godesberg 126; Karlsbad 121–123; Lauchstädt 120–121; Meinberg 126; Pyrmont 117–120; Rehburg 124; Wiesbaden 128–129; Wilhelmsbad 123–124

Reden, Marie Eleonore Elisabeth von 210

Rehburg 7, 34; beggars at 47; health and sickness at 7; Kestner's spa diary for 71–72, 208–210; landscape and interior space of 144–145; noble-bourgeois interactions in 209–210; print culture at 70; remodeled to conform to new spa ideal 124; social tone of 217

Reichard, Heinrich August Ottokar: *Passagier auf der Reise* 92n134

Reinerz 48, 57n161, 178n49

Reise nach den Badeörtern Karlsbad, Eger und Töplitz 177n31, 216, 232, 237, 251

Rem, Lucas 27, 29, 200

Renchtal spa cluster 48, 149

Rippoldsau 42, 149

Ritter, Rosa Dorothea *see* Lindenthal, Freifrau von

Ritzebüttel *see* Cuxhaven

Romans 25

Ronneburg 213

Rosenburg, castle 153, *154*

Rousseau, Jean-Jacques: *Julie, or the New Heloise* 100

Rügen 162, 182n114

rulers *see* princes

Rys, Simon Louis de 123

Sagard 182n114

salons 191–192

Salzbrunn 48, 57n161, 178n49

satire 78, 80–84

Sattelzeit see watershed period

Saxon Switzerland, spas in 9, 149, 150, 155, 287

Schäfer, Andreas 50n23

Schandau 42, 48, 57n159, 149–150, 178n46

Scheidemantel, Friedrich Christian Gottlieb 3–4
Scherf, Johann Christian Friedrich 216
Schinznach 72
Schlangenbad 48; landscape at 109, 111, 148–149, 155; patrons of 34–36
Schlüsselgeldbücher 53nn81–82
Schmid, Ludwig Friedrich Christoph 12, 208–209, 289
Schönborn, Friedrich Karl von (prince-bishop of Würzburg) 35
Schopenhauer, Adele 60, 148, 233
Schopenhauer, Johanna 4–5, 39–40, 244–246, 187n184, 253; "Badeleben in Karlsbad" ("Spa Life in Karlsbad") 146; *Die Brunnengäste (The Spa Guests)* 81
Schott, Peter 104, 202
Schreiber, Aloys: *Handbuch für Reisende am Rhein (Handbook for Travelers Along the River Rhine)* 78
Schulz, Joachim Christoph Friedrich 256; *Reise eines Liefländers (Journey of a Livonian)* 170, 214, 232, 254, 264–265
Schütte, Johann Heinrich: *Amusemens des eaux de Cleve (Amusements at the Waters of Kleve)* 72, 107, 203
Schwalbach 29, 33, 43–44, 48–49, 284; *Amusemens* publications about 73–74; landscape at 155; noble-bourgeois interaction at 233; as urban space 108, 109
Schwalbacher Sommer-wehrende Perpetuum mobile, Das 73, 199
Schwalbach Perpetuum Mobile Lasting All Summer, The see Schwalbacher Sommer-wehrende Perpetuum mobile, Das
Schwarz, Sophie *see* Becker, Sophie
sea, perceptions of 162–164, 287–288
seaside resorts 156–157, 283, 288; daily routine at 173–174; discourse about 158, 162–167; Lichtenberg on 157–158; *see also* Doberan-Heiligendamm; Föhr; Norderney
seating arrangements 206–207, 210, 218, 233–234
Senckenberg, Renatus Leopold Christian Karl von 69
Seven Years' War 4, 29
Severin, Carl Theodor 160, 162

Seydewitz, Johann Christoph Heinrich von 159–160
showers 27, 27, 284
Sichersreuth *see* Alexandersbad
Sierstorpff, Caspar Heinrich von 32
Silesian spa cluster 33–34, 48, 149, 287
sociability 191–192
social class: differentiation within spa clusters by 48–49; hierarchy of spas and 42–47; separation at spas by 199–204, 262–263, 289; spas open to each 5–6, 199
social equality at spas: bourgeois demands for 195, 204–206; practices and limits of 206–211; in spa discourse 211–218
social tone 213, 215–218, 229, 266, 290
Soden 57n157, 153
Sommerfrische see summer retreat
Spa (town) 44, 72
spa freedom 205–206, 213–215, 290
spa gifts 104, 202
spa king 249
spa lists 40–42
spa physicians *see* physicians, spa
spa uniform 235–236, 236
Sponagel, George Christian 78; *Meine viertägigen Leiden im Bade zu Pyrmont (My Four-Day Sufferings in the Spa of Pyrmont)* 79–80; *Des Vetters Feldzug in die Seebäder von Doberan (The Cousin's Military Campaign to the Seaside Resort of Doberan)* 79–80
Sporck, Franz Anton von (count) 37–38
Sporck, Franziska Apollonia von (countess) 37
Sporck, Johann von (count) 37
Springsfeld, Gottlob Carl: *Abhandlung vom Carlsbade* 92n135
spring temple 116, 123–124
Stary Zdrój *see* Altwasser
Stein, Heinrich Friedrich Karl Baron (*Reichsfreiherr*) vom: Pyrmont-Ohsen circle and Nassau castle of 61
Strube, Julius Melchior 59
Sulzbach 48, 178n47
Sulzer, Johann Caspar 202
summer retreat 167
Świeradów-Zdrój *see* Flinsberg
Switzerland, spa discourse and 143–144, 149, 166
Szczawno-Zdrój *see* Salzbrunn

Taunus spa cluster 48–49, 155
Teinach 31–32, 34, 36, 47, 149, 207
Teplice *see* Teplitz
Teplitz 31, 43, 48, 130, *131*, 153, 251
Tharand 48, 57n159, 178n46
Thirty Years' War 4, 29, 44, 48
Tilling, Johann Christian: *Nachricht vom Carlsbade* (*News from Karlsbad*) 73
time at the spa: daily routine 167, 170–174, 288; spa season and visit length 167–168
Ton see social tone
Tönnisstein 32–33
Töplitz *see* Teplitz
tourism 101–102, 283
tourist gaze 15, 101, 283
towns: landscape and 142; princely spas and 35
Tralles, Balthasar Ludwig: *Ode* 73, 199, 202–203
Trampel, Johann Erhard 49
Travemünde 162–163

Überkingen 32
Ulm 32
uniform *see* spa uniform
Unschuldiger Zeitvertreib im Carlsbad 73, 203
urban space, spa as 104–114, 133–134, 286

visitors to spas 41–47, 284
Vogel, Samuel Gottlieb 158–162, 169, 173, 288
Voigts, Jenny von 60–61, 255
Vulpius, Christiane *see* Goethe, Christiane von
Vulpius, Johann Friedrich 260

Waitz, August Christian 117
Waldersee, Franz von 65
Warmbrunn 48, 57n161, 178n49
Warnstedt, Friedrich von: *Die Insel Föhr und das Wilhelminen See-Bad* (*The Island of Föhr and the Wilhelmine Seaside Resort*) 165–166
War of the Bavarian Succession 69
watershed period 9–10, 15, 283, 291
Weber, Christoph 124
Weimar court theater 46
Welcker, Johann Peter 109, 111
wells, drinking *28*, 28
Wiesbaden 5, 25, 29, *108*, 285; landscape and urban space of

108, 128–129, 155, 287; noble-bourgeois interactions in 208–209; patrons of 34–35; spa lists of 40; visitors to 42, 46, 48–49
Wiesenbad 57n159, 178n46
Wildbad 29; Alpine euphoria and 149; bathing practices at 27, 200; Eberhard II of Württemberg attacked in 25; landscape and urban space of 111; patrons of 34; town charter granted to 33
Wilhelm I (landgrave of Hesse-Kassel) *see* Wilhelm IX (count of Hanau)
Wilhelm IX (count of Hanau): as enlightened ruler 252; Masonic Congress of Wilhelmsbad and 67; as patron of spas 31, 34–35, 39, 123; on the unattractive location of Ems 108
Wilhelmina Caroline (countess of Hanau) 108, 252
Wilhelminen-Seebad *see* Föhr
Wilhelmsbad 30–31; healing power of waters at 3, 51n46; Jews accommodated at 263; layout and amenities offered at *123*, 123–124, *124*, *125*; Masonic Congress of 66–67; palace at 130; weekend visits common at 46; Wilhelm IX of Hanau and 34–35, 123, 252
Willebrand, Johann Peter: *Nachrichten von einer Carlsbader Brunnenreise* (*News from a Spa Visit to Karlsbad*) 6, 63, 121, 247–248
Wipfeld 48
Wolkenstein 57n159, 178n46
work at spas 169–170
Wörlitz Park 100

Zeitung für die elegante Welt 74, 265
Zimmermann, Johann Georg Ritter von 60–61; *Über Friedrich den Großen und meine Unterredung mit ihm* (*On Frederick the Great and My Conversation with Him*) 67–68
Zinnendorf, Johann Wilhelm Kellner von 67
Zirkel see circles, social
Zobel, Baron (*Freiherr*) von 35
Zobelet, Mademoiselle 210
Zwierlein, Conrad Anton 235

For Product Safety Concerns and Information please contact our EU
representative GPSR@taylorandfrancis.com
Taylor & Francis Verlag GmbH, Kaufingerstraße 24, 80331 München, Germany